Gene Amplification and Analysis

Volume 4
Oncogenes

Gene Amplification and Analysis

Jack G. Chirikjian and Takis S. Papas, *Series Editors*

Gene
Amplification
and Analysis

Volume 4
Oncogenes

Editors:
Takis S. Papas, Ph.D.
National Cancer Institute, Bethesda, Maryland

George F. Vande Woude, Ph.D.
Litton Bionetics, Frederick, Maryland

ELSEVIER
NEW YORK • AMSTERDAM • LONDON

Elsevier Science Publishing Company, Inc.
52 Vanderbilt Avenue, New York, New York 10017

Sole distributors outside the United States and Canada:

Elsevier Science Publishers B.V.
P.O. Box 211, 1000 AE Amsterdam, the Netherlands

Library of Congress Cataloging in Publication Data
Oncogenes.

   (Gene amplification and analysis, ISSN 0275-2778 ;
v. 4)
   Includes index.
   1. Oncogenes. I. Papas, Takis S. II. Vande Woude,
George F. III. Series. [DNLM: 1. Cell Transformation,
Neoplastic. 2. Oncogenes. 3. Oncogenic Viruses.
W1 GE184N v.4 / QZ 202 0542]
RC268.4.05 1986   616.99′4071   86-16704
ISBN 0-444-01116-1
ISSN 0275-2778

Current printing (last digit)

10 9 8 7 6 5 4 3 2 1

Manufactured in the United States of America

Contents

Preface

This series has been established to rapidly convey information of topical interest to scientists and students of recombinant genetics and molecular biology. Oncogenes, the fourth volume in the series, represents an exciting area of intensive research activity that has intruded into all of the traditional cancer research disciplines. During the past several years we have witnessed a rapid evolution as critical points were reached in many different research areas requiring a common language to permit a universal dialogue and allow the cross-fertilization of ideas. Only the language of molecular biology could satisfy this compelling requisite and with astonishing speed it has woven a common thread cohesively bonding the varied research disciplines and effectively focusing them into the arena of oncogenes, and cellular growth-factors and receptors.

Oncogenes were first discovered as part of the genome of acute transforming retroviruses. These viruses were characterized via their ability to cause transformation of cells in culture or their ability to form tumors rapidly in infected newborn animals. By the mid '70s there was compelling evidence to suggest that new information was present in these viruses but it was not immediately clear that the different acute transforming viruses possessed novel or unique genetic information. Once it became understood that such unique oncogene(s) could be harbored by retroviruses, there was a movement en masse back to the laboratory freezer to recover the many "treasures" that had been stored away in prior years (dating back, in several instances, more than half a century). These faithful investigators were much more convinced than many of their colleagues that these treasures would prove to be of extreme importance to the cancer research community. The number of these genes described to date now totals upwards of 40 and may well reach into the hundreds before long, particularly as the definition of oncogenes expands to encompass the properties of each new class that is isolated and identified as such. Consider, for example, the number portended should the majority of growth factors and their receptors be included in this category and thus considered as oncogenes; appreciating at the same time the limited number of assays we presently have for detecting them. Not suprisingly, therefore, oncogenes have only been recognized and identified as portions of retroviral genomes or by DNA transfection/transformation assays. The number of oncogenes will also be expected to substantially increase if genes identified at breakpoints of critical, nonrandom chromosomal translocations, such as BclI and BclII, become included.

It is becoming highly improbable that a specific cellular oncogene is responsible for establishing cancer in a single cell type. In this connection the acute transforming retroviruses are unique since, they are able to malignantly transform a variety of host cell types directly. Perhaps this feat is accomplished by virtue of the retroviral transcription control elements which cannot be sufficiently modulated by the host cell; perhaps as well, the ability of the virus through successive rounds of replication and infection optimizes its genetic information providing the host cell with a proliferative (and selective) advantage. The activation of the cellular oncogene is, however, much more restricted. First, a mutation or rearrangement must be introduced into a single gene which then confers upon the cell some selective growth advantage. The probability of introducing additional alterations within the same gene which then can increase its transforming potential precludes its occurence. For this reason it is more probable that a second or independent oncogene activation event occurs, causing the afflicted cell to proliferate malignantly. There are currently many efforts directed at trying to understand the mechanism of action of these genes, as transforming genes, but it is quite likely that we will first have to define their normal activity as proto-oncogenes, before we can even begin to understand how they contribute to the transformation event.

The contributors to this volume have provided reviews of several select aspects in the area of molecular oncology. We have attempted to provide sufficient diversity in the subject matter in order to capture the imagination of the young investgators and to encourage them to begin studying this exciting area. The chapters are also meant to provide useful references for our many colleagues. We are therefore grateful for our colleagues' contributions, acknowledging their efforts and eagerness to undertake this responsibility in such a rapidly expanding field. In particular the editors would especially like to acknowledge the editorial assistance of Ms. Pamela Green, whose daily and dutiful functions of coordinating, typing and editing, coupled with her gentle prodding, enabled us to meet our anticipated deadlines.

Takis S. Papas
George F. Vande Woude
April 21, 1986

Contributors

Numbers in brackets indicate the page on which the author's contribution begins.

S. A. Aaronson, Laboratory of Cellular and Molecular Biology, Bldg. 37, Rm. 1E24, National Cancer Institute, National Institutes of Health, Bethesda, Maryland 20205(161)

R. Ascione, Laboratory of Molecular Oncology, National Cancer Institute, Frederick Cancer Research Facility, Frederick, Maryland 21701(109, 207, 253)

M. A. Baluda, Department of Pathology, UCLA School of Medicine, Los Angeles, California 90024(73)

M. Barbacid, NCI-Frederick Cancer Research Facility, P.O. Box B, Building 539, Frederick, Maryland 21701(21)

A. H. Beggs, Department of Biology, The Johns Hopkins University, Baltimore, Maryland 21218(177)

D. Blair, Laboratory of Molecular Oncology, Bldg. 469, Rm. 117, National Cancer Institute, Frederick Cancer Research Facility, Frederick, Maryland 21701(239)

Z-Q. Chen, Laboratory of Molecular Oncology, National Cancer Institute, Frederick Cancer Research Facility, Frederick, Maryland 21701(53)

D. J. Clanton, Laboratory of Molecular Oncology, National Cancer Institute, Frederick Cancer Research Facility, Frederick, Maryland 21701(53)

W. Colby, Genetech, Inc., 460 Pt. San Bruno Blvd., South San Francisco, California 94080(39)

J. B. Cohen, Genetech, Inc., 460 Pt. San Bruno Blvd., South San Francisco, California 94080(39)

C. Croce, The Wistar Institute, 36th at Spruce Street, Philadelphia, Pennsylvania 19104(143)

M. Dean, LBI-Basic Research Program, Bldg. 469, Frederick, Cancer Research Facility, Frederick, Maryland 21701(239)

P. Duesberg, Department of Molecular Biology, University of California, 229 Stanley Hall, Berkeley, California 94740(109)

R. J. Fisher, Laboratory of Molecular Oncology, National Cancer Institute, Frederick Cancer Research Facility, Bldg. 469, Rm. 206, Frederick, Maryland 21701(109,253)

C. Flordellis, Dana Farber Cancer Institute, 44 Binney St., Boston, Massachussetts 02115(109)

S. Fujiwara, Laboratory of Molecular Oncology, National Cancer Institute, Frederick Cancer Research Facility, Bldg. 469, Rm. 206, Frederick, Maryland 21701(109,253)

N. A. Giesse, Laboratory of Cellular and Molecular Biology, Bldg. 37, Rm. 1E24, National Cancer Institute, National Institutes of Health, Betheda, Maryland 20205(161)

M. Gonzatti-Haces, LBI-Basic Research Program, Bldg. 469, Frederick Cancer Research Facility, Frederick, Maryland 21701(239)

S. Hattori, Laboratory of Molecular Oncology, National Cancer Institute, Frederick Cancer Research Facility, Bldg. 469, Frederick, Maryland 21701 (53)

H. Igarashi, Laboratory of Cellular and Molecular Biology, Bldg. 37, Rm. 1E24, National Cancer Institute, National Institutes of Health, Bethesda, Maryland 20205(161)

A. Iyer, LBI-Basic Research Program, Bldg. 469, Frederick Cancer Research Facility, Frederick, Maryland 21701(239)

N. C. Kan, Laboratory of Molecular Oncology, National Cancer Institute, National Institutes of Health, Bldg. 469, Rm. 205, Frederick, Maryland 21701(109)

K. Kaul, LBI-Basic Research Program, Bldg. 469, Frederick Cancer Research Facility, Frederick, Maryland 21701(239)

K. Kelly, Immunology Branch, Building 10, Room 4B-17, National Cancer Institute, National Institutes of Health, Bethesda, Maryland 20205(197)

C. R. King, Laboratory of Cellular and Molecular Biology, Bldg. 37, Rm. 1E24, National Cancer Institute, National Institutes of Health, Bethesda, Maryland 20205(161)

J. A. Lautenberger, Laboratory of Molecular Oncology, National Cancer Institute, National Institutes of Health, Bldg. 469, Rm. 205, Frederick, Maryland 21701(53,109)

F. Leal, Laboratory of Cellular and Molecular Biology, Bldg. 37, Rm. 1E24, National Cancer Institute, National Institutes of Health, Bethesda, Maryland 20205(161)

A. D. Levinson, Genetech, Inc., 360 Pt. San Bruno Blvd., South San Francisco, California 94080(39)

J. S. Lipsick, Department of Pathology, UCLA School of Medicine, Los Angeles, California 90024 (73)

P. C. Nowell, The Wistar Institute, 36th at Spruce Street, Philadelphia, Pennsylvania 19104(143)

S. J. O'Brien, Laboratory of Viral Carcinogenesis, National Cancer Institute, Bldg. 569, Frederick Cancer Research Facility, Frederick, Maryland 21701(207)

T. S. Papas, Laboratory of Molecular Oncology, National Cancer Institute, National Institutes of Health, Bldg. 469, Rm. 102, Frederick, Maryland 21701(53,109,207,253)

M. Park, LBI-Basic Research Program, Bldg. 469, Frederick Cancer Research Facility, Frederick, Maryland 21701(239)

J. T. Parsons, Department of Microbiology, University of Virginia School of Medicine, Charlottesville, Virginia 22908(1)

S. J. Parsons, Department of Microbiology, University of Virginia School of Medicine, Charlottesville, Virginia 22908 (1)

M. Psallidopoulos, Laboratory of Molecular Oncology, National Cancer Institute, Frederick Cancer Research Facility, Bldg. 469, Rm. 205, Frederick, Maryland 21701(109)

E. P. Reddy, Department of Molecular Oncology, Roche Research Center, Hoffman-La Roche Institute, Nutley, New Jersey 07110(99)

K. C. Robbins, Laboratory of Cellular and Molecular Biology, Building 37, Room 1E24, National Cancer Institute, National Institutes of Health, Bethesda, Maryland 20205(161)

T. Robins, LBI-Basic Research Program, Bldg. 469, Frederick Cancer Research Facility, Frederick, Maryland 21701(239)

D. Rosson, Department of Molecular Oncology, Roche Research Center, Hoffmann-La Roche Institute, Nutley, New Jersey 07110(99)

N. Sacchi, Laboratory of Molecular Oncology, National Cancer Institute, Frederick Cancer Research Facility, Bldg. 469, Rm. 206, Frederick, Maryland 21701(207), 253)

K. Samuel, Program Resources, Inc., Bldg. 469, Frederick Cancer Research Facility, Frederick, Maryland 21701 (109)

G. A. Scangos, Department of Biology, The Johns Hopkins University, Baltimore, Maryland 21218(177)

A. Seth, LBI-Basic Research Program, Bldg. 469, Frederick Cancer Research Facility, Frederick, Maryland 21701(109, 253)

T. Shih, Laboratory of Molecular Oncology, National Cancer Institute, Frederick Cancer Research Facility, Frederick, Maryland 21701(53)

S. Sukumar, NCI-Frederick Cancer Research Facility, P.O. B, Building 539, Frederick, Maryland 21701(21)

Y. Tsujimoto, The Wistar Institute, 36th at Spruce Street, Philadelphia, Pennsylvania 19104(143)

L. S. Ulsh, Laboratory of Molecular Oncology, National Cancer Institute, Frederick Cancer Research Facility, Frederick, Maryland 21701(53)

B. Underwood, Immunology Branch, Bldg. 10, Rm. 4B-17, National Cancer Institute, National Institutes of Health, Betheda, Maryland 20205(197)

R. Van Beneden, Laboratory of Molecular Oncology, National Cancer Institute, Frederick Cancer Research Facility, Bldg. 469, Rm. 205, Frederick, Maryland 21701(109)

G. F. Vande Woude, LBI-Basic Research Program, Frederick Cancer Research Facility, Frederick, Maryland 21701(239)

D. K. Watson, Laboratory of Molecular Oncology, National Cancer Institute, Frederick Cancer Research Facility, Bldg. 469, Rm. 205, Frederick, Maryland 21701(109,207,253)

V. Wilkerson, Department of Microbiology, University of Virginia School of Medicine, Charlottesville, Virginia 22908(1)

D. Yu, Genetech, Inc., 460 Pt. San Bruno Blvd., South San Francisco, California 94080(39)

H. Zarbl, NCI-Frederick Cancer Research Facility, P.O. B, Building 539, Frederick, Maryland 21701(21)

R-P. Zhou, Department of Molecular Biology, University of California, 229 Stanley Hall, Berkeley, California 94740(109)

1

Structural and Functional Motifs of the Rous Sarcoma Virus
Src Protein

J. Thomas Parsons, Victoria Wilkerson and Sarah J. Parsons

Department of Microbiology
University of Virginia School of Medicine
Charlottesville, VA 22908

.

I. INTRODUCTION

The discovery of oncogenes and the proposal that oncogene activation may play a pivotal role in the establishment of neoplasms have prompted considerable interest in the biochemical function of oncogene encoded proteins[1,2]. Exploitation of molecular cloning and DNA sequencing techniques has lead to the identification of a large number of oncogenes and their normal cellular counterparts, proto-oncogenes. DNA sequences information has provided the deduced amino acid sequence for many of these gene products, thereby lending considerable insight into their structures. Analysis of individual oncogene sequences has revealed interesting and provocative relationships between cellular proto-oncogene encoded proteins and their oncogenic viral counterparts. For example, the viral protein encoded by the oncogene (erb B) of the retrovirus, avian erythroblastosis virus (AEV), represents a truncated form of the epidermal growth factor (EGF) receptor[3]. Similarly, the product of the fms oncogene of SM FeSV is an altered form of the macrophage colony stimulating factor (CSF I) receptor[4]. Molecular genetics has also provided another powerful tool for the analysis of oncogene encoded proteins, specifically, the utilization of in vitro mutagenesis techniques to define important functional and structural domains. In this review we describe the application of this technology to study the src gene of the avian retrovirus, Rous sarcoma virus (RSV), and the src product, pp60src. The src gene of RSV encodes a membrane-associated phosphoprotein of 60 kd, pp60src [5], that exhibits tyrosine protein kinase activity both in vitro and in vivo[6,7,10]. Expression of the src protein is a prerequisite for cellular transformation by RSV and is required for all of the manifestations accompanying the establishment of the neoplastic phenotype[8]. In addition, the observed increases in intracellular phosphotyrosine levels and the appearance of phosphotyrosine modified proteins in transformed cells lead directly to the conclusion that tyrosine phosphorylation of specific cellular target proteins is a critical step in RSV-mediated transformation[7,9]. Considerable information has been obtained regarding the molecular architecture of the src protein, including the characterization of several post-translational modifications (Figure 1). Pp60src contains two sites of phosphorylation, a serine residue at position 17, which is phosphorylated by the cAMP dependent protein kinase system[11], and tyrosine 416, which appears to be phosphorylated by the

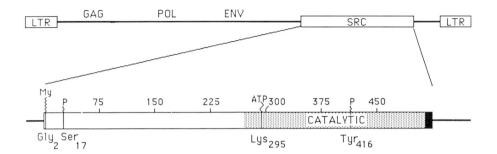

Figure 1. Important structural features of the RSV src gene.
The schematic diagram denotes the sites within pp60src for: myristylation,
(My); phosphorylation, (P); ATP binding, (ATP). The "catalytic" domain
(see text) is indicated by the stippled region. The region of sequence
divergence between viral and cellular src is indicated by the dark (■)
shading.

auto-catalytic activity of pp60[src] itself[12,13]. The src protein also undergoes a unique covalent modification at the amino terminus, the addition of
myristic acid to the penultimate glycine residue[14,15]. Current evidence
supports the idea that the membrane localization of the src protein is a
consequence of this covalent modification[16,17].

Comparison of the amino acid sequence of the src protein with the sequences of other known tyrosine protein kinases reveals a structural
homology within the carboxy terminal half of the src molecule that is
shared with other oncogene encoded tyrosine protein kinases as well as
normal growth factor receptors[18,19,20,21]. In contrast, the amino terminal half of the src protein shares little homology with most of the other
members of the tyrosine kinase family, the exceptions being the fgr, yes
and abl oncogene proteins, which exhibit a limited homology with pp60src in
this region. A variety of evidence suggests that the conserved regions of
the different tyrosine kinases represent the catalytic domain (Figure 1).[2]

In this review we summarize data obtained in our laboratory during the
past several years regarding the structural organization of the domains
of the pp60[src] protein. In addition we review the evidence from other
laboratories and speculate as to how these domains are integrated in the

overall topological structure of the <u>src</u> protein. Experimental details regarding the isolation and characterization of the mutants described in this review have been reported elsewhere[22,25,26].

II. Materials and Methods

A. <u>Cells, viruses, plasmids and antibodies.</u>

Cultures of primary chicken embryo cells were prepared from gs-negative embryos (Spafas) and maintained in culture as previously described[22]. Viral DNA used for mutagenesis was derived from a nonpermuted molecular clone of Prague A-RSV inserted into a pBR322 plasmid vector (pJD100) (Figure 2). Mutagenesis was performed on a subgenomic clone of RSV containing a <u>SalI-BamHI</u> fragment of pJD100, which includes the 3' portion

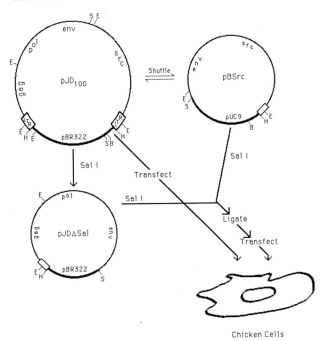

Figure 2. Construction of infectious RSV vectors.

The derivation of individual plasmids is described in detail in the text. Restriction enzyme sites for the following enzymes are indicated: E, Eco RI; S, <u>Sal</u> I; H, <u>Hind</u> III; and B, <u>Bam</u> HI. Chicken cells were transfected with either pJD100 or with a ligated mixture of pBSrc and pJD Δ <u>Sal</u>, each previously digested with the enzyme <u>Sal</u> I, as described in the text.

of _env_, all of _src_, and the 3' LTR, inserted into a pUC9 plasmid vector (Figure 2). Transfection of chicken embryo cells required reconstitution of the mutagenized subgenomic fragment into an intact viral genome. This was accomplished by either ligation of the _SalI-BamHI_ _src_ fragment into an appropriately modified form of pJD100 or by digestion of the mutagenized pBSrc and a viral complementation vector, pJD Δ _Sal_ (Figure 2). Ligated DNA (1-2μg) was then applied to cultures of cells as described previously[22]. Transfected cells produced high titers of mutant virus, which were then used for subsequent experiments. For detection of _src_ proteins, either polyclonal rabbit anti-_src_ sera[23] or monoclonal antibody[23] to pp60src was used.

B. Restriction enzyme digestion and agarose gel electrophoresis.

Restriction enzymes were purchased from New England Biolabs, Inc., Beverly, MA, Bethesda Research Laboratories, Gaithersburg, MD, or P. L. Biochemicals, Piscataway, NJ, and used as recommended by the supplier. DNA restriction fragments were purified either from low-gelling temperature agarose (Seaplaque, FMC Corp., Marine Colloids Div., Rockland, ME) or by adsorption to and elution from DEAE-membrane paper (Schleicher and Schuell, Keen, NH). Synthetic DNA linkers were purchased from Bethesda Research Laboratories, Gaithersburg, MD.

C. Construction of deletion mutants.

For a detailed discussion of the construction of specific mutations the reader is referred to the appropriate references as discussed in the Results section.

D. Immunoprecipitation and polyacrylamide gel analysis of labeled cell proteins.

Labeling of cultures with [^{35}S]-methionine or [^{32}P]-orthophosphage and immunoprecipitation of labeled _src_ proteins were performed as described[22,24]. Equal amounts of protein extract were immunoprecipitated to allow quantitation of wild type of mutant _src_ proteins. Immune complex kinase assays were performed as described previously[25,26]. Phosphorylation of angiotensin II was determined following the addition of 3mM [Val5]-angiotensin II (Sigma, St. Louis, MO) and 5 μCi of γ-^{32}P labeled ATP to 50 μl of immune complex in 10 mM Tris-HCl, pH 7.5, 5 mM MgCl$_2$. The reaction was carried out for 20 minutes at 22°C and terminated by the addition of ice-cold TCA to a final concentration of 4%. After centrifugation, the acid-soluble, labeled peptide was collected on Whatman P81 phosphocellulose paper, washed and counted by liquid scintillation.

III. Results

A. Targeting of mutations within the src gene.

To test the hypothesis that the transforming activity of the src protein is governed by a functional tyrosine protein kinase and to define important structural and functional domains which might be important in the regulation of the tyrosine kinase activity we have introduced defined mutations into the src gene of RSV using conventional techniques of site-directed mutagenesis. The techniques include the introduction of deletions, point mutations and linker insertions. Figure 3 summarizes the structure of the mutations analyzed to date. These include deletion mutations within the amino-terminal one-half of the src protein (section III.B), point mutations within an amino acid sequence conserved among virtually all tyrosine kinases (section III.C), and insertion mutations adjacent to a highly conserved leu residue, leu_{516}, close to the carboxy-terminus (section III.C).

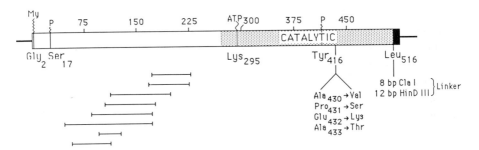

Figure 3. Summary of site-directed mutations in the src gene.
The important structural features of the src gene product, pp60src, are indicated as described in Figure 1. Deletion mutations within the src gene are indicated by the solid line (⊢——◀). Point mutations are indicated by denoting the amino acid changes introduced as a consequence of the mutation. The position of linker insertion mutations are indicated by denoting the relative position of the linker.

B. Analysis of amino terminal mutations.

Bryant and Parsons[22] first reported that a deletion within the src gene which resulted in the removal of amino acid residues 173 to 227 yielded a mutant of RSV that was temperature sensitive for morphological transformation of chicken cells in culture. The initial characterization of this

mutant suggested that the deletion was at or near a region of the src
protein necessary for functional activity[22]. Since a number of ts mutants
of RSV, selected by conventional biological techniques, had been mapped to
the 5' one-half of the src gene[27], we proceeded to define further the properties of this amino terminal domain required for transformation using the
techniques of site-directed mutagenesis. Figure 4 depicts the structure of
a series of overlapping deletion mutations spanning the region of the src
gene encoding amino acid residues 38 to 225. These deletions were created
using a combination of linker insertion and linker joining techniques. The
construction and detailed characterization of these mutants have been

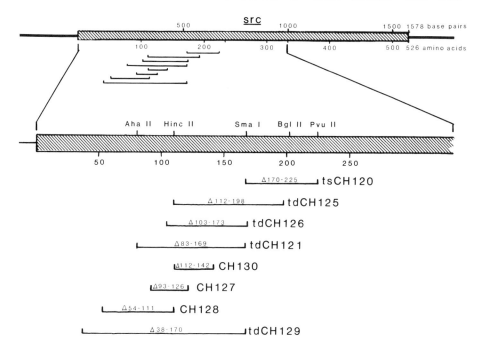

Figure 4.   Summary of deletion mutations within the 5' end of the src
            gene.
Deletions introduced with the src gene are indicated by the solid lines;
the amino acid residues removed as a consequence of the deletions are denoted above the line. The altered biological phenotypes induced by the
individual mutant viruses are also shown, td, transformation defective;
ts; temperature sensitive transformation. Relevant restriction sites within the src gene are included for reference.

described in detail elsewhere[28]. Transfection of chicken cells with an appropriately reconstructed, infectious RSV vector (see Materials and Methods) bearing each of the individual mutations was carried out to determine the phenotype of the engineered viral mutations. Deletion of amino acid residues 54-111 (CHd1128), 93-126 (CHd1127), or 112-142 (CHd1130) did not alter the transforming properties of the mutant src gene. In contrast, deletion of residues 83-169 (CHd1121), 103-173 (CHd1126) or 112-198 (CHd1124) yielded virus that was defective for transformation, i.e., the infected cells retained a normal phenotype and normal growth properties. The deletion of residues 170-225 (CHts120) yielded a virus that was temperature sensitive for transformation, inducing the transformed phenotype upon growth at 35°C but not at 41°C. This phenotype was identical to that orginally described by Bryant and Parsons[22] for the mutant CHts119. The biological properties of the above mutants established that a region of the src protein encompassing residues 38 to 142 could be removed without compromising the ability of the src protein to mediate cellular transformation. In contrast, deletion mutations impinging upon a region encoding residues 142 to 169 resulted in the inactivation ofthe transforming function. These results confirmed our earlier hypothesis that a region within the amino acid terminal one-half of pp60src contains a domain required for functional transforming activity.

To analyze the biochemical properties of the mutant proteins, cells, infected with individual mutants, were labeled with ^{32}P, extracts were immunoprecipitated with monoclonal antibody to pp60src and the immunoprecipitated proteins were characterized by polyacrylamide gel electrophoresis[22,23,25]. Each of the deletion mutants encoded a structurally altered protein whose size was consistent with the size of the engineered deletion. Furthermore, partial protease mapping of the mutant proteins with Staphylococcus aureus V8 protease coupled with phosphoamino acid analysis revealed that each was phosphorylated on both serine and tyrosine residues[26]. To measure the intrinsic protein kinase activity of the src proteins encoded by the individual mutants, immune complexes were prepared from infected cell extracts and the autophosphorylation activity as well as the kinase activity with two exogenous substrates, casein and the tyrosine containing peptide, angiotensin II, was measured. As shown in Table 1, immune complexes from cells infected with each of the transformation conpetent deletion mutants exhibited kinase activities virtually identical to that of immune complexes

Table 1. In vitro kinase activity of mutant src proteins.

Mutant[a]	Auto phosphorylation	Casein	Angiotensin II
uninfected	0.02	0.03	0.16
WT PrRSV	1.0	1.0	1.0
tsCH120	1.0, 0.3[b]	1.0, 0.4[b]	0.8,0.4[b]
tdCH121	0.4	0.4	0.5
tdCH125	0.2	0.4	n.d.
tdCH126	0.4	0.3	0.5
CH127	1.7	1.6	1.2
CH128	0.9	0.9	0.7
tdCH129	0.2	n.d.	n.d.
CH130	0.9	0.9	0.8
tdCHpm 26	0.05	0.04	n.d.
tdCHpm 9	0.1	0.08	n.d.
tdCHpm 6	0.09	0.01	n.d.
tdCHpm 65	0.06	0.05	n.d.
CHpm 59	1.05	1.0	n.d.
tdCHis 1545-C	0.05	0.04	n.d.
tdCHis 1545-H	0.07	0.06	n.d.

[a]Cell extracts, prepared from uninfected, wild type RSV, and mutant infected cells, were immunoprecipitated with excess antibody to the src protein and autophosphorylation, casein and angiotensin phosphorylation were measured in the immune complex kinase assay. Values are expressed relative to that obtained with wild type infected cells (1.0). The prefix (td) denoted a transformation defective phenotype, (ts), denotes a temperature sensitive phenotype.

[b]kinase activity at non-permissive temperature (41°C).

[c]n.d.: not done.

from wild type RSV infected cells. In contrast, the kinase activity recovered in immune complexes from cells infected with transformation defective mutants was reproducibly lower (40 to 20% of wild type levels). Immune complexes from CHts120 infected cells exhibited wild type levels of kinase activity when prepared from cells grown at 35°C but reduced levels when cells were grown at 41°C. Additional experiments have shown that cells infected with the transformation defective deletion mutants exhibit elevated but not wild type levels of total phosphotyrosine, contain elevated levels of phosphotyrosine labeled 36 kd protein (a major target for pp60src phosphorylation[31,32]) and have an unaltered distribution of membrane associated src protein[28]. In summary, our experiments suggest that the src protein contains a region, tentatively localized a residues 142 to 169, whose native structure is absolutely required for functional transformation. This domain maps outside the domain specifying catalytic activity, yet appears to be essential for pp60[src] mediated transformation.

C. Analysis of carboxy terminal mutations.

The carboxy terminal one-half of the src protein is evolutionarily related to other tyrosine protein kinases, based on the overall degree of amino acid sequence homology among these proteins[2]. Figure 5 illustrates this homology by comparing the amino acid sequence of the src protein with that of other oncogene proteins, growth factor receptors, and more distantly related yeast[29] and Drosphila[30] proteins. Inspection of these homologies reveals that among the most highly conserved sequences is the sequence ala_{430}-pro_{431}-glu_{432}-ala_{433} (Figure 5). To investigate the role of these highly conserved sequences in maintaining src function and to probe in a more general fashion of the topological constraints of the tyrosine kinase domain, we have engineered a number of point mutations and linker insertion mutations within this region.

Using the previously described techniques for sodium bisulfite mutagenesis, we isolated single point mutations within a sequence defined by a Bgl I restriction site (Figure 6). Analysis of individual, mutagenized plasmids by Bgl I restriction enzyme analysis, direct DNA sequencing and transfection of chicken cells led to the identification of four point mutations encoding single amino acid changes within this sequence (Figure 6). The mutant CHpm26 contained a single C to T change, altered the codon for Ala_{430} (GCC) to Val (GTC); CHpm9 contained a single C to T change, altering the codon for Pro_{431} (CCC) to Ser(TCC); CHpm6 contained two G and A alterations, changing the codon for Glu_{432} (GAG) to Lys (AAA); and CHpm65 contained a single G to A change, altering the codon for Ala_{433} (GCA) to Thr (ACA).

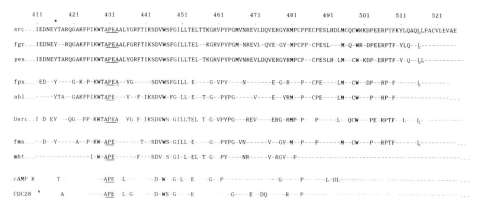

Figure 5. Comparison of a portion of the amino acid sequence from viral
tyrosine kinase oncogenes and other structurally related gene
products.

The deduced amino acid sequence for src[35] are compared with the sequences
of other viral oncogene products fgr, yes, fps, abl, fms, and mht and with
the deduced amino acid sequences of Drosophila melanogaster src, Dsrc, the
yeast cell division control gene, CDC 28, and cAMP kinase. The amino acid
numbers denote the sequence of pp60src; the site of tyrosine phosphorylation
in pp60src is denoted by the (*); the highly conserved amino acid sequences
ala (A)-pro(P)-glu(E)-ala(A) and leu$_{516}$ are underlined.

```
                    ... 430 431 432 433 ...
                ...Ile lys trp thr ala pro glu ala ala leu ...

                ...ATC AAG TGG ACA GCC CCC GAG GCA GCC CTC ...
                             ( -- Bgl I -- )
```

Mutant		Transformation	Protein Kinase
CHpm 26	............T.......... (val)	–	–
CHpm 9	............T........... (ser)	–	–
CHpm 6	............A.A......... (lys)	–	–
CHpm 65	............A........... (thr)	–	–
CHpm 59	.............G........... (glu)	+	+

Figure 6. Nucleotide sequence of point mutations within the src gene.
Alterations induced by bisulfite mutagenesis at the Bgl I restriction site
in the src gene are indicated. The cellular phenotype of individual mutants
was determined by DNA transfection of chicken cells as described in the text.

CHpm59 contained a G to A change in the third base of the codon for Glu432 and therefore does not alter the amino acid sequence at this position.

In addition to these point mutations, linker insertion mutations were isolated after introduction of either an 8 base pair Cla I or a 12 bp Hind III linker at a Pvu II site, 32 bp (nucleotide 1545) from the TAA termination codon of the src gene (Figure 7). These mutations alter the structure adjacent to leu516, a highly conserved amino acid residue present in most of the active tyrosine protein kinases (see Figure 5). The mutant CHis 1545-H contained an insertion of two Hind III linkers resulting in the inframe insertion of 8 amino acids. The mutant CHis 1545-C contained a single 8 base pair Cla I linker resulting in a frame shift mutation which encoded 18 unrelated amino acids at the carboxy terminus of the src protein (Figure 7).

Wild type pp60src amino acid residues 512 TO 526.

..leu gln ala gln LEU leu pro ala cys val leu glu val ala glu ***
..CTG CAG GCC CAG CTG CTC CCT GCT TGT GTG TTG GAG GTC GCT GAG TAA GTA CGA GGC GTG ACC...

CHis 1545-C

..leu gln ala gln his arg cys cys ser leu leu val cys trp arg ser leu ser lys tyr glu ala ***
..CTG CAG GCC CAG cat cga tgC TGC TCC CTG CTT GTG TGT TGG AGG TGG CTG AGT AAG TAC GAG GCG TGA...

CHis 1545 H

.leu gln ala gln pro lys leu gly pro ser leu gly leu leu pro ala cys val leu glu val ala glu ***
..CTG CAG GCC CAG ccc aag ctt ggg ccc aag ctt ggg CTG CTC CCT GCT TGT GTC TTG GAG GTC GCT GAG TAA..

Figure 7. Nucleotide sequence of mutations within the 3' terminus of the RSV src gene.
Insertions of synthetic oligonucleotides are designated by lowercase letters. Sequence alterations were identified by digestion with restrictions endonuclease and by direct DNA sequence analysis.

Transfection of chicken cells with genomic plasmids bearing each of the individual mutations revealed that the point mutations, pm26, pm9, pm6 and pm65 were defective for transformation. In addition, each of the linker insertion mutations, is1545-H, and is1545-C was also defective for transformation. In contrast, both wild type and the pseudo-mutant pm59 readily induced morphological transformation of chicken cells. To determine the

level of src-specific tyrosine protein kinase activity expressed in cells
infected with the individual mutants, immune complex kinase activity was
measured in extracts from cells infected with both wild type and mutant
virus. Table 1 summarizes the results of several experiments measuring
both autophosphorylation and the phosphorylation of the exogenous substrate
casein. Immune complexes from mutant infected cells consistently exhibited
reduced levels of kinase activity, ranging from 0.05 to 2% of the level
observed in immune complexes from wild type infected cells. The precise
level of activity may in fact be lower, since it is difficult to ascertain
the amount of kinase activity due to contamination of the immune complexes
with pp60[c-src]. In a parallel set of experiments, measurement of the level
of tyrosine specific phosphorylation of the 36 kd protein (a major target of
pp60[src] [31,32]) in mutant infected cells revealed a substantial reduction
in in vivo tyrosine kinase activity compared to wild type infected cells[25].
These data document that mutations within the carboxy terminal domain of the
src protein exhibit profound effects on tyrosine protein kinase activity
in vitro and in vivo, and conconmitantly on the transforming potential of
the mutant src protein.

IV. Discussion

A. pp60[src] contains distinct functional domains.

Several lines of evidence support the hypothesis that the src protein is
composed of multiple structural and functional domains. First, the comparison of the deduced amino acid sequences of a number of retroviral-encoded
tyrosine protein kinases and growth factor receptors reveals substantial
sequence homology within regions corresponding to the putative tyrosine
kinase domain (Figure 1). This sequence homology rapidly diverges at a
point upstream of the consconsus ATP binding site[33], suggesting that for
each oncogene protein the amino terminal sequences encode structurally and
functionally distinct domains. In the case of the receptors for the growth
factors, EGF[3] and insulin[37], and the retrovirus-encoded analogues of receptors (the erb B and fms proteins[3,4]), these sequences encode a transmembrane
domain and an extracellular ligand binding domain. However in the case of
the oncogene encoded proteins, src, fps/fes, abl, fgr and yes, the function
of these upstream sequences remains unresolved. The oncogene proteins encoded by fps/fes, abl, fgr, and yes contain amino terminal gag related sequences, a result of fusion of portions of the gag gene with the respective

oncogene sequence[18,19,20,34]. The gag sequences may play an important role in altering either the functional specificity of the gag-onc fusion proteins or their intracellular location and/or stabilization.

The analysis of site-directed mutations within the src gene indicates that the amino terminal region of pp60src contains at least two structural domains required for functional activity. The first of these putative domains is defined by alterations within the extreme amino terminus of the src protein (residues 2-15). Such mutations greatly reduce the efficiency of transformation but appear not to reduce its intrinsic tyrosine protein kinase activity of the mutant protein. These mutations include point mutations that convert the penultimate glycine residue to either alanine or glutamic acid[17,38] and deletions mutations that remove residues 2 to 15[16]. Biochemical analysis of cells infected with these mutations has shown that mutant src proteins lacking amino terminal myristylation do not stably associate with the plasma membrane. Therefore, myristylation of the amino terminal sequence of the src protein appears to play a major role in its intracellular distribution and functional activity[36].

The second putative domain is defined by introduction of deletions into a region encoding residues 15 to 169. Mutations that remove residues 15-149 do not alter the ability of the src gene product to mediate cellular transformation[39] (Figure 3). In each case the structurally altered src protein appears to localize to the plasma membrane and to retain wild type levels of tyrosine protein kinase activity[28,39]. In contrast, deletions which impinge upon the sequence encoding residues 143 to 169, result in the loss of transforming ability and yield structurally altered src proteins with reduced tyrosine protein kinase activity (Table 1). These mutations therefore appear to define a domain required for functional transformation. As we will discuss below, the phenotype of these mutants suggests that this domain may play a critical role in determining the selection of target proteins for the src protein.

B. The role of carboxy terminal sequences in src function.

A large body of biochemical and genetic evidence supports the notion that the carboxy terminal one-half of the src protein contains the kinase catalytic domain. The observation that point mutations within a highly conserved sequence of this domain result in both the loss of transforming potential and protein kinase activity is consistent with this view. The carboxy terminal limits of this domain are defined by linker insertion mutations near the carboxy terminus (within eleven amino acids). As illustrated above, insertion mutations adjacent to leu$_{516}$ exhibit profound effects on transformation and kinase activity. It would appear from these results that maintainence of the three dimensional structure of the src protein requires a substantial contribution from these distal carboxy terminal sequences. In this context two points should be noted. First, leu$_{516}$ marks the boundary of amino acid sequence divergence between v-src and c-src. Secondly, sequences immediately downstream from leu$_{516}$ in c-src include potential site(s) for tyrosine phosphorylation (missing from v-src due to the recombinational replacement of these sequences). It is interesting to speculate that the kinase domain of the cellular src protein may be subject to regulation via this site whereas, because of sequence alteration, the virus encoded src protein may be insensitive to regulation. A similar structural modification is observed in the EGF receptor and its retroviral homologue, the v-erb B protein. A major site of tyrosine phosphorylation within the EGF receptor resides in a sequence close to its carboxy terminus. This sequence however is deleted in the transforming protein (a truncated form of the EGF receptor), suggesting that the presence of this phosphorylation site may influence the normal control of EGF receptor function.

C. The role of amino terminal sequences in src function.

   The two amino terminal structural features of the src protein defined by mutagenesis studies, namely the site of myristylation and the putative amino acid 150-169 region, clearly play an important role in src function. The requirement for myristylation appears directly linked to the need to insert the src protein in a membrane compartment. Presumably this membrane localization reflects the requirement for juxaposition of the src protein with important cellular targets. At this time the identity of these targets remains unknown, but could possibly represent intrinsic membrane proteins such as growth factor recpetors, or enzymes involved in the maintenance of cytoskeletal structures or components of the phosphatidyl inositol turnover pathway. In this regard Chen et al. have recently suggested that the presence of pp60^{src} at specific sites in the plasma membrane results either directly or indirectly in the activation of extra cellular proteases, an event that could directly contribute to the metastatic properties of src transformed cells[40]. In addition, Purchio et al. have shown tha phorbol ester treatment of RSV transformed cells gives rise to the site-specific phosphorylation of the src protein on an amino terminal serine residue[41]. Finally, Yonemoto et al. have shown that pp60[c-src] complexed with polyoma middle T antigen undergoes a unique amino terminal tyrosine phosphorylation[42]. This phosphorylation appears to play a role in the activtion of middle T associated pp60c-src kinase activity.

The signficance of the functional domain defined by mutations impinging on sequences within amino acid residues 143 to 169 remains less clear. However in light of our current knowledge, two possibilities must be considered. First, it is possible that transformation defective deletion mutations alter the intrinsic protein kinase activity of the src protein, thereby reducing the transforming potential of the gene product. We feel that this possibility is unlikely since the residual kinase activity measured in cells infected with these transformation defective mutants excedes that observed in many RSV transformed mammalian cell lines. Therefore it would appear unlikely that these quantitative differences could explain the phenotypic changes observed. Secondly, one can argue that the regions encompassing residues 150 to 169 define a portion of the src protein required for target protein binding or substrate recognition. This region is highly conserved between viral and avian cellular src proteins as well as with the human cellular src protein[43]. The fact that amino terminal modifications appear to alter src kinase activity[42] lends further support to the target recognition role for this domain. Clearly, the analysis of additional mutants and the availability of purified mutant src protein should permit the testing of such an hypothesis.

C. Prospectus.

Site-directed mutagenesis of the src gene has provided the molecular virologist with unique and useful insights into the structure and function of an important viral oncogene product as well as its normal cellular counterpart. However, these genetic engineering techniques have not succeeded in providing the answers to important biological and biochemical questions. What remains to be carried out is a systematic analysis of the enzymatic properties of mutant proteins as well as a complete ultrastructural analysis of the src protein. The elucidation of a three dimensional structure of the src protein will undoubtedly provide the information needed to understand the complex and important functions of this oncogene protein.

V. Summary.

Site-directed mutagenesis techniques have been utilized to define important structural and functional domains within the RSV src gene product, pp60^{src}. Deletion mutations within the amino terminal one-half of the src gene which impinge upon a region of the src protein delineated by amino acid residues 143 to 169 yielded transformation defective viruses. Src proteins encoded by such RSV mutants exhibited diminished tyrosine protein kinase activity in vitro and only slightly reduced levels of in vivo tyrosine protein kinase activity. We speculate that these structurally altered proteins are defective for target protein recognition. Point mutations and linker insertion mutations within the putative catalytic domain of pp60^{src} served to block the transforming activity of mutant viruses. Mutant viruses encode src proteins that exhibited substantially reduced levels of tyrosine protein kinase activity both in vitro and in vivo.

VI. Acknowledgements.

We thank our many colleagues for the interest and support during the course of these experiments. We wish to especially acknowledge the technical assistance of B. Creasy, D. McCarley, A. Coffman and R. Renaud. We also thank M. Weber, D. Benjamin, J. Morgan, D. Bryant, M. Heaney and G. Gilmartin for the many helpful discussion. J.T.P. is supported by a Faculty Research Award from the American Cancer Society. S.J.P.is a Scholar of the Leukemia Society of America. These studies were supported by Public Health Service grants CA29243 and CA27578 awarded by the National Cancer Institute and grant NP-462G from the American Cancer Society.

VII. References.

1. Bishop, J. M. (1983) Annu. Rev. Biochem. 52, 301-354.
2. Bishop, J. M. (1985) Cell 42, 23-38.
3. Ullrich, A., Coussens, L., Haflick, J. S., Dull, T. J., Gray, A., Tom, A. W., Lee, J. Yarden, Y. Liberman, T. A. Schlessinger, J. Downward, J. Mayes, E. L. V., Whittle, N., Waterfield, M. D., and Seeburg, P. H. (1984) Nature 309, 418-425.
4. Sherr, C. J., Rettenmier, C. W., Sacca, R., Roussel, M., Look, A. T., and Stanley, E. R. (1985) Cell 41, 665-676.
5. Brugge, J. S., and Erikson, R. L. (1977) Nature 269, 346-348.
6. Collet, M. S. and Erikson, R. L. (1978) Proc. Natl. Acad. Sci. U.S.A. 75, 2021-2024.

7. Cooper, J. A., and Hunter, T. (1981) Mol. Cell Biol. 4, 1213-1220.

8. Hanafusa, H. (1977) in Compr. Virol (H. Fraenkel-Konrat and R. R. Wagner, eds.) Plenum Publishing Corp., New York, 10, 410-483.

9. Cooper, J. A., Reiss, N. A., Schwartz, R. J., and Hunter, T. (1983) Nature 302, 218-223.

10. Hunter, T. and Sefton, B. (1980) Proc. Natl. Acad. Sci. U.S.A. 77, 1311-1315.

11. Collett, M. S., Erikson, E. and Erikson, R. L. (1979) J. Virol. 29, 770-781.

12. Smart, J. E., Oppermann, H., Czernilofsky, A. P., Purchio, A. F., Erikson, R. L., and Bishop, J. M. (1981) Proc. Natl. Sci. U. S. A. 78, 6013-6017.

13. Sugimoto, Y. Whitman, M., Cantley, L., and Erikson, R. L. (1984) Proc. Natl. Acad. Sci. U. S. A. 81, 2117-2121.

14. Garber, E. A., Krueger, J. G., Hanafusa, H., and Goldberg, A. R. (1983) Nature 302, 161,163.

15. Sefton, B., Trowbridge, I. S., Cooper, J. A., and Scolnick, E. M. (1982) Cell 31, 465-474.

16. Cross, F. R., Barber, E. A., Pellman, D., and Hanafusa, H (1984) Mol. Cell. Biol. 4, 1834-1842.

17. Kamps, M. P., Buss, J. E., and Sefton, B (1985) Proc. Natl. Sci. U.S.A. 82, 4625-4628.

18. Kitamura, N., Kitamura, A., Toyoshima, K., Hirayama, Y., and Yoshida, M. (1982) Nature 297, 205-208.

19. Reddy, E. P., Smith, M. J., and Srinivason, A. (1983) Proc. Natl. Sci. U.S.A. 80, 3623-3627.

20. Shibuya, M., and Hanafusa, H. (1982) Cell 30, 787-795.

21. Hampe, A., Gobet, M., Sherr, C. J., and Gabbert, F. (1982) Cell 30, 775,785.

22. Bryant, D., and Parsons, J. T. (1982) J. Virol. 44, 683-691.

23. Parsons, S. J., McCarley, D. J., Ely, C. M., Benjamin, D., and Parsons, J. T. (1984) J. Virol. 51, 273-278.

24. Parsons, S. J., Riley, S. C., Mullen, E. E., Brock, E. J., Benjamin, D. C., Kuehl, W. M., and Parson, J. T. (1979) J. Virol. 27, 227-238.

25. Byrant, D., and Parsons, J. T. (1984) Mol. Cell. Biol. 4, 862-866.

26. Wilkerson, V. W., Bryant, D. L., and Parsons, J. R. (1985) J. Virol. 55, 314-321.

27. Fincham, V., Chiswell, D. J., and Wyke, J. A. (1982) Virology 116, 72-83.

28. Wilkerson, V. W., and Parsons, J. T. (1985) submitted for publication.

29. Lorincz, A. T., and Reed, S. I. (1984) Nature 307, 183-185.

30. Hoffman, F. M., Fresco, L. D., Hoffman-Falk, H., and Shilo, B. Z. (1984) Cell 35, 393-401.

31. Radke, K., Gilmore, T., and Martin, G. S. (1980) Cell 21, 821-828.

32. Erikson, E., and Erikson, R. L. (1980) Cell 21, 829-836.

33. Barker, W. C., and Dayhoff, M. O. (1982) Proc. Natl. Acad. Sci. U.S.A. 79, 2836-2839.

34. Naharro, G., Robbins, K. C., and Reddy, E. P. (1984) Science 223, 63-66.

35. Schwartz, D. R., Tizard, R., and Gilbert, W. (1982) Cell 32, 853-869.

36. Schultz, A. M., Henderson, L. E., Oroszlan, S., Garber, E. A., and Hanafusa, H. (1985) Science 227, 427-429.

37. Ullrich, A., Bell, J. R., Chen, E. Y., Herrra, R., Petruzzelli, L. M., Dull, T. J., Gray, A., Coussens, L., Liao, Y-C., Tsubokawa, M., Masom, J. (1985) Nature 313, 756-761.

38. Pellman, D., Garber, E. A., Cross, F. R., and Hanafusa, H. (1985) Proc. Natl. Acad. Sci. U.S.A. 82, 1623-1627.

39. Cross, F. R., Garber, E. A., and Hanafusa, H. (1985) Mol. Cell Biol. 5, 2789-2795.

40. Chen, W.-T., Chen, J.-M., Parsons, S. J., and Parsons, J. T. (1985) Nature 316, 156-158.

41. Purchio, A. F., Shoyab, M., and Gentry, L. E. (1985) Science 229, 1393-1395.

42. Yonemoto, Y., Jarvis-Morar, M., Brugge, J. S., Bolen, J. B., and Israel, M. A. (1985) Proc. Natl. Acad. Sci. U.S.A. 82, 4568-4572.

43. Anderson, S. K., Gibbs, C. P., Tanaka, A., Kung, H-J. and Fujita, J. (1985) Mol. Cell. Biol. 5, 1122-1129.

2

Activation of _ras_ Oncogenes by Chemical Carcinogens

Mariano Barbacid, Saraswati Sukumar, and H. Zarbl

Developmental Oncology Section
LBI-Basic Research Program
NCI-Frederick Cancer Research Facility
P.O. Box B
Frederick, MD   21701

22

I. INTRODUCTION

One of the most significant advances in recent cancer research has been the identification and subsequent characterization of oncogenes in human tumors. Oncogenes were initially identified as the transforming principle of acute transforming retroviruses (v-onc genes) and were subsequently shown to be altered versions of normal cellular genes, generically designated as proto-oncogenes[1]. Oncogenes are known to acquire their malignant properties by a number of different mechanisms[2]. Viral oncogenes, for example, arose by recombination between cellular proto-oncogenes and the genome of nontransforming retroviruses[1]. Proto-oncogene activation may also result by enhancer activation[3,4], point mutations[5-7], chromosomal translocations[8,9], gene amplification[10], and insertional mutagenesis[11,12]. Such a wide spectrum of activating mechanisms would indeed be expected for genes involved in neoplasia considering the vast number of viral, chemical, and physical agents that have been implicated in the origins of cancer.

The role of proto-oncogenes in the normal cell remains, for the most part, unknown. It is generally believed that proto-oncogenes code for proteins functional in the regulation of cell differentiation and/or proliferation. Recent findings demonstrating a high degree of similarity between certain oncogenes and growth factors or growth factor receptors corroborate this general hypothesis[13-15]. Activation of such regulatory proteins by mutations, overexpression, or expression in inappropriate cells would be expected to result in uncontrolled growth, the hallmark of transformed cells.

Gene transfer assays have made it possible to demonstrate the presence of oncogenes in human cancers as well as in chemically induced animal tumors[2,16]. Within the limits of sensitivity of these assays, the presence of activated proto-oncogenes does not appear to be a pathogenomic indicator of cancer cells. Although a significant fraction (15-20%) of human tumors have oncogenes capable of inducing the malignant transformation of cell lines of rodent origin, there is not apparent correlation with the pathological parameters of the tumor. In contrast, some carcinogen-induced animal model tumor systems exhibit a good correlation (70-90%) between oncogene activation and tumor development[17]. The discrepancy between the frequency of transforming genes in human and carcinogen-induced animal tumors suggests that oncogene activation may be more related to the etiology of cancer and the genetic background of the host than to the pathology of the tumor. The majority of the oncogenes detected in gene transfer experiments have been found to be members of the ras gene family[18-21], first identified as the transforming principle of several strains of murine sarcoma virus[22,23]. The following report summarizes the data from ours as well as other laboratories pertaining to the mechanism of activation and involvement of ras oncogenes in human and carcinogen-induced animal tumors.

II. MATERIALS & METHODS

Mnl I Restriction Fragment Length Polymorphisms

In order to detect Mnl I restriction fragment length polymorphisms (RFLP) in H-ras-1 oncogenes, forty micrograms of DNA isolated from normal breasts and carcinogen-induced mammary carcinomas were digested for sixteen hours with 40 units of Mnl I using conditions recommended by the supplier (New England Biolabs, Inc.). Digests ere electrophoresed (18 hours at 40 V) in horizontal 2.8% agarose gels (w/v) and blotted to either zeta-probe™ blotting membranes (Bio-Rad Laboratories) or nitrocellulose as described by Southern[24]. Membranes were hybridized under stringent conditions (50% formamide, 5 x SSC, and 42°C) for 72 hours with 10^7 cpm/ml of ^{32}P-labelled probe obtained by nick translation of the 120 bp Hpa II-Sac I DNA fragment described in Figure 1A. Blots were exposed for 24 hours to Kodak XAR-5 film at -70°C in the presence of intensifier screens.

Synthetic Oligonucleotide Probes

Synthetic oligonucleotide probes were used to determine the point mutations responsible for malignant activation of the H-ras-1 locus in carcinogen-induced rat mammary carcinomas. DNAs were isolated from NIH/3T3 cells co-transfected with the normal H-ras-1 gene and pSV2-neo[25] and selected for growth in the presence of G418. Fifty micrograms of each DNA were digested with 400 units of Hind III using conditions recommended by the supplier (New England Biolabs, Inc.). Digests were electrophoresed (12 h at 50 V) in horizontal agarose (0.7% w/v) gels which were subsequently prepared for hybridization as previously described[26]. Dried gels were prehybridized for 1 h in hybridization buffer containing 500 µg/ml of sonicated herring sperm DNA and subsequently hybridized for 18 h at the discriminating temperature previously determined for each individual oligonucleotide probe. [^{32}P]-labelled oligonucleotide probes were used at a concentration of 5 ng/ml (specific activity of ~2 x 10^9 cpm/µg) or 1.5 ng/ml (specific activity of ~7 x 10^9 cpm/µg) depending on the labelling protocol utilized (see below). Hybridized gels were then washed with constant agitation as follows: 300 ml (four changes) of 6 x SSC for 15 min each at room temperature and 400 ml of 6 x SSC for 30 min at room temperature. Then 500 ml of 6 x SSC at 2°C above the hybridization temperature were poured onto the gel and allowed to cool to room temperature for 30 min. Finally the gel was rinsed with 200 ml of 6 x SSC at room temperature, dried and exposed to Kodak XAR-5 film for 18 h at -70°C in the presence of intensifier screens.

Oligonucleotide Labelling

High specific activity probes ($\sim$7 x 10^9 cpm/μg) were synthesized as previously described[27,28]. An octamer complementary to the 3' end of the template nonadecamers was quantitatively phosphorylated at its 5' end under conditons described above. After phenol extraction, the phosphorylated primer was purified by gel filtration on Sephadex G-25 columns (Superfine) eluted in water. The octamer primer was then annealed to the nonadecamer templates in 50 mm NaCl-10 mM Tris-HCl (pH 8.0) - 1 mM EDTA at final concentrations of 50 ng/ml of template (7.5 μM) and 100 ng/ml of primer (30 μM) by heating to 80°C and cooling slowly to 4°C. Primer extension reactions were done in a final volume of 10 μl containing 0.1 mM dATP, 0.1 mM TTP, 5 mM β-mercaptoethanol, 50 mM NaCl, 25 mM Tris-HCl (pH 7.5), 10 mM $MgCl_2$, 1 μl of annealed primer and template mixture (30 pmoles and 7.5 pmoles, respectively), 30 pmoles each of [$\alpha^{32}P$]dCTP and [$\alpha^{32}P$]dGTP (Amersham, at 3000 Ci/mmole, evaporated to dryness), and DNA Polymerase I Klenow Fragment at a final concentration of 0.5 U/μl (New England Biolabs). Reaction mixtures were incubated at 0°C for 90 min. 10 μl of formamide containing xylene cyanol and bromophenol blue marker dyes were then added and the samples were boiled for 5 min. The labelled nonadecamer probes were then separated from the unlabelled template by electrophoresis in a denaturing 20% polyacrylamide gel[26]. The positions of nonadecamer probes were determined by autoradiography, the bands excised and eluted by washing gel slices three times for 1-3 hours each with 300 μl of 0.9 M NaCl, 0.18 M Tris-HCl (pH 8.0) and 6 mM EDTA. Eluted probes were added directly to hybridization mixtures.

III. RESULTS

H-ras-1 Oncogenes in Carcinogen-Induced Mammary Carcinomas

Treatment of female rats with a single dose of carcinogen during their sexual development leads to the efficient and reproducible induction of mammary carcinomas[29,30]. We have previously shown that each of nine mammary carcinomas induced by NMU in Buf/N rats contained a transforming H-ras-1 oncogene[31]. These observations have now been generalized[32]. 79% (30 of 38) of those DNAs isolated from NMU-induced mammary carcinomas of Buf/N rats were capable of inducing morphological transformation of NIH/3T3 cells in gene transfer experiments due to the presence of H-ras-1 oncogenes. Similar results (18 of 25 or 72%) were obtained with tumors induced in Sprague-

Dawley rats, a random-bred strain. Transforming H-ras-1 genes were also identified in mammary tumors induced by DMBA (7,12-dimethylbenz(a)anthracene), a different carcinogen. In this case, however, only five of twenty-six DNAs contained this oncogene. The results with DMBA-induced contrast the high frequency of oncogene activation observed in NMU-induced tumors. The reason for this difference remains to be determined. However, they illustrate the role that the inducing etiological agent plays in determining the molecular pathways that lead to neoplastic transformation.

Mechanisms of Activation of H-ras-1 Oncogenes in NMU-Induced Tumors

ras oncogenes have been shown to acquire their transforming properties by missense mutations in codons 12, 13, 59, 61, and 63[5-7,33-35]. Codons 12, 13, and 61 have been shown to be responsible for the malignant activation of ras genes in both human and animal tumors[2,16]. Codon 59 has been implicated in the activation of the retroviral oncogenes[36,37]. Finally, codon 63 has only been identified in in vitro mutagenesis experiments[35]. Some of these mutations alter sequences specifically recognized by restriction endonucleases, thus leading to the generation of diagnostic RFLPs. RFLP have been successfully utilized to identify oncogenes in human tumor DNAs[38]. We have utilized this experimental approach to identify the point mutations responsible for the specific activation of the H-ras-1 locus in NMU-induced mammary carcinomas[32].

Figure 1 depicts the generation of a polymorphic Mnl I DNA fragment generated by mutations affecting the second and third nucleotides of codon 12 (residues 35 and 36) and the two coding deoxyguanosines of codon 13 (residues 37 and 38). The first exon of the normal H-ras-1 allele spans two Mnl I DNA fragments of 206 and 74 base pairs (bp). Elimination of this Mnl I cleavage site generates a single 280 bp Mnl I DNA fragment. Wild type (206 bp) and polymorphic (280 bp) DNA fragments can be identified by Southern blot analysis utilizing the 120 bp Hpa II-Sac I DNA fragment depicted in Figure 1A as a radioactive probe. Figure 1B shows two representative experiments. Most of the tumors tested exhibited the polymorphic 280 bp Mnl I DNA fragment diagnostic of a mutated H-ras-1 gene. In addition to this polymorphic fragment, each tumor DNA exhibited the normal 206 bp Mnl I DNA fragment, indicative of heterozygocity at this locus. The stronger intensity of the latter (Figure 1B) is probably contributed by the normal H-ras-1 alleles of the accompanying stroma.

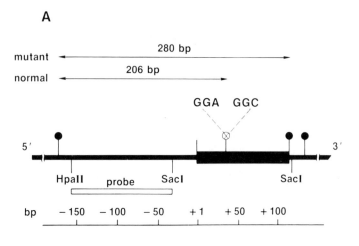

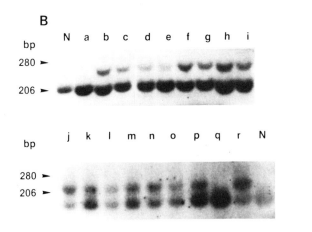

Figure 1. A) Strategy for detection of Mnl I restriction fragment length polymorphisms (RFLP) created by mutations within the twelfth or thirteenth codons of the rat H-ras-1 locus. Wild-type Mnl I restriction sites (●) in the vicinity of the first exon (solid box, nucleotides +1 to +111) are indicated. The position of the polymorphic Mnl I site (GAGG, ⊗ , nucleotides +35 to +38) relative to the sequences of the normal twelfth (GGA) and thirteenth (GGC) codons is shown. Arrows span the normal (206 bp) and polymorphic (280 bp) Mnl I restriction fragments detected by the 120 bp Hpa II-Sac I probe.

B) DNA isolated from normal breasts (N) and NMU-induced mammary carcinomas (a-r). Arrows indicate the positions of the normal (206 bp) and the polymorphic (280 bp) Mnl I restriction fragments.

In total, 61 NMU-induced tumors of 71 tested, scored as positive in the Mnl I RFLP assay (Table I). The 61 Mnl I RFLP positive tumors included 32 from Buf/N rats and 23 from Sprague-Dawley. Of these 55 mammary carcinomas known to contain H-ras-1 oncogenes by molecular assays, only 48 (30 from Buf/N rats and 18 from Sprague-Dawley) scored positive in gene transfer assays (see above). These results indicate that gene transfer assays underestimate the number of existing oncogenes. None of twenty-six normal breasts obtained from eighteen Buf/N and six Sprague-Dawley rats exhibited the Mnl I RFLP (Table I). More importantly, four of these normal breasts were obtained from animals carrying one or more mammary carcinomas. These observations rule out the possibility that the high frequency of Mnl I RFLPs might be due to random mutagenesis, and thus, suggest a close association between mutagenesis in this specific domain of the H-ras-1 locus and tumor development.

G → A Mutations in NMU-Induced H-ras-1 Oncogenes

To establish the role of ras oncogenes in the development of neoplasia, it is necessary to define the stage at which they become activated. Induction of rat mammary carcinomas by a single dose of NMU, does not proceed through identifiable pre-neoplastic stages in which the presence of ras oncogenes could be demonstrated[29,30]. However, this animal tumor system possesses two important properties. First, initiation of carcinogenesis is a well defined process that is completed within hours following administration of NMU. Second, the mutagenic properties of NMU have been well characterized. NMU is a direct acting alkylating agent that preferentially induces G → A mutations as a consequence of its ability to methylate the O^6 position of deoxyguanosine residues[39-41]. In an effort to establish whether H-ras-1 oncogenes were directly activated by NMU during initiation of the carcinogenesis we examined whether the diagnostic Mnl I RFLP's shown above were generated by G → A mutations.

For this purpose, we utilized oligonucleotide probes capable of detecting specific point mutations in genomic DNA. We synthesized nonadecamers to identify substitutions in position 35. This residue is the only nucleotide of the Mnl I cleavage site that can alter the coding properties of the critical twelfth codon of the H-ras-1 gene. Oligomers included Ha19-G^{35} [5' TGGGCGCTGG*AGGCGTGGG-3', where the underlined nucleotides define the diagnostic Mnl I cleavage site and G* is the deoxyguanosine residue located in position 35]; while Ha19-A^{35} and Ha19-T^{35} had position 35 (G*) substituted by either a deoxyadenosine (Ha19-A^{35}) or a thymidine (Ha19-T^{35}). The cor-

Table I. Malignant Activation of the H-ras-1 Locus in NMU-Induced Mammary
Carcinomas of Rats[a]

Strain	Mammary Carcinomas		Normal Breasts	
	Tested	H-ras-1 Oncogene	Tested[b]	H-ras-1 Oncogene
Buf/N	38	32 (84%)	18	0
Sprague-Dawley	25	23 (92%)	8	0
Fischer 344	8	6 (75%)	-	-
TOTAL	71	61 (86%)	26	0

[a]As determined by the Mnl I RFLP assay.
[b]Includes four Buf/N and two Sprague-Dawley normal breasts obtained from
tumor-bearing animals.

responding Ha19-C^{35} oligonucleotide was not synthesized because a G^{35} → C^{35}
transversion would have created a polymorphic Pst I cleavage site which
could not be detected in any of the tumors tested (data not shown). The
specificity of each of these three nonadecamers were verified by hybridization to plasmids containing the normal rat H-ras-1 gene (pH-ras-1) and a
transforming allele (pNMU-1) previously shown to carry an activating
G^{35} → A mutation[31] (Figure 2).

The oligonucleotide probes were hybridized to Hind III cleaved DNAs isolated from the representative NIH/3T3 transformants obtained from each of
the NMU-induced mammary carcinomas that scored positive in gene transfer experiments. NIH/3T3 transformants were initially selected because they contain slightly amplified oncogene sequences and lack the normal H-ras-1 rat
allele. Results of representative experiments are depicted in Figure 3.
At the discriminating temperature, each of the NIH/3T3 transformants tested
hybridized to Ha19-A^{35} but not to Ha19-G^{35} or Ha19-T^{35}, indicating that
their transforming H-ras-1 oncogenes carried identical G → A transitions in
position 35. As expected, DNA isolated from NIH/3T3 cells containing multiple copies of the normal H-ras-1 proto-oncogene (which was co-transfected
with pSV2neo[25]) hybridized to Ha19-G^{35}, but not to the Ha19-A^{35} or Ha19-T^{35}
oligonucleotide probes (Figure 3).

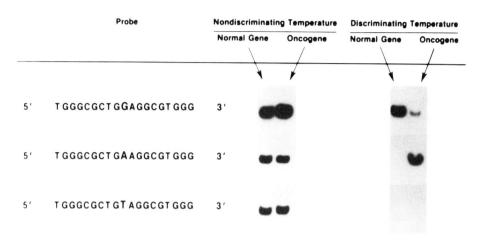

Figure 2. Synthetic nonadecamer probes corresponding to the nucleotide residues 26 to 44 in the first exon of the normal H-ras-1 locus as well as those for $G^{35} \rightarrow A$ and $G^{35} \rightarrow T$ mutations were synthesized. Probes were hybridized to Hind III-digested DNA from plasmids containing the normal (pH-ras-1) and transforming (pNMU-1) alleles of the rat H-ras-1 locus[31]. Nondiscriminating temperature was 42°C; the discriminating temperature was 65°C.

In order to eliminate any possible artifact during transfection procedures we identified the mutated H-ras-1 oncogenes directly in tumor tissue (Figure 4). Panel A depicts the results obtained when Bam HI digested tumor DNA were hybridized with the nonadecamer probe Ha19-G^{35}, which specifically detects the normal H-ras-1 locus. This oligonucleotide probe hybridizes with the expected 10 kbp Bam HI fragment in DNA isolated from both normal breast tissue (N) and mammary carcinomas (a-k). The detection of a normal H-ras-1 allele in tumor DNA corroborates the results obtained in the Mnl I RFLP assay (see Figure 1) and are indicative of heterozygocity of the H-ras-1 locus in these tumors. Panel B shows the results obtained when Bam HI digested tumor DNAs were hybridized with the nonadecamer probe Ha19-A^{35}, which specifically detects H-ras oncogenes harboring $G \rightarrow A$ transitions to the second deoxyguanosine residue of codon 12. The Ha19-A^{35} probe hybridized with two Bam HI fragments. The first of these is a 12 kbp fragment that was detec-

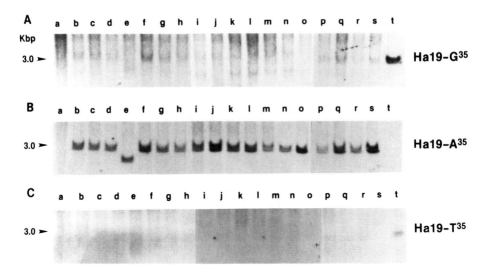

Figure 3. Use of synthetic oligonucleotide probes to determine the specific point mutations responsible for malignant activation of the H-ras-1 locus in NMU-induced rat mammary carcinomas. DNAs were isolated from NIH/3T3 cells (a), representative NIH/3T3 transformants derived from NMU-induced mammary carcinomas (b to s), and NIH/3T3 cells co-transfected with the normal H-ras-1 gene and pSV2-neo and selected for growth in the presence of G418 (t). A) Hybridization with probe Ha19-G35 (5'TGGGCGCTGGAGGCGTGGG 3'); B) Hybridization with probe Ha19-A35 (5'TGGGCGCTGAAGGCGTGGG 3'); C) Hybridization with probe Ha19-T35 (5'TGGGCGCTGTAGGCGTGGG 3'). Arrowheads indicate the expected 3.0 kbp Hind III DNA fragment of H-ras-1, which contains all coding sequences except the first 12 nucleotides (16).

ted in DNA from both normal breast and breast carcinomas. Hybridization of the probe with the 12 kbp fragment was more frequently detected in DNA from Fischer 344 rats (N and h-k) than in Sprague-Dawley rats (N and d-g) or Buf/N rats (N and a-c), and presumably represents a polymorphism in the H-ras-2 pseudogene locus. The second fragment detected by the Ha19-A35 probe is the expected 10 kbp Bam HI fragment containing the H-ras-1 onco- gene. This fragment was not detected in DNA from normal breast (N) or in

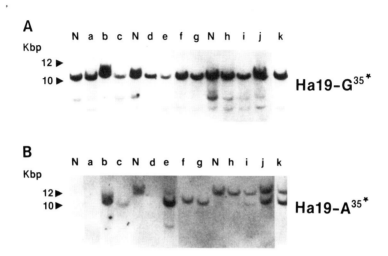

Figure 4. Use of high specific activity nonadecamer probes to determine specific point mutations responsible for the malignant activation of the H-ras-1 locus in NMU-induced rat mammary carcinomas. DNAs were isolated from normal breast tissue (N), from NMU-induced tumors that did not have activated H-ras-1 oncogenes (a, d, and h) and tumors which did have activated H-ras-1 oncogenes (b, c, e-g, and i-j). A) Hybridization with probe Ha19-G^{35}* (~7 x 10^9 cpm/μg), and B) hybridization with probe Ha19-A^{35}* (~6 x 10^9 cpm/μg). Arrowheads indicate the expected 10 kbp and 12 kbp Bam HI fragments which contain all of the coding sequences of the H-ras-1 gene and H-ras-2 pseudogene, respectively.

DNA from mammary tumors that had been previously shown not to have activated H-ras-1 oncogene (lanes a, d, and h) using DNA mediated NIH/3T3 cell transfection assays and the Mnl I RFLP assay. The Ha19-A^{35} probe did, however, detect the 10 kbp fragment in those tumors that were shown to have activated H-ras-1 oncogenes by transfection assays or the Mnl I RFLP assay (lanes b, c, e-g, and i-j). These results unequivocally demonstrate the presence of the activating G^{35} A mutations of H-ras-1 oncogenes in DNA isolated from tumor tissues.

DMBA-Induced H-ras-1 Oncogenes are Activated by Mutations in the 61st Codon

The striking specificity of the above findings strongly suggests that the activating $G^{35} \rightarrow A$ transitions were the direct consequence of the mutagenic activity of NMU. However, alternative explanations must also be considered. For instance, it is possible that this mutation may confer a selective growth advantage to the neoplastic mammary cells. Alternatively, mammary cells may have repair systems that preferentially introduce deoxyadenosine residues. To address this fundamental question, we examined the mutations responsible for the activation of H-ras-1 oncogenes in mammary carcinomas induced by DMBA. This carcinogen forms large adducts with deoxyguanosine and deoxyadenosine residues leading to the induction of excision repair mechanisms, which occassionally generate point mutations of undefined specificity[42]. DNA from representative NIH/3T3 transformants derived from each of five DMBA-induced mammary carcinomas known to contain a transforming H-ras-1 oncogene, efficiently hybridized to the Ha19-G^{35} probe but not to the Ha19-A^{35} or Ha19-T^{35} probes. These results indicate that H-ras-1 oncogenes in DMBA-induced tumors were not activated by point mutations in either the twelfth or adjacent codons. In agreement with these observations, none of these oncogenes exhibit the polymorphic Mnl I RFLP.

Previous studies have indicated that ras genes may also acquire transforming properties as a result of missense mutations in the sixty first codon. It was, therefore, plausible that H-ras-1 oncogenes present in DNBA-induced mammary tumors were activated as a result of point mutations within the sixty-first codon. In order to examine this possibility, we utilized a nonadecamer probe complementary to the sixty-first codon (CAA) and flanking sequences of the normal rat H-ras-1 locus. DNA from transformants derived from DMBA-induced tumors failed to hybridize to the nonadecamer probe using hybridization conditions that will not allow for detection of sequences with single base mismatches. These results indicated that each of the five H-ras-1 oncogenes present in the DMBA-induced tumors harboured mutations in the region of the sixty-first codon.

Mixed sequence oligonucleotides capable of detecting all mutations in the deoxycytosine residue of codon sixty-one (CAA), failed to hybridize to DNA from any of the five transformants. Four of the transformants hybridized to the oligomer probe which detected point mutations in the second residue (deoxyadenosine) of codon sixty-one. One transformant hybridized to the oligomer probe which detected transversions in the third residue (deoxyadenosine) of codon sixty-one. These results indicate that H-ras-1 oncogenes of DMBA-induced tumors were activated by point mutations in either of the deoxyadenosine residues of codon 61 (CAA). These findings, summarized in Figure 5, rule out the possibility that the G^{35} , A mutations present in each of the NMU-induced H-ras-1 oncogene are the result of either positive growth selection or specific repair systems. Instead they indicate that malignant activation of the H-ras-1 locus in NMU-induced mammary carcinomas is the result of the direct mutagenic effect of NMU on this locus.

III. DISCUSSION

In spite of the wealth of information regarding ras oncogenes, their role in human neoplasia remains to be defined. Based on the apparent simplicity with which these genes acquire transforming properties[5-7] and on the fact that ras gene activation does not correlate with the histopathology of any type of human neoplasia[16], it has been speculated that ras oncogenes may only play a circumstantial role in carcinogenesis. The reproducible and specific activation of H-ras-1 oncogenes in 61 of 71 NMU-induced mammary

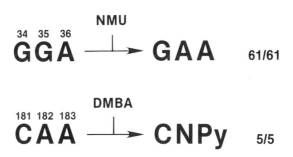

Figure 5. Mutagenesis of H-ras-1 oncogenes in NMU and DMBA-induced mammary carcinomas of rats. 61 H-ras-1 oncogenes present in NMU-induced mammary carcinomas acquired their transforming properties by a G : A transition in the second nucleotide (position 35) of codon 12 (GGA). 5 H-ras-1 oncogenes present in DMBA-induced mammary carcinomas exhibited normal codon 12. Instead, their activating mutations were localized in either of the two deoxyadenosine residues (positions 182 and 183) of codon 61 (CAA). N means any nucleotide other than A, and Py menas a pyrinidine (C or T) residue.

carcinomas of rats strongly argues against this possibility[32]. Instead, it favors the concept that malignant activation of this ras locus is a necessary step in the development of these mammary carcinomas.

Additional support for the hypothesis that ras oncogenes play a major role in carcinogenesis has been provided by similar studies in other animal tumor systems. For instance, ras oncogenes have been reproducibly detected in DMBA-induced mouse skin carcinomas[43,44], in X-ray and NMU-induced mouse thymomas[45] and in MCA-induced fibrosarcomas[46]. More recently, an EGF receptor-related oncogene, designated neu, has been identified in each of four ethylnitrosourea induced neuroblastoma cell lines[47], indicating that reproducible activation of oncogenes is not limited to members of the ras gene family, but instead might be a general property of tumors sharing a common genetic background, and perhaps more importantly, a defined etiology. Although the molecular basis for these observations are unknown, it is likely that malignant activation of a given locus might be determined, at least in part, by its role in those cells that become the target for carcinogenesis.

To establish the role that ras genes play in the multistep process of carcinogenesis requires precise definition of the stage at which they become activated. In vitro studies have suggested that ras oncogenes may play a role in tumor progression based on the fact that transformation of primary embryo fibroblast by ras oncogenes require acquisition of continuous cell proliferating capacity[48-50], a property that can be paralleled with the early stages of tumor development. However, we must take notice that these results were obtained with senescent fibroblasts. Therefore, any attempt to generalize them to in vivo systems must be taken with caution.

Studies obtained with in vivo animal model systems suggests a rather different picture. Induction of skin carcinomas in mice by a single dose of DMBA followed by repeated application of the tumor promotor TPA proceeds through well defined preneoplastic stages including induction of multiple papillomas. Only a few of these papillomas will eventually evolve into malignant carcinomas. Balmain and co-workers have shown that transforming H-ras genes exist in the majority of these papillomas indicating that these oncogenes were activated early in tumor development and that additional secondary changes are necessary to achieve the full malignant phenotype characteristic of carcinomas[44].

Induction of rat mammary carcinomas by NMU does not proceed through identifiable preneoplastic stages[29]. However, efficient induction of mammary carcinomas can be readily achieved by a single dose of NMU[30,31]. This compound is highly unstable under physiological conditions, therefore, its mutagenic effect must occur within hours following adminstration. Therefore, our findings indicating that H-ras-1 oncogenes are directly activated by NMU imply that malignant activation of this oncogene must be concomitant with the initiation of the carcinogenic process. Considering the well documented property of these oncogenes to induce neoplastic transformation in a variety of in vitro and in vivo systems, our findings strongly suggest that activation of ras oncogenes plays a fundamental role in the initiation of carcinogenesis.

In spite of the tremendous progress achieved in the molecular characterization of oncogenes and in studies leading to the establishment of their role in animal tumor systems, extrapolation of these findings to human neoplasia must be done with caution. The etiology of most human cancers is still unknown. Humans are not exposed to the high doses of carcinogen generally utilized to induce animal tumors. It is generally accepted that human tumors might be induced by chronic exposure to subcarcinogenic doses of a variety of carcinogens. Our results suggest that tumor etilogy and perhaps the physiological status of the target cells at the time of the carcinogenic insult, are the most relevant factors to determine the activation of transforming ras genes by single point mutations. Therefore, it is very likely that some environmental carcinogens might initiate human tumors by activating ras oncogenes. However, it is also possible that in certain cases ras gene activation may occur during tumor progression due to errors in the replication machinery. Although it is evident that many questions remain to be answered, studies summarized in this report illustrate how molecular characterization of transforming genes in experimentally induced tumors have provided very important clues in unveiling the molecular basis of human neoplasia.

IV. ACKNOWLEDGEMENTS

Research sponsored by the National Cancer Institute, DHHS, under contract No. N01-C0-23909 with Litton Bionetics, Inc. The contents of this publication do not necessarily reflect the views or policies of the Department of Health & Human Services, nor does mention of trade names, commercial products, or organizations imply endorsement by the U.S. Government.

V. REFERENCES

1. Bishop, J.M. (1985) Cell 42, 23-38.
2. Varmus, H.E. (1984) Annu. Rev. Genet. 18, 553-612.
3. Hayward, W.S., Neel, B.G., Astrin, S.M. (1981) Nature 290, 475-479.

4. Blair, D.G., Oskarsson, M.K., Wood, T.G., McClements, W.L., Fischinger, P.J., Vande Woude, G.F. (1981) Science 212, 941-943.
5. Tabin, C.J., Bradley, S.M., Bargmann, C.I., Weinberg, R.A., Papageorge, A.G. et al. (1982) Nature 300, 143-149.
6. Reddy, E.P., Reynolds, R.K., Santos, E., Barbacid, M. (1982) Nature 300, 149-152.
7. Taparowsky, E., Suard, Y., Fasano, O., Shimizu, K., Goldfarb, M.P., Wigler, M. (1982) Nature 300, 762-765.
8. Klein, G. (1983) Cell 32, 311-315.
9. Rowley, J.D. (1983) Nature 301, 290-292.
10. Alitalo, K. (1984) Medical Biology 62, 304-317.
11. Nusse, R., van Odyen, A., Cox, D., Fung Y.K.T., Varmus, H. (1984) Nature 307, 131-135.
12. Shen-Ong, G.L.C., Potter, M., Mushinski, J.F., Lavu, S., Reddy, E.P. (1984) Science 226, 1077-1080.
13. Doolittle, R.F., Hunkapiller, M.W., Hood, L.E., DeVare, S.G., Robbins, K.C., Aaronson, S.A., Antoniades, H.N. (1983) Science 221, 275-276.
14. Waterfield, M.D., Scrace, G.J., Whittle, N., Strooban, P., Johnson, A., Wasteson, A., Westermark, B., Heldin, C.H., Huany, J.D., Duel, T.F. (1983) Nature 304, 35-39.
15. Downward, J., Yarden, Y., Mayes, E., Scrace, G., Totty, N., Stockwell, P., Ullrich, A., Schlessinger, J., Waterfield, M.D. (1984) Nature 300, 521-527.
16. Barbacid, M. (1985) In: Important Advances in Oncology 1986 (DeVita, V.T., Hellman, S., Rosenberg, S., eds.), 3-22.
17. Barbacid, M. (1986) In: Accomplishments in Cancer Research 1985 (Fortner, J.G., Rhoads, J.E., eds.), J.B. Lippincott Company (Philadelphia, PA). In press.
18. Der, K.C., Krontiris, T., Cooper G. (1982) Proc. Natl. Acad. Sci. U.S.A. 79, 3637-3640.
19. Parada, L.F., Tabin, C.J., Shih, C., Weinberg, R.A. (1982) Nature 297, 474-478.
20. Santos, E., Tronick, S.R., Aaronson, S.A., Pulciani, S., Barbacid, M. (1982) Nature 298, 343-347.
21. Shimizu, K., Nakatsu, Y., Sekiguchi, M., Hokamura, K., Tanaka, K., Terada, M., Sugimura, T. (1985) Proc. Natl. Acad. Sci. U.S.A. 82, 5641-5645.

22. Ellis, R.W., DeFeo, D., Shih, T., Gonda, M., Young, H.A., Tsuchida, N., Lowy, D., Scolnick, E.M. (1981) Nature 292, 506-511.
23. Andersen, P.R., DeVare, S.G., Tronick, S.R., Ellis, R.W., Aaronson, S.A., Scolnick, E.M. (1981) Cell 26, 129-136.
24. Southern, E.M. (1985) J. Mol. Biol. 98, 503-517.
25. Southern, P.J., Berg, P. (1982) J. Molec. Appl. Genetics 1, 327-341.
26. Kidd, V.J., Wallace, R.B., Itakura, K., Woo, S.L.C. (1983) Nature 304, 230-234.
27. Studnecki, A.B., Wallace, R.B. (1984) DNA 3, 7-15.
28. Bos, J.L., Verlaan-de Vries, M., Jansen, A.M., Veeneman, G.H., van Boom, J.H., van der Eb, A.J. (1984) Nucleic Acids Res. 12, 9155-9163.
29. Gullino, P.M., Pettigrew, H.M., Grantham, F.H. (1975) J. Natl. Cancer Inst. 54, 401.
30. McCormick, D.L., Adamowski, C.B., Fiks, A., Moon, R.C. (1981) Cancer Res. 41, 1690.
31. Sukumar, S., Notario, V., Martin-Zanca, D., Barbacid, M. (1983) Nature 300, 658-661.
32. Zarbl, H., Sukumar, S., Arthur, A.V., Martin-Zanca, D., Barbacid, M. (1985) Nature 315, 382-385.
33. Yuasa, Y., Srivastava, S.K., Dunn, C.Y., Rhim, J.S., Reddy, E.P., Aaronson, S.A. (1983) Nature 303, 775-779.
34. Taparowsky, E., Shimizu, K., Goldfarb, M., Wigler, M. (1983) Cell 34, 581-586.
35. Fasano, O., Aldrich, T., Tamanoi, F., Taparowsky, E., Furth, M., Wigler, M. (1984) Proc. Natl. Acad. Sci. U.S.A. 81, 4008-4012.
36. Dhar, R., Ellis, R.W., Shih, T.Y., Oroszlan, S., Shapiro, B., Maizel, J., Lowy, D., Scolnick, E. (1982) Science 217, 934-937.
37. Tsuchida, N., Ryder, T., Ohtsubo, E. (1982) Science 217, 937-939.
38. Santos, E., Martin-Zanca, D., Reddy, E.P., Pierotti, M.A., Della Porta, G., Barbacid, M. (1984) Science 223, 661-664.
39. Loveless, A. (1969) Nature 223, 206-207.
40. Eadie, J.S., Conrad, M., Toorchen, D., Topal, M.D. (1984) Nature 308, 201-203.
41. Loechler, E.L., Green, C.L., Essigmann, J.M. (1984) Proc. Natl. Acad. Sci. U.S.A. 81, 6271-6275.
42. Singer, B., Kusmierek, J.T. (1982) Ann. Rev. Biochem. 51, 655-693.
43. Balmain, A., Pragnell, I.B. (1983) Nature 303, 72-74.

44. Balmain, A., Ramsden, M., Bowden, G.T., Smith, J. (1984) Nature 307, 658-660.

45. Guerrero, I., Calzada, P., Mayer, A., Pellicer, A. (1984) Proc. Natl. Acad. Sci. U.S.A. 81, 202-205.

46. Eva, A., Aaronson, S.A. (1983) Science 220, 506.

47. Schechter, A.L., Stern, D.F., Vaidyanathan, L., Decker, S.J., Drebin, J.A., Greene, M.I., Weinberg, R.A. (1984) Nature 312, 513-516.

48. Land, H., Parada, L.F., Weinberg, R.A. (1983) Nature 304, 596-602.

49. Ruley, H.E. (1983) Nature 304, 602-606.

50. Newbold, R.F., Overell, R.W. (1983) Nature 304, 648-651.

3

Sequences 3' of the Human c-Ha-<u>ras</u>1 Gene Positively

Regulate its Expression and Transformation Potential

Wendy W. Colby, Justus B. Cohen, Deborah Yu and Arthur D. Levinson

Department of Molecular Biology
Genetech, Inc.
460 Point San Bruno Blvd.
South San Francisco, CA 94080

I. INTRODUCTION

Cellular _ras_ genes constitute a highly conserved family first identifed by
homology with the transforming genes of certain oncogenic retroviruses (for
reviews, see 1-3). There are three known members of the human _ras_ family:
c-Ha-_ras_ and c-Ki-_ras_, cellular homologues of the transforming genes of Harvey and Kirstein murine sarcoma viruses respectively, and N-_ras_, first identified as an activated transforming gene in a neuroblastoma[1]. These genes encode related polypeptides of 21,000 daltons (p21) that are localized in the
plasma membrane[4,5], bind guanine nucleotides[6], and possess weak GTPase activity[7-9]. In a large number of tumor cells _ras_ genes contain mutations that
endow them with oncogenic potential as determined from experiments involving
DNA-mediated gene transfer[1]. These activating mutations typically affect
the coding portions of the gene at codons specifying amino acids 12 and 61[1].
Studies involving _in vitro_ mutagenesis of the c-Ha-_ras_1 gene at codon 12 have
demonstrated that while all amino acids except glycine and proline can activate the transforming potential of p21, certain amino acids at this position
allow the polypeptide to induce greater phenotypic changes in cellular morphology than others; these differences can, however, be masked by increased
expression levels of the gene[10]. When elevated amounts of p21 are present,
more fully transformed phenotypes are observed as assessed by cellular morphology, saturation density, and growth in agar. We found that the expression level of weakly-transforming activated Ha-_ras_ genes (e.g. pRas(lys-12))
was affected by sequences in the 3' non-coding region. These sequences
facilitate expression of the Ha-_ras_ gene, apparently reflecting the contributions of an associated enhancer element.

II. MATERIALS AND METHODS

A. Bacterial strains and plasmid manipulations. Bacterial transforma-
tions and plasmid isolations were performed as described[11] using Escherichia
coli strain 294[12]. Vectors were constructed with appropriate enzymes used
according to manufacturer's (New England Biolabs) instructions. Plasmid
p19E-CAT-H, from which other CAT vectors were made, was derived from the previously desribed Hepatitis B virus (HBV) vector p342E[13]. Full details of
its construction will be presented elsewhere; briefly, the vector contains
a polylinker derived from plasmid pUC13[14], followed by an enhancer-less SV40
early promoter, the chloramphenicol acetyl tranferase (CAT) gene derived
from pSV1-cat[15] and HBsAg 3' untranslated sequences from p342E from which
the HBV enhancer[16] was removed. The 1730-bp SphI-BamHI restriction fragment from the 3' end of the human c-Ha-_ras_ gene was cloned in either orientation 5' of the SV40 promoter sequences, or 3' of the HBV poly A site following the CAT gene.

B. Growth and labelling of cells. Rat-1 and COS[17] cells were grown in Dulbecco modified Eagle (DME) medium supplemented with 10% fetal bovine serum. Primary Fisher rat embryo fibroblasts were prepared and maintained in DME medium supplemented with 10% FBS. For isotopic labelling, cells were plated in 35mm dishes, pre-incubated in methionine-free media for 1 hr, and grown for 3 hr in 1 ml of methionine-free media containing 160 μCi [35S]-methionine (Amersham). Lysates were prepared and immunoprecipitated with anti-p21 polyclonal rabbit serum or preimmune serum as described[10]. Immunoprecipitated proteins were analysed by electrophoresis on 12.5% SDS-polyacrylamide gels[18] and visualized by fluorography after treatment with EnHance (New England Nuclear).

C. Transfections. Secondary cultures of embryonic rat cells were transfected with 5 μg of the ras plasmids and 5 μg of a myc plasmid (pLTRmyc) in the presence of 35 μg sheared salmon sperm DNA. pLTRmyc (kindly provided by W. Lee and H. Varmus) contains exons 2 and 3 of a translocated human c-myc gene under the transcriptional control of a Moloney murine leukemia virus promoter[19]. Cells were transfected by the calcium phosphate procedure[20] for 5 hr and refed with maintenance medium. After 48 hr, cultures were transferred to 10 cm dishes and fed every 3-4 days with DME medium supplemented with 5% FBS. Dishes were stained 15 days after replating and scored for foci. Rat-1 co-transfections were performed as described[10] using 10 μg of ras plasmid with 0.5 μg of a vector (pSVE-Neo-Bal6)[10] encoding neomycin resistance. Cells expression the transfected neo sequences were selected by growth in the presence of the antibiotic G418 as described[10]. These were propagated as mass cultures; in addition, subclones were isolated for analysis in selected experiments.

D. CAT assays. CAT assays were performed as described[21]. Briefly, COS cells were plated onto 60mm dishes and transfected with 3 μg of the appropriate DNA. Cells were harvested, extracts prepared, and reactions performed as described except that 10 μl extract was used for each reaction and incubation was for 30 min. at 37°C.

III. RESULTS

We have previously described the construction of plasmids that encode altered human c-Ha-ras1 genes[10]. These were used to study the transformation potential of p21s with various amino acids at position-12. The plasmids contained the presumptive promoter element of the Ha-ras gene[22,23], the four coding exons, and sequences extending approximately 1000-bp 3' of the polyadenylation site employed in the processing of the primary transcript[22]. We found that all amino acids except glycine and proline activated the transforming potential of p21; certain amino acids (e.g. valine, leucine), however, appeared to be stronger inducers of the protein's transforming activity than others (e.g. lysine, tryptophan)[10]. We unexpectedly found that the efficiency with which these vectors could transform Rat-1 cells was significantly reduced compared to vectors containing additional 3' flanking sequences that complete the 6.6-kb BamHI restriction fragment encompassing the Ha-ras gene[10]. To investigate the influence of these sequences on the transformation potential of activated Ha-ras genes, we transfected Rat-1 cells with plasmids containing either the 6.6-kb BamHI restriction fragment spanning an activated (lys-12 or trp-12) Ha-ras gene (pRas(lys-12) or pRas(trp-12)), or truncated versions lacking the 3' terminal 1730 nucleotides (pRas(lys-12)Δ or pRas(trp-12)Δ)(Fig. 1). This region was previously found to contain a 28-bp pyrimidine-rich repeat present in 29 copies[22], deletions and expansion in which are thought to account for the restriction fragment length

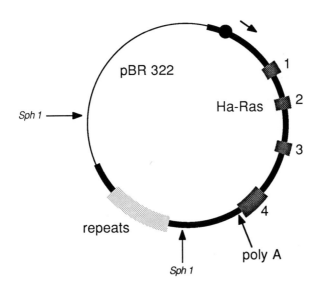

Figure 1. Plasmid vectors containing human Ha-ras genes. Depicted is the 6.6-kb BamHI restriction fragment encompassing the human H-ras gene (heavy line), inserted onto the BamHI site of pBR322. Also shown are the positions of the four coding exons, the polyadenylation site employed in the processing of the transcribed RNA, the 28-bp repeats, and the approximate locations of the promoter and RNA initiation sites. The 3' truncations were achieved by removing sequences between the two SphI sites.

polymorphisms observed at this locus in the human population[24]. The different ras gene constructs were introduced into the cells by CaPO4-mediated
transfection in the presence of a vector encoding G418 (neo) resistance;
cells expressing the neo marker were selected by the addition of G418 to
the culture medium. In all experiments at least 50 independent drug-resis-
tant colonies appeared, and we examined in detail both mass populations of
transfected cells and individual clones. As shown in Fig. 2, cells derived
form transfections using the Ha-ras vector pRas(lys-12)Δ exhibit a morphology similar to Rat-1 cells, although they will, if not passaged for 3 weeks,
from foci that overgrow the monolayer. In contrast, cells transfected with
the Ha-ras(lys-12) gene containing the additional 3' sequences (pRas(lys-12))
are more fully transformed as judged by morphology (Fig. 2.). These cells
display the spindly and refractile morphology characteristic of transformed
cells, and rapidly overgrow the monolayer at high cell densitites. This phenotype is similar to that displayed by cells transformed with pRas(val-12),
the form of the activated ras gene found in the T24 bladder carcinoma cell[22]
(Fig. 2). Mass populations of G418-resistant cells derived from pRas(trp-12)
and pRas(trp-12)Δ-transfections displayed similar morphological differences (data not shown).

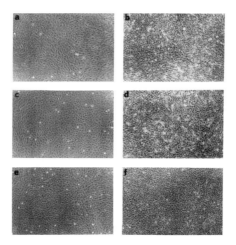

Figure 2. Phase contrast photomicrographs (x80) of transfected Rat-1 cells.
Subclones were derived from G418-resistant cultures co-transfected with
pBR322 (panel a); pRas(val-12)(clone #1) (panel b); pRas(lys-12)Δ (clone
#1) (panel c); pRas(lys-12)(clone #1)(panel d); pRas(lys-12)Δ (clone #2)
(panel e); pRas(lys-12)Δ (clone #4) (panel f).

We characterized subclones of cells derived from cultures transfected with either pRas(lys-12) or pRas(lys-12)Δ plasmids with regard to two additional transformation-responsive phenotypic traits. First, we determined the density to which they grew at saturation; second, we evaluated their ability to grow in an anchorage independent manner. Table 1 illustrates the results of these studies. While cells transfected with pRas(lys-12)Δ achieve a saturation density similar to that of control Rat-1 cells, cells transfected with pRas(lys-12) grow to considerably (~three-fold) higher densities, comparable to cells transfected with the complete 6.6-kb activated (val-12) Ha-ras gene derived from T24 bladder carcinoma cells[22]. To examine the ability of the transfected cells to grow without anchorage support, the efficiency with which the various cell lines formed colonies in agar was determined. As seen in Table 1, cells transfected with activated ras genes containing the additional 3' sequences grow much more efficiently in agar than cells transfected with the 3' deletion mutants.

TABLE I

Growth Properties of ras-Transfected Cells

Cell line	Saturation density*	Agar growth†
Rat-1	2.9	<.0001
Rat-1(pRas(lys-12Δ))#1	2.7	0.003
Rat-1(pRas(lys-12Δ))#2	2.9	0.007
Rat-1(pRas(lys-12)#1	7.2	.22
Rat-1(pRas(lys-12)#4	8.8	.19
Rat-1(pRas(val-12)#12	9.3	.24

*Cells derived from individual subclones (Fig. 2) were seeded at initial densitites of $2x10^4$ cells onto multiple 60mm dishes in DME medium supplemented with 10% fetal bovine serum. Cells were trypsinized and counted using a hemacytometer every three days; plateau values are presented (cells/60mm dish ($x10^{-6}$)).

†10^4 cells were plated onto agar in 60mm dishes; the percentage of seeded cells forming colonies of >30 cells was determined by microscopic evaluation after 14 days.

The above results strongly suggest that 3' sequences modulate the transformation potential of activated ras genes. To evaluate this further, we
utilized the primary rat embryo fibroblasts assay in which transformation
depends on the concerted action of two distinct oncogenes[25,26]. Embryonic
rat cells were transfected with a vector containing the human myc proto-
oncogene under viral promoter control[19], together with activated ras genes
either containing or lacking the 3' sequences. As shown in Table 2, no
transformation of primary rat cells was observed following transfection with
activated ras genes alone, or with the myc gene alone. Similarly, no transformation was observed with the myc gene was transfected in combination with
a non-activated ras gene (gly-12). Foci, however, were observed after co-
transfection of cells with the myc gene and the T24 bladder carcinoma-derived
(val-12) Ha-ras oncogene. Notably the number of foci was strongly dependent
upon the presence of the 3' sequences (Table 2), again establishing that se-
qeunces 3' of the human c-Ha-ras gene augment the transformation potential of
activated derivatives. We also transfected embryonic rat cells with the
lys-12 ras mutant together with the myc oncogene. This altered ras gene also
promoted the immortalization and transformation of these cells, extending our
earlier findings with this mutant[10]. As with the val-12 version of the Ha-
ras gene, the efficiency of focus formation was markedly dependent upon the
presence of the Ha-ras 3' sequences.

TABLE II

Transformation of Secondary Rat Embryo Fibroblasts

Transfected DNA	Foci
pLTRmyc + pRas(gly-12)	0
pLTRmyc + pRas(gly-12)Δ	0
pLTRmyc + pRas(val-12)	77
pLTRmyc + PRas(val-12)Δ	10
pLTRmyc + pRas(lys-12)	89
pLTRmyc + pRas(lys-12)Δ	2
pLTRmyc	0
pRas(val-12)	0
carrier	0

Secondary Fisher rat embryo fibroblasts were transfected with the various
Ha-ras vectors and pLTRmyc as indicated. Dishes were stained after 18 days
and scored for foci.

The findings presented above document that sequences 3' of the Ha-ras coding exons contribute in a significant way to the oncogenic potential of activated derivatives. To determine if these sequences act to increase the level of the encoded protein, we labelled two transformed subclones derived from transfections with either pRas(lyl-12) or pRas(lys-12)Δ with [^{35}S]-methionine. Cell extracts were prepared and immunoprecipitated with antisera prepared against bacterially derived p21[7]. As depicted in Fig. 3, low levels of p21 are present in both subclones of cells transfected with the Ha-ras 3' deletion mutants (lanes b, c); much higher levels are present in subclones derived from transfections with vectors containing the additional 3' sequences (lanes d, e). Only very small amounts of p21, reflecting endogenous synthesis, are detected in non-transfected cells (lane a).

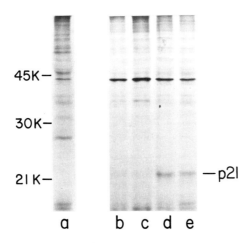

45K—

30K—

21 K—   —p2l

a   b c d e

Figure 3. Expression of p21 in transfected cell lines. Extracts of cells labelled with [^{35}S]-methionine were immunoprecipitated with rabbit anti-p21 serum. Extracts were derived from cell lines: lane a, Rat-1; lane b, Rat-1(lys-12Δ)#1; lane c, Rat-1(lys-12Δ)#2; lane d, Rat-1(lys-12)#1; lane e, Rat-1(lys-12)#4.

These results establish that sequences residing 3' of the Ha-ras gene increase the steady state level of the encoded protein, which could account for the increased oncogenic potential of activated ras gene derivatives carrying these sequences. We considered the possibility that these sequences harbor an enhancer function that acts to positively regulate the Ha-ras promoter. While the localization of an enhancer to a region 3' of the coding region of a cellular gene would represent a novel finding, it would realize the potential of enhancers to act from great distances as determined from gene reconstruction experiments. To explore this possibility, we employed a transient expression system using chloramphenicol acetyltransferase (CAT)-based vectors that respond to the presence of enhancer sequences. Mammalian cells lack endogenous CAT activity, and accurate and quantitative procedures are available to measure levels of the enzyme present in transfected cells. We inserted the 1730-bp restriction endonuclease fragment located 3' of the human Ha-ras gene that encompasses the repeated sequences (see above) in either orientation 5' or 3' of the simian virus 40 (SV40) early promoter-CAT transcription unit of plasmid p198E-CAT-H. In this plasmid (Fig. 4) expression of the CAT gene is under the control of the SV40 early promoter from which its own enhancer sequences have been removed. Proper processing of the transcribed RNA is ensured by the presence of appropriate sequences derived from Hepatitis B virus

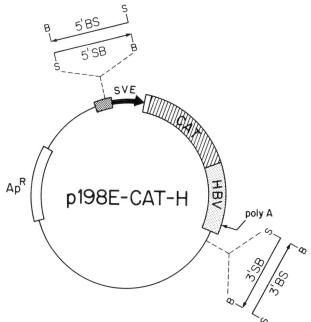

Figure 4. Construction of Ha-ras/CAT vectors. The 1730-bp SphI-BamHI fragment (denoted SB) derived from the 3' end of the human Ha-ras gene (nucleotides 4725-6454[22]; was inserted in either orientation (SB or BS) into cloning sites of p198E-CAT-H (see Materials and Methods) either 5' of the SV40 promoter or 3' of the CAT sequences. p198E-CAT-H, a derivative of pSV1-cat (13C), directs the synthesis of CAT under the control of the SV40 early promoter from which the normal enhancer element was removed.

48

(HBV)[27]. Fig. 4 indicates the positions at which the Ha-<u>ras</u>-linked sequences were inserted. The various plasmids were introduced into COS cells by calcium phosphate-mediated DNA transfection; cellular extracts were prepared 36-48 hr. later and assayed for the level of CAT activity present. Representative results are shown in Fig. 5. CAT activity is measured as the extent to which radioactively labelled chloramphenicol is converted to its mono- and diacetylated forms upon incubation with the cellular extracts. The parental plasmid p198E-CAT-H shows low, but detectable CAT activity (lane 2) that is well above the level detected in mock-transfected cells or cells transfected with CAT vectors lacking a promoter (lane 1). Using a vector containing the complete SV40 promoter/enhancer unit (p348E-CAT-H), somewhat higher levels of CAT activity are observed (lane 3). Notably, the highest levels of CAT activity are present in extracts prepared from cells transfected with plasmids lacking SV40 enhancer sequences, but containing the <u>ras</u> associated sequences (lanes 4-7). It is apparent that high levels of CAT are assured by the presence of the <u>ras</u> sequences at locations independent of position and orientation, properties consistent with their role as enhancer elements.

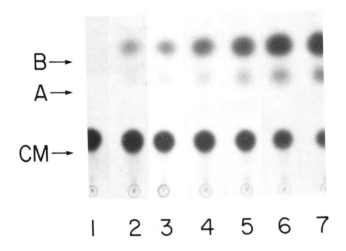

Figure 5. Transient expression of the CAT gene using CAT/Ha-<u>ras</u> vectors. Depicted are the assay results using extracts prepared from COS cells transfected with p0-cat (lacking promoter sequences) (lane 1); p198E-CAT-H (lane 2); p348-CAT-H (lane 3); p198E-CAT-H-Ras(5'SV) (lane 4); p198-CAT-H-Ras(4'BS) (lane 5); p198E-CAT-Ras(3'SB) (lane 6); p198E-CAT-H-Ras(3'BS) (lane 7).

III. DISCUSSION

Evidence is accumulating that the products of cellular ras genes play an important role in normal growth control[28-32]. As such, the expression of these genes is likely regulated according to the needs of the cell. In an effort to define elements that mediate this control, we have begun to characterize sequences within and surrounding the human c-Ha-ras gene that may be so involved. Relatively little is known about the structure of the 5' end of the Ha-ras gene. From a comparison of the nucleotide sequences of the cellular and viral genes, we suggested that human c-Ha-ras possesses a 5' untranslated exon[22]. If true, this positions the prommoter at least 1230 nucleotides upstream of the first coding exon[22]. Indeed, recent evidence seems to verify this supposition: the 5' end of mature Ha-ras mRNA was localized by primer extension to the predicted region[23]. We focused our efforts on the role of sequences residing 3' of the Ha-ras gene, between 1000 and 2700 nucleotides beyond the point at which mature messenger transcripts end. We have found that such sequences exert a profound influence on the transformation potential of activated ras genes. Cells transfected with activated Ha-ras genes containing the additional 3' sequences, relative to cells transfected with corresponding genes lacking such sequences, were: i) more transformed by morphological criteria; ii) able to grow to higher saturation densities; iii) much better able to grow much better without anchorage support. These sequences also contributed in a strongly positive fashion to the ability of ras genes to promote the transformation of secondary rat cells in collaboration with an active myc gene.

Efficient transcription of many eukaryotic genes depends on the presence of a transcriptional enhancer[32]. Such elements were originally identified as long-range activators of gene transcription, distinguishing them from previously described upstream promoter elements of eukaryotic genes. While the majority of enhancers characterized to date have been localized to regions upstream of genes, their ability to function in other positions prompted us to examine the 3' ras sequences for enhancer function. Our results establish that these sequences facilitate the expression of a heterologous gene (CAT) under the control of a foreign promoter (SV40). Furthermore, these sequences mainifest themselves in a manner independent of position and orientation, properties consistent with a role as an enhancer of transcription. While we have not carried out extensive studies to examine the extent to which the Ha-ras associated enhancer functions in a tissue-specific manner, preliminary indications suggest that the sequences facilitate expression from the SV40 promoter to only a limited extent in several cell types (unpublished data). It should be noted that while these sequences exhibit properties of enhancer elements, it is possible that additional control elements are present within the 1730-bp restriction endonuclease fragment analyzed. For example, the presence of transcriptional termination signals could additionally act to facilitate expression of the Ha-ras gene.

Our results further emphasize the importance of quantitative effects in the transformation process by ras genes. While all amino acids except proline and glycine at position-12 activate the protein's transformation potential, differences were discernable among the transformation-competent forms. As such (for example), p21(lys-12) was found to be a less potent transforming protein in Rat-1 cells than p21(val-12)[10]. From this study it is apparent that these differences can be obscured by increased levels of p21, levels that can be achieved without access to strong heterologous promoters or enhancers as required for the mainifestation of transforming activity by p21 (gly-12)[34]. Previous efforts have provided indications that increased ras gene expression, in addition to the well-documented role of mutated ras genes, may be a factor in the development of some tumors. For example, amplification of the Ki-ras locus has been found in cell lines derived from tumors[35,36], and in an unmanipulated solid tumor[37], although in at least one instance these amplified copies contain mutational alterations known to be of an activating type[36]. Furthermore, increased levels of ras gene transcription have been observed in certain preneoplastic tumors[38], while increased p21 levels have been documented in majority of human colon and mammary carcinomas[39]. Perhaps most astonishing is the report by Krontiris et al.[24], who presented that the susceptibility to cancer in humans is linked to the presence of an unusual number of 28-bp repeats that are associated with, or linked to, the enhancer activity we describe. While further work is clearly necessary to evaluate the significance of this finding, it is conceivable that the activity of the ras-associateed enhancer correlates with those unusual alleles that predispose individuals toward the development of tumors; if so, it is conceivable that this genetic susceptibility toward cancer may result from an enhanced expression of c-ras genes.

IV. REFERENCES

1. Varmus, H.E. (1984) Annu. Rev. Genet. 18, 553-612.
2. Gibbs, J.B., Sigal, I.S. and Scolnick, E.M (1985) Trends in Biochem. Sci. 10, 350-353.
3. Levinson, A.D. (1986) Trends in Genet., in press.
4. Willingham, M. et al. (1980) Cell 19, 1006-1014.

5. Scolnick, E.M., Papageorge, A.G. and Shih, T.Y. (1979) Proc. Natl. Acad. Sci. U.S.A. 76, 5355-5359.

6. Shih, T.Y. et al. (1982) J. Virol. 42, 253-261.

7. McGrath, J.P. et al. (1984) Nature 310, 644-649.

8. Sweet, R.W. et al. (1984) Nature 311, 273-275.

9. Gibbs, J.B. et al. (1984) Proc. Natl. Acad. Sci. U.S.A. 81, 5704-5708.

10. Seeburg, P.H., Colby, W.W., Capon, D.J., Goeddel, D.V. and Levinson, A.D. (1984) Nature 312, 71-75.

11. Maniatis, T., Fritsch, E.F. and Sambrook, J. (1982) Molecular Cloning: A Laborator Manual. Cold Spring Harbor Laboratory, Cold Spring Harbor, N.Y.

12. Backman, K., Ptashne, M. and Gilbert, W. (1976) Proc. Natl. Acad. Sci. U.S.A. 73, 4174-4178.

13. Crowley, C.W., Liu, C.-C. and Levinson, A.D. Mol. Cell Bio. 3, 44-55.

14. Messing, J. (1983) Meth. In Enzym. 101, 20-78.

15. Gorman, C.M., Moffat, L.F. and Howard, B.H. (1982) Mol. Cell. Biol. 2, 1044-1051.

16. Shaul, Y., Rutter, W.J. and Laub, O. (1985) EMBO J. 4, 427-430.

17. Gluzman, Y. (1981) Cell 23, 175-182.

18. Laemmli, U.K. (1970) Nature 227, 680-685.

19. Lee, W.M.F., Schwab, M., Westaway, D. and Varmus, H.E. (1985) Mol. Cell. Biol. 5, 3345-3356.

20. Wigler et al. (1980) Proc. Natl. Acad. Sci. U.S.A. 77, 3567-3571.

21. Gorman, C.M., Rigby, P.W.J. and Lane, D.L. (1985) Cell 42, 519-526.

22. Capon, D.J. et al. (1983) Nature 301, 33-37.

23. Ishii, S., Merlino, G.T. and Pastan, I. (1985) Science 230, 1378-1381.

24. Krontiris, T.G., DiMartino, N.A., Colb, M. and Parkinson, D.R. (1985) Nature 313, 369-374.

25. Land, H., Parada, LF. and Weinberg, R.A. (1983) Nature 304, 596-602.

26. Ruley, E. (1983) Nature 304, 602-606.

27. Simonsen, C.C. and Levinson, A.D. (1983) Mol. Cell. Biol. 3, 2250-2258.

28. Stacey, D.W. and Kung, H.-F. (1984) Nature 310, 508-511.

29. Feramisco, J.R. et al. (1984) Cell 38, 109-117.

30. Mulcahy, L.S., Smith, M.R. and Stacey, D.W. (1985) Nature 313, 241-243.

31. Moda, M. et al. (1985) Nature 318, 73-75.

32. Bar-Saqi, D. and Feramisco, J.R. (1985) Cell 42, 841-848.

33. Serfling, E., Jasin, M. and Schaffner, W. (1985) Trends In Gen. XX.

34. Chang, E.H., Furth, M.E., Scolnick, E.M. and Lowy, D.R. (1982) Nature 297, 479-484.

35. Schwab, M. et al. (1983) Nature 303, 497-501.
36. Taya, Y. et al. (1984) EMBO J. 3, 2943-2946.
37. Pulciani, S. et al. (1985) Mol. Cell. Biol. 5, 2836-2841.
38. Spandidos, D.A. and Kerr, I.B. (1984) Br. J. Cancer 49, 681-688.
39. Hand, P.H. et al. (1984) Proc. Natl. Sci. U.S.A. 81, 5227-5231.

4

Structure and Function of p21 _ras_ Proteins

Thomas Y. Shih, Seisuke Hattori[†], David J. Clanton,
Linda S. Ulsh, Zhang-qun Chen, James A. Lautenberger and Takis S. Papas

Laboratory of Molecular Oncology,
Division of Cancer Etiology,
National Cancer Institute,
National Institutes of Health,
Frederick, MD. 21701

[†]Dept. of Pure and Applied Sciences,
University of Tokyo,
Tokyo 153, Japan

I. INTRODUCTION

As is very often the case in many areas of medical research, the quest for understanding the abnormalities in human diseases has resulted in the discovery of many life processes that are important for the normal functioning of organisms. This also appears to be happening in basic cancer research. Attempts to understand the fundamental abnormality of cancer cells, have resulted in the discovery of a group of genes now known as oncogenes, whose normal function may be for the control of cell proliferation during the normal growth and development of organisms, a subject long elusive to students of basic cell biology.

Cancer in a sense is a collection of many different diseases affecting various organs and tissues of the body, and perhaps there are also quite diverse causes for different types of malignant diseases. But the fundamental cellular abnormality characterizing all kinds of cancers is uncontrolled cell growth. Cancer cells have undergone a process of transformation from the normal phenotype to a malignant phenotype of autonomous growth. Recent advances in cancer research have identified a group of oncogenes approximately 20 to 30 in number, whose inappropriate expression may be important in human cancer, and whose normal function may constitute the central mechanism of controlling cell growth. Oncogenes were first identified in a group of oncogenic retroviruses which induce tumors in animals and very often are also capable of transforming cells in tissue culture. Extensive genetic and molecular biological studies on these viruses, especially the avian sarcoma viruses which have served as the prototype viruses for most studies, have concluded that the capability of oncogenic retroviruses to transform cells is due to the presence of oncogenes within their viral genomes, and the immediate agents of these oncogenes are the transforming proteins encoded by these genes.

Oncogenic proteins can be classified into four categories according to their biochemical properties. The first group is the protein kinases, most of which phosphorylate proteins on tyrosine residues. The members of this group include src, fes/fps, abl, yes, ros, fgr, erbB, raf/mht, fms, rel and mos; the latter may have serine kinase and/or ATPase activities. The second group of oncogenic proteins, including myc, myb, fos, and ski, are located in cell nuclei; their function may be in the control of nuclear activities. That the normal function of cellular oncogenes may be involved in the control mechanisms of cell growth is most clearly exemplified by the third category. This includes the sis gene, which is or is closely related to the gene of platelet-derived growth factor (PDGF). It is particularly significant in this connection to a growth factor that the previously mentioned erbB protein is an homologue of the epidermal growth factor (EGF) receptor, and the fms protein is a receptor for macrophage colony stimulaing factor (CSF-1).

The fourth group, the p21 ras proteins, is guanine nucleotide binding proteins which are probably related to the family of G-proteins having roles in cellular signal transduction. Although the cellular function of oncogene proteins is still not completely understood, it may be fruitful to view this group of proteins in the perspective of a superfamily of growth-related gene products, which may function as a group constituting a pathway(s) for processing growth control signals, very much like a metabolic pathway in processing metabolites. Cancer, after all, is a malfunction of cellular growth control. Many excellent reviews have been written on this exciting subject[61,50,24,3,29]. In this chapter, we wish to focus our attention on the recent studies of the structure and function of p21 ras proteins. Other chapters in this volume will deal with aspects of ras oncogenes in human and experimental animal tumors.

II. The ras gene family

The ras gene family encodes a group of closely related 21,000 dalton proteins, p21, in most vertebrates. In the human genome, there are three distinct c-ras genes (reviewed in 48). The c-ras[H] locus, which is homologous to the v-ras gene of Harvey murine sarcoma virus (Ha-MuSV) and the bas gene of Balb sarcoma virus, is located on chromosome 11. The c-ras[K] gene, which is homologous to a closely related Kirsten murine sarcoma virus (Ki-MuSV) v-ras gene, is on chromosome 12; and the c-ras[N] gene which was originally identified in a neuroblastoma cell line and has, as yet, no known viral counterpart, is located on chromosome 1. Ras genes have been found in most vertebrates, in insects such as Drosophila malanogaster, and in unicellular organisms such as yeast cells. Perhaps ras genes are present in virtually all eukaryotes although no definitive report has yet documented their presence in the plant kingdom. We can not even rule out the possible existence of these genes in prokaryotes whose genes may have diverged to such an extent that they can no longer be readily recognized by most molecular probes for ras genes. Figure 1 compares the primary amino acid sequences of ras proteins of different members of the gene family, and of evolutionarily diverse groups of organisms. Several important and useful insights into the structure and function of p21 ras proteins can be

56

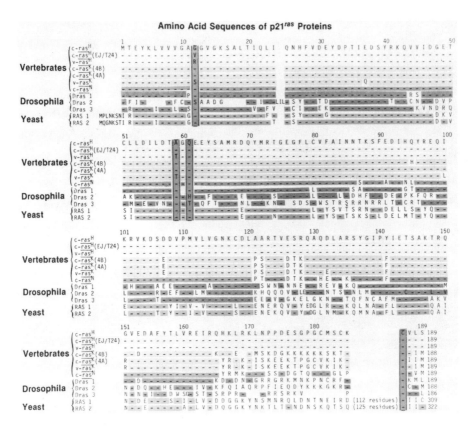

Figure 1. Comparison of amino acid sequences of ras proteins. Amino acid sequences deduced from DNA sequences of different ras genes of evolutionarily divergent organisms are compared. The dash indicates amino acid residues identical to c-ras[H] p21, and homologous regions are shaded. Boxed residues #12 and #61 are hot spots for mutations in tumors; #59, the autophosphorylation site; and #186, the palmitylation site. The amino acid symbols are: A, Ala; R, Arg; N, Asn; D, Asp; C, Cys; E, Glu; Q, Gln; G, Gly; H, His; I, Ile; L, Leu; K, Lys; M, Met; F, Phe; P, Pro; S, Ser; T, Thr; W, Trp; Y, Tyr; V, Val. Data were taken from c-ras[H], Capon et al.[6]; v-ras[H], Dhar et al.[13]; c-ras[K], Shimizu et al.[52], McGrath et al.[37]; v-ras[K], Tsuchida et al.[59]; c-ras[N], Taparowsky et al.[57]; Dras 1, 2, 3, Newman-Silberberg et al.[42]; RAS 1 and 2, Powers et al.[45].

Three H-, K- and N-ras genes of the vertebrate gene family all encode similar p21 proteins of 189 amino acid residues. From a differential splicing of an alternative fourth exon of the c-ras^K gene, K-ras gene encodes an additional protein of 188 amino acid residues, c-ras^K(4B). These amino acid sequences are deduced from DNA sequences of ras genes, and it should be pointed out here that the actual N-termini and C-termini of these proteins produced in eukaryotic cells have not yet been determined. The p21 proteins of these three human ras genes share extensive amino acid sequence homology with the exception of some divergence at the C-terminal regions, i. e., residues 165 to 185, and to a lesser extent from residues 121 to 141. Even more remarkable than the conservation of p21 structures within the gene family is the conservation of the structure of the same gene among different organisms. The amino acid sequence of c-ras^H gene of man, for example, is identical to that of the murine species from which these murine sarcoma viruses acquired their viral oncogenes. As seen in Fig. 1, stringent conservation of ras protein structure extends to insects and yeast, however in the latter, an additional 112 to 125 amino acid residues are inserted at the C-terminal heterologous region.

Several important features of p21 proteins are depicted in Fig. 1 and will be discussed later in more detail. Single point mutations of amino acid 12, 13, 59 or 61 are responsible for proto-oncogene activation found in numerous human and animal tumors and sarcoma viruses. The cysteine-186 is conserved in all ras genes, and is the site of palmitylation of p21.

A group of proteins collectivly known as G-proteins share very similar guanine nucleotide binding properties with p21, and perhaps also perform their different cellular functions by a similar biochemical mechanism. It is interesting to note that ras genes may belong to this extended gene family although most of these genes are not oncogenes. These G-proteins include regulatory G proteins of adenylate cyclase[25,4], transducin of retina rod outer segments[25,40,55,64], the recently identified rho gene[33], and perhaps also the genes for elongation factors, EF-Tu[1] and EF-G[42], of the protein synthesis system.

III. Biosynthesis and the membrane binding domain

Fig. 2 illustrates the pathway of p21 biosynthesis. Pulse-chase experiments indicate that p21 is synthesized in the free cytosol in a precursor form, the pro-p21, and shortly after synthesis it is processed and associated with the plasma membrane accompanied by a slight increase (approximately 1,000 daltons) in electrophoretic mobility on SDS-polyacrylamide gels[51].

58

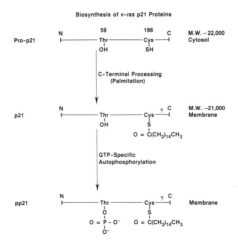

Biosynthesis of v-*ras* p21 Proteins

Figure 2. Biosynthetic pathway of p21 ras proteins. Shortly after its synthesis in the free cytosol, the pro-p21 is palmitylated at cysteine-186, and phosphorylated at threonine-59. These processed products are associated with the plasma membrane. Question marks indicate the precise C-terminus and N-terminus have not yet been determined.

Post-translational processing of p21 appears to be a common pathway for the synthesis of all ras proteins[60]. Sefton et al. demonstrated that part of the processing event involves acylation of p21[47]. The importance of p21 acylation to its transforming function is most clearly demonstrated by Willumsen et al., using a series of genetic mutations located near the p21 C-terminus[62,63]. Studies of these mutants indicate that cysteine-186 is essential, although not sufficient, for p21 processing. Recently, we have employed the p21 overproduced in E. coli, which is not acylated and is an equivalent of pro-p21, to identify the acylation site by comparative peptide mapping with acylated p21 on high performance liquid chromatography (HPLC)[9]. The unique precursor peptide of p21 overproduced in E. coli, which is different from the processed product, is identical to a synthetic tetrapeptide containing cysteine-186 of p21. The acylated hydrophobic peptide of the processed p21 has been isolated by HPLC, which after cleavage with hydroxylamine, co-chromatographs precisely with the synthetic precursor peptide. Thus, chemical evidence establishes that cysteine-186 is indeed the acylation site. Interestingly, in contrast to src proteins and many other cellular and viral proteins, which are myristylated on their N-termini[47,5,38], the fatty acid associated with p21 is palmitic acid, although p21 can be metabolically labeled with either ^{3}H-palmitate or ^{3}H-myristate, which is two carbons shorter than the former. The specifity of the enzymatic mechanism of p21 palmitylation may be different from N-terminal myristylation of other proteins. It is interesting to note that the palmitylation site, which is four amino acid residues from the C-terminus, is conserved not only in all ras genes (Fig. 1) but is also present in the membrane associated members of the extended family of ras related proteins such as the α sub-unit of transducin[40,55,64] and the rho protein[34]. It appears that this C-terminal tetrapeptide may also define the membrane binding domain of these proteins. The question marks in Fig. 2, however, indicate that there still is some uncertainty as to the exact C-termini of these proteins. There may be some heterogeneity due to further proteolytic removal of terminal residues after palmitylation at cysteine-186; therefore, the hydrophobic peptide we have identified may be an intermediate species in p21 processing[9]. Also undetermined are the exact N-termini of p21 proteins. The amino terminal residues are blocked by other undetermined modifications from Edman degradation (Oroszlan et al., unpublished observation). From pulse labeling of p21 by ^{35}S-methionine and chasing with an excess of unlabled amino acid, we have determined that the p21 has an intracellular half life of approximately 20 hr, and the phosphorylated forms which are presence in v-ras p21s of Ha-MuSV and Ki-MuSV, have a much longer half life of 56 hr[60].

IV. Biochemical properties

In cells transformed by viral or cellular ras oncogenes, p21 is present in extremely small amounts (in the order of one part per 10,000 or less), precluding any detailed characterization of its biochemical properties. Recently, we and others have succeeded in expressing high levels of biochemically active ras proteins in E. coli[31,27,18,54]. Using a novel pJL6 expression vector[30], p21 of v-ras[H] oncogene is expressed as a fusion protein with the N-terminal portion of the bacteriophage λ cII protein under the transcriptional control of the λ p_L promoter inducible by inactivation of a temperature-sensitive repressor[31]. The scheme for construction of this plasmid is shown in Fig. 3. In this construct, the 4 N-terminal amino acid residues of p21 are replaced by 14 amino acid residues from the cII protein. Fig. 4 shows a comparison of this chimeric p21 protein with other G-proteins. It is significant to point out that the fusion point precedes the box of homologous sequences starting from lysine-5, which as we shall discuss later, is part of the GTP binding domain, so that the p21 overproduced in E. coli possesses full biochemical activities[23].

A.

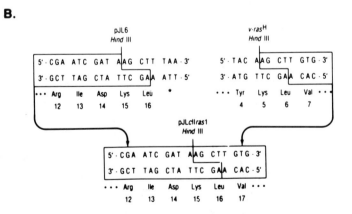

Figure 3. Construction of the pJLcIIrasI plasmid overproducing p21 as a fusion protein in E. coli. Reproduced from Lautenberger et al.[31].

N-TERMINAL SEQUENCES OF p21 ras AND G-PROTEINS

c-H-<u>ras</u>   (1-22)   M T E Y|K L V V V G A G̲|G V|G V|G K S A L|T I|Q|
v-H-<u>ras</u>   (1-22)   M T E Y|K L V V V G A|R G V|G K S A L|T I|Q|
v-H-<u>ras</u>   (1-32) MVRANKRNEAL R I D|K L V V V G A|R̲ G V|G K S A L|T I|Q|
(<u>E. coli</u>) | | | | | |
α Transducin (27-48)   A K T V|K L L L L G A G|E S|G K S T I|V K|Q|
α G₀   A K D V|K̲ L L̲ L̲ L G A̲ G̲|E S|G K S T I|V K|O̲|
EF-Tu   (9-30)   K P N V N|V̲|G T|I̲ G̲|H V D H|G̲ K T T L̲|T A A

Figure 4. Comparison of N-terminal sequences of p21 with G-proteins. The
junction point of the chimeric p21 protein between residues 4 and 5 precedes
the boxed homologous regions of G-proteins. The following Dayhoff conserva-
tive categories are used: C; S, T, P, A, G; N, D, E, Q; H, R, K; M, I,
L, V; and F, Y, W[12]. Amino acid symbols see Fig. 1. Sequences are from
transducin α , Medynski <u>et</u> <u>al</u>.[40]; α subunit of G₀ from brain, Hurley <u>et</u>
<u>al</u>.[25]; EF-Tu, Arai <u>et</u> <u>al</u>.[1].

The p21 produced in this manner constitutes approximately 10% of the
total <u>E. coli</u> proteins. After cell lysis, approximately 50% of the p21
can be recovered in the supernatant fraction of high speed centrifugation.
p21 has been isolated with over 95% purity in the presence of 25% glycerol

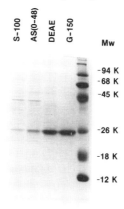

Figure 5. Purification of p21 overproduced in E. coli. p21 is purified
from the high speed supernatant (S-100) of <u>E. coli</u> lysate by ammonium sulfate
fractionation (AS), DEAE-Sephacel chromatography (DEAE) and Sephadex G-150
gel filtration (G-150). The purity of proteins is determined by Coomassie
blue staining of a sodium dodecyl sulfate-polyacrylamide gel. The same
amount of total proteins was applied to each lane.

but without the use of any detergent or protein denaturant, as shown in Fig. 5. The procedure involves high speed centrifugation, ammonium sulfate precipitation, DEAE-Sephacel chromatography and Sephadex G-150 gel filtration. Fig. 6 shows that three biochemical activities with specificity to guanine nucleotides are co-purified with p21. It binds GTP or GDP with high affinity (K_d=1-10 x 10^{-8} M) and high specificity, with virtually no binding of GMP or nucleotides of other bases. It has a GTPase activity with a very low turnover number (0.2 mmol GTP hydrolyzed per mol p21 per min for the v-ras[H] p21 of Ha-MuSV)[23], which is at least 10-fold lower than that of p21 of proto-oncogenes[18,36,54]. p21s of Ha-MuSV or Ki-MuSV also exhibits an autokinase activity due to the presence of threonine-59 mutations, which generate the phosphoryl acceptor sites[49]. This autokinase, in contrast to GTPase, is increased by mutations that activate proto-oncogenes[17]. Using the Scatchard plot analysis on highly purified proteins, we[23] and others[34] have concluded that p21 has a single site per molecule for binding either GTP or GDP, with approximately the same affinity. The dissociation constant, K_d, is on the order of 1 x 10^{-8} M. As shown in Fig. 7, using immunochemical probes, we[23] concluded that the same site is also responsible for the associated GTPase and autokinase, since these activities are specifically affected by the same monoclonal antibody (Y13-259)[16].

We have also studied the sensitivity of sulfhydryl groups of this highly purified v-ras[H] p21 to a thiol specific reagent, N-ethylmaleimide (NEM)[22].

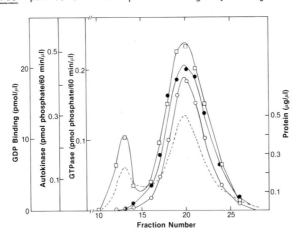

Figure 6. Co-purification of GTP/GDP binding, autokinase, and GTPase with p21. The final step of p21 purification from a Sephadex G-150 column is shown here. Symbols: o , ^{3}H-GDP binding activity; • , autokinase activity; □ , GTPase activity; ----, protein concentration. Reproduced from Hattori et al.[23].

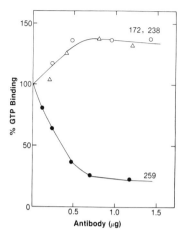

Figure 7. <u>Specific inhibition of GTP binding activity of p21 by a mono-</u>
<u>clonal antibody.</u> The ^{3}H-GTP binding activity of the highly purified p21
was assayed after preincubation with anti-p21 monoclonal antibodies[16],
 • , Y13-259; o , Y13-238, and Δ , YA6-172. Reproduced from Hattori <u>et</u>
<u>al.</u>[23].

Approximately 70% of GTP binding and autokinase activities of p21 were
inactivated by NEM; and excessive amounts of GTP or GDP protected p21
activities from NEM inactivation. The reaction can be described as, where

$$GTP(GDP) \cdot p21 \underset{1 \times 10^{-8} M}{\overset{K_d}{\longleftrightarrow}} GTP(GDP) + p21 \overset{+ NEM}{\longrightarrow} p21\text{-}NEM + GTP(GDP)$$

NEM irreversibly alkylates p21, presumably the nucleotide-free form of the
protein. Thiol titration revealed approximately two fast reactive cysteines;
the susceptibility of one of them was modulated by GTP binding. A total of
4 or 6 residues became titratable upon complete denaturation with 6 M guanidine hydrochloride or reduction with dithiothreitol, respectively. This
observation and a previous study of p21 electrophoretic mobility in reducing
vs. nonreducing gels[53], suggests the presence of a disulfide linkage
within the p21 molecule. The GTP-modulated sulfhydryl group was identified
as cysteine-80 by comparative peptide mapping and sequence analysis of the
purified peptide. We shall come back to this point when we discuss in
detail the GTP-binding domain.

V. The GTP binding domain.

As mentioned previously, the p21 proteins of ras genes have a highly conserved amino acid sequence. Of particular significance for defining the GTP binding domain of the ras proteins is the extensive sequence homology found between p21 and the family of G-proteins, which also bind GTP or GDP. There are at least three regions of homology, i. e., residues 5-27; 58-73; and 109-120[21,32,55,40,25,64,33]. X-ray crystallography of EF-Tu has revealed the structure of its GDP binding site, which involves four peptide loops, connecting β sheets and α helices, that are in direct contact with the nucleotide ligand[28,26]. The homologous regions in p21s are residues 10-16, 57-63, 115-128 and 144-160, as shown in Fig. 8[35,26]. Of key importance to this proposed structure is the asparagine-116 of p21, which, in EF-Tu, is in a position to form a hydrogen bond with the oxygen atom at the 6 position of the guanine ring. Perhaps the aspartate-119 of p21 also forms a bond with nitrogen-1 or nitrogen-2 of guanine. We have constructed a series of point mutations of the v-ras[H] oncogene in this homologous region by oligonucleotide-directed mutagenesis, resulting in single amino acid substitutions[10]. Mutations of the v-ras[H] gene at asparagine-116 of p21 to lysine or tyrosine abolish GTP binding activity, whereas mutations at the adjacent 117th or 118th positions do not. These observations strongly suggest that the guanine base binding site is conserved between p21 and EF-Tu. In another class of mutations at the autophosphorylation site, alterations of threonine-59 to a closely related serine or the unphosphorylable alanine drastically decrease or eliminate the autokinase activity, further suggesting that the 57-63 peptide loop, which in EF-Tu contains the Mg^{++} pocket, is the phosphate contact point for GTP or GDP. These speculations are consistent with the fact that unlike mutations at asparagine-116, which eliminate the binding completely, mutations at threonine-59 alter the autokinase and GTPase. The same situation may be also true for the peptide loop consisting of amino acid 10-16. Mutations at glycine-12 change p21 enzymatic activities but have little effect on binding affinity[15]. These mutations also disallow the special conformation these glycine residues assume[44]. The observation that the anti-peptide antisera against this peptide loop inhibit GTP binding is consistent with the model in Fig. 8, which shows that this peptide loop is in contact with the nucleotide[11]. Although the gross structure of the GDP binding domain appears to be conserved between p21 and EF-Tu, it is worth noting that there is considerable amino acid sequence divergence among members of different G-proteins. Employing a sulfhydryl reagent, we have found that the reactivity of a cysteine residue of p21, modulated by GTP binding, is more closely related to that of EF-G than EF-Tu, suggesting differences in the fine structure of the GTP-binding domain[22,43,39,20].

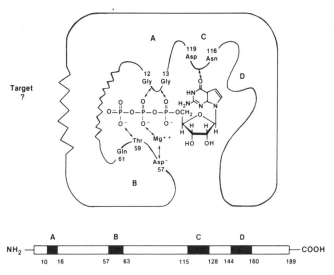

Figure 8. The GTP binding domain of p21 ras proteins. The detailed structure of the GTP binding site is the result of many studies described in the text. The four peptide loops which constitute the GTP binding domain are shown in the p21 linear structure below. Arrows indicate interactions of specific amino acid residues with GTP. The zigzag regions suggest possible conformational changes of p21 upon binding with GTP and following its hydrolysis to GDP, functioning as an on/off switch for its interaction with targets.

The common structure of the GTP binding domain is conserved among members of G-proteins. However, different G-proteins have unique regions perhaps for interacting with specific target macromolecules in signal transduction, e. g., the regulatory G_s and G_i proteins interact with subunits of adenylate cyclase whereas p21 does not[4]. Within the ras gene family, there is a short membrane binding domain at the C-terminus of p21. Most of the other sequences are highly conserved, as shown in Fig. 1, except for a so-called "hinge" region separating these two domains, which exhibits considerable sequence divergence among different ras proteins. This hinge region, residues 165-185 of vertebrate ras proteins, is considerably longer in yeast

ras proteins. Deletions of this region appear not to affect the transforming activity of the v-ras oncogene[62]. However, the normal function of
this region of ras proteins remains an enigma, since this sequence is completely conserved between ras[H] genes of man and murine species for example.

VI. Crucial roles of GTP binding to ras function.

Although it is clear that p21 is required for transformation induced by
ras oncogenes and perhaps plays a role in cellular proliferation in normal
growth and development, crucial p21 properties required for these cellular
functions are not clearly delineated. Recently, we and others have identified antibodies that inhibit p21 GTP binding activity in vitro[23,11]. Upon
microinjection of these antibodies into cells transformed by ras oncogenes,
transient reversion to the normal phenotype can be observed[41,14]. These
studies suggest that p21 in vitro activities may be responsible for its in
vivo function. Our recent studies using site-directed mutagenesis to dis-
sect the structure-function relationship have demonstrated that GTP binding
is crucial for ras gene fucntion[10]. The proviral DNA with mutations at
asparagine-116 of p21, which has lost its GTP binding activity, is unable
to transform NIH-3T3 cells even in the presence of a strong viral LTR and
activating mutations at arginine-12 and threonine-59 of the v-ras[H] oncogene[8].
Mutations for example at amino acid 12, 13, 59 or 61, which activate
proto-oncogenes, decrease the GTPase and increase the autokinase activities,
but do not alter the GTP binding affinity to a great extent. It appears
that both the proto-oncogenes and activated oncogenes have essentially the
same basic property of GTP binding, and the purpose of proto-oncogene activation may be to increase the potency of this basic function. This apprent-
ly can be achieved by mutations which decrease the GTP hydrolyzing activity,
or alternatively, by mass action to increase the protein level by enhanced
transcription, for example, by viral LTR or other cellular enhancers.
Therefore, the arguments for the quantitative[56,46,58] vs. qualitative[2,7]
mechanisms of proto-oncogene activation are not necessarily mutually ex-
clusive.

The precise cellular role of ras proteins, however, is still one of the
major unresolved problems in oncogene research. The similarity of the biochemical properties of p21 to the group of G-proteins would suggest that
p21 may function in an analogous manner in cellular signal transduction[19].
Fig. 9 shows a working model for the possible mechanism of p21 function.
Like the regulatory G-proteins in the adenylate cyclase system, p21 may
serve as a coupling factor for mediating transduction of extracellular

messages through their receptor systems to intracellular effectors, resulting in stimulating cell division[41], [14]. This coupling function is turned on and off by the switch of binding GTP ligand and its hydrolysis to GDP. It is interesting to notice from the detailed crystal structure of EF-Tu[28], [26], that the α and β phosphates of GDP are pointing inward rather than outward to the bottom of the GDP binding pocket (both the guanine base and

A Working Model for p21 ras Proteins

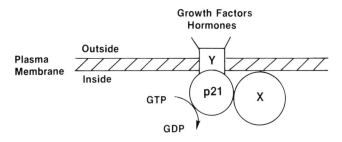

p21 : Membrane Signal Transducer
X : Cellular Effector
Y : Transmembrane Receptor

Figure 9. <u>A working model for the function of p21 ras proteins.</u> p21 is shown as a coupling factor for transduction of growth control signals from extracellular factors across the plasma membrane to intracellular effectors. The binding of guanine nucleotide serves as an on/off switch for these interactions. The cellular effector (X) and the transmembrane receptor (Y) are hypothetical at present.

phosphoryl groups are held by the binding pocket, with the ribose moiety exposing to the exterior), as if the binding of GTP with an extra γ phosphate would force a conformational change of the protein molecule as depicted in Fig. 8. Perhaps this change in the p21 conformation by the binding of different ligands would alter its interactions with target macromolecules and thus regulate the flow of signal transduction. Cancer research is a facinating subject at this atomic level of resolution.

VII. Summary

Cancer is a malfunction of cellular growth control. The discovery of oncogenes, first in transforming retroviruses, and later in human and animal tumors, may have uncovered the key to understanding one of the most elusive subjects of basic cell biology, namely, the controlling mechanisms of cell growth. The ras gene family encodes a group of closely related 21,000 dalton (p21) proteins with special affinity for guanine nucleotides. Other cellular proteins with similar biochemical properties, collectively known as G-proteins, include the regulatory G proteins of adenylate cyclase, the α subunit of transducin of retina rod outer segments, the recently identified rho gene proteins, and perhaps also the elongation factors, EF-Tu and EF-G, of the protein synthesis system. These G-proteins have roles in cellular signal transduction; by analogy p21 may have a similar cellular function in mediating the flow of growth control signals. Recent progress in the cloning and sequencing of these genes, overproduction of gene products in E. coli, protein engineering, detailed biochemical characterization, and the molecular structure determined by high resolution X-ray crystallography, have helped to elucidate in great detail the structure and function of p21 ras proteins. p21 appears to have a small membrane binding domain at the C-terminus, which contains a palmitylation site at cysteine-186, four amino acid residues from the end. Separated by a variable "hinge" region, most of the rest of ras amino acid sequences are highly conserved in nature. Four regions of extensive sequence homology among G-proteins constitute the GTP/GDP binding domain. In the crystal structure of EF-Tu, four peptide loops connecting β sheets and α helices form the pocket for binding GDP. Studies using site-directed mutagenesis and immnochemical probes, indicate that the basic structure of the GDP binding site is conserved between p21 and EF-Tu. Furthermore, these studies also conclude that GTP binding is crucial for p21 ras cellular function. Although the precise target molecules for p21 are still unknown, the finding of the on/off switch function for ras genes have provided a better understanding of the mechanism of proto-oncogene activation, and may also provide further impetus to explore means of cancer intervention by interfering with the switch function.

VIII. REFERENCES

1. Arai, K., Clark, B. F. C., Duffy, L., Jones, M. D., Kaziro, Y., Laursen, R. A., L'Italien, J., Miller, D. L., Nagarkatti, S., Nakamura, S., Nielsen, K. M., Petersen, T. E., Takahashi, K. and Wade, M. (1980). Proc. Natl. Acad. Sci., USA, 77, 1326-1330.
2. Blair, D. G., Oskarsson, M., Wood, T. G., McClements, W. L., Fischinger, P. J. and Vande Woude, G. F. (1981). Science, 212, 941-943.

3. Bishop, J. M. (1983). Ann. Rev. Biochem., 52, 301-354.

4. Beckner, S. K., Hattori, S. and Shih, T. Y. (1985). Nature (London), 317, 71-72.

5. Buss, J. E. and Sefton, B. M. (1985). J. Virol., 53, 7-12.

6. Capon, D. J., Chen, E. Y., Levinson, A. D., Seeburg, P. H. and Goeddel, D. V. (1983). Nature (London), 302, 33-37.

7. Chang, E. H., Furth, M. E., Scolnick, E. M. and Lowy, D. R. (1982). Nature (London), 297, 479-483.

8. Chang, E. H., Maryak, J. M., Wei, C. M., Shih, T. Y., Shober, R., Cheung, H., Ellis, R. W., Hager, G. L., Scolnick, E. M. and Lowy, D. R. (1980). J. Virol., 35, 76-92.

9. Chen, Z. Q., Ulsh, L. S., DuBois, G. and Shih, T. Y. (1985). J. Vriol., 56, 607-612.

10. Clanton, D. J., Hattori, S. and Shih, T. Y. (1985). Submitted for publication.

11. Clark, R., Wong, G., Arnheim, N., Nitecki, D. and McCormick, F. (1985). Proc. Natl. Acad. Sci., USA, 82, 5280-5284.

12. Dayhoff, M. O. (1978). Atlas of Protein Sequence and Structure, 5, 345-352.

13. Dhar, R., Ellis, R. W., Shih, T. Y., Oroszlan, S., Shapiro, B., Maizel, J., Lowy, D. and Scolnick, E. M. (1982). Science, 217, 934-937.

14. Feramisco, J. R., Clark, R., Wong, G., Arnheim, N., Milley, R. and McCormick, F. (1985). Nature (London), 314, 639-641.

15. Finkel, T., Der, C. J. and Cooper, G. M. (1984). Cell, 37, 151-158.

16. Furth, M. E., Davis, L. J., Fleurdelys, B. and Scolnick, E. M. (1982). J. Virol., 43, 294-304.

17. Gibbs, J. B., Ellis, R. W. and Scolnick, E. M. (1984). Proc. Natl. Acad. Sci., USA, 81, 2674-2678.

18. Gibbs, J. B., Sigal, I. S., Poe, M. and Scolnick, E. M. (1984). Proc. Natl. Acad. Sci., USA, 81, 5704-5708.

19. Gilman, A. G. (1984). Cell, 36, 577-579.

20. Girshovich, A. S., Bochkareva, E. S., Pozdnyakov, V. A. and Ovchinnikov, Yu. A. (1978). FEBS Letters, 85, 283-286.

21. Halliday, K. R. (1984). J. Cyclic Nucleotides and Protein Phosphorylation Research, 9, 435-448.

22. Hattori, S., Copeland, T. D., Oroszlan, S. and Shih, T. Y. (1985). Submitted for publication.

70

23. Hattori, S., Ulsh, L. S., Halliday, K. and Shih, T. Y. (1985). Mol. Cell. Biol., 5, 1449-1455.

24. Hunter, T. (1984). Scientific American, 251, 70-79.

25. Hurley, J. B., Simon, M. I., Teplow, D. B., Robishaw, J. D. and Gilman, A. G. (1984). Science, 226, 860-862.

26. Jurnak, F. (1985). Science, 230, 32-36.

27. Lacal, J. C., Santos, E., Notario, V., Barbacid, M., Yamazaki, S., Kung, H. F., Seamans, C., McAndrew, S. and Crowl, R. (1984). Proc. Natl. Acad. Sci., USA, 81 5305-5309.

28. la Cour, T. F. M., Nyborg, J., Thirup, S. and Clark, B. F. C. (1985). The EMBO Journal, 4, 2385-2388.

29. Land, H., Parada, L. F. and Weinberg, R. A. (1983). Science, 222, 771-778.

30. Lautenberger, J. A., Court, D. and Papas, T. S. (1983). Gene, 23, 75-84.

31. Lautenberger, J. A., Ulsh, L., Shih, T. Y. and Papas, T. S. (1983). Science, 221, 858-860.

32. Leberman, R. and Egner, U. (1984). The EMBO Journal, 3, 339-341.

33. Madaule, P. and Axel, R. (1985). Cell, 41, 31-40.

34. Manne, V., Yamazaki, S. and Kung, H. F. (1984). Proc. Natl. Acad. Sci., USA, 81, 6953-6957.

35. McCormick, F., Clark, B. F. C., la Cour, T. F. M., Kjeldgaard, M., Norskov-Lauritsen, L. and Nyborg, J. (1985). Science, 230, 78-82.

36. McGrath, J. P., Capon, D. J., Goeddel, D. V. and Levinson, A. D. (1984). Nature (London), 310, 644-649.

37. McGrath, J. P., Capon, D. J., Smith, D. H., Chen, E. Y., Seeburg, P. H., Goeddel, D. V. and Levinson, A. D. (1983). Nature (London), 304, 501-506.

38. Marchildon, G. A., Casnellie, J. E., Walsh, K. A. and Krebs, E. G. (1984). Proc. Natl. Acad. Sci., USA, 81, 7679-7682.

39. Marsh, R. C., Chinall, G. and Parmeggiani, A. (1975). J. Biol. Chem., 250, 8344-8352.

40. Medynski, D. C., Sullivan, K., Smith, D., Van Dop, C., Chang, F. H., Kung, B. K. K., Seeburg, P. H. and Bourne, H. R. (1985). Proc. Natl. Acad. Sci., USA, 82, 4311-4315.

41. Mulcahy, L. S., Smith, M. R. and Stacey, D. W. (1985). Nature (London), 313, 241-243.

42. Neuman-Silberberg, F. S., Schejter, E., Hoffmann, F. M. and Shilo, B. Z. (1984). Cell, 37, 1027-1033.

43. Ovchinnikov, Y. A., Alakhov, Y. B., Bundulis, Y. P., Bundule, M. A., Dovas, N. V., Kozlou, V. P., Motuz, L. P. and Vinokurov, L. M. (1982). FEBS Letters, 139, 130-135.

44. Pincus, M. R. and Brandt-Rauf, P. W. (1985). Proc. Natl. Acad. Sci., USA, 82, 3596-3600.

45. Powers, S., Kataoka, T., Fasano, O., Goldfarb, M., Strathern, J., Broach, J. and Wigler, M. (1984). Cell, 36, 607-612.

46. Reddy, E. P., Reynold, R. K., Santos, E. and Barbacid, M. (1982). Nature (London), 300, 149-152.

47. Schultz, A. M., Henderson, L. E., Oroszlan, S., Garber, E. A. and Hanafusa, H. (1985). Science, 227, 427-429.

48. Sefton, B., Trowbridge, I. S., Copper, J. A. and Scolnick, E. M. (1982). Cell, 31, 465-474.

49. Shih, T. Y., Stokes, P. E., Smythers, G. W., Dhar, R. and Oroszlan, S. (1982). J. Biol. Chem., 257, 11767-11773.

50. Shih, T. Y. and Weeks, M. O. (1984). Cancer Investigation, 2, 109-123.

51. Shih, T. Y., Weeks, M. O., Gruss, P., Dhar, R., Oroszlan, S. and Scolnick, E. M. (1982). J. Virol., 42, 253-261.

52. Shimizu, K., Birnbaum, D., Ruley, M. A., Fasano, O., Suard, Y., Eglund, L., Taparowsky, E., Goldfarb, M. and Wigler, M. (1983). Nature (London), 304, 497-500.

53. Srivastava, S. K., Yuasa, Y., Reynolds, S. H. and Aaronson, S. A. (1985). Proc. Natl. Acad. Sci., USA, 82, 38-42.

54. Sweet, R. W., Yokoyama, S., Kamata, T., Feramisco, J. R., Rosenberg, M. and Gross, M. (1984). Nature (London), 311, 273-275.

55. Tanabe, T., Nukada, T., Nishikawa, Y., Sugimoto, K., Suzuki, H., Takahashi, H., Noda, M., Haga, T., Ichiyama, A., Kangawa, K., Minamino, N., Matsuo, H. and Numa, S. (1985). Nature (London), 315, 242-245.

56. Tabin, C. J., Bradley, S. M., Bargmann, C. I., Weinberg, R. A., Papageorge, A. G., Scolnick, E. M., Dhar, R., Lowy, D. R. and Chang, E. H. (1982). Nature (London), 300, 143-149.

57. Tapararowsky, E., Shimizu, K., Goldfarb, M. and Wigler, M. (1983). Cell, 34, 581-586.

58. Taparowsky, E., Suard, Y., Fasano, O., Shimizu, K., Goldfarb, M. and Wigler, M. (1982). Nature (London), 300, 762-765.

59. Tsuchida, N., Ryder, T. and Ohtsubo, E. (1982). Science, 217, 937-939.

72

60. Ulsh, L. S. and Shih, T. Y. (1984). Mol. Cell. Biol., 4, 1647-1652.
61. Vande Woude, G. F., Levine, A. J., Topp, W. C. and Watson, J. D. (Eds.) (1984). Cancer Cells: Oncogenes and Viral Genes. Cold Spring Harbor Laboratory Press, Cold Spring Harbor, New York.
62. Willumsen, B. M., Christensen, A., Hubbert, N. L., Papageorge, A. G. and Lowy, D. R. (1984). Nature (London), 310, 583-586.
63. Willumsen, B. M., Norris, K., Papageorge, A. G., Hubbert, N. L. and Lowy, D. R. (1984). The EMBO Journal, 3, 2581-2585.
64. Yatsunami, K. and Khorana, H. G. (1985). Proc. Natl. Acad. Sci., USA, 82, 4316-4320.

5

The _myb_ Oncogene

Joseph S. Lipsick and Marcel A. Baluda

Jonsson Comprehensive Cancer Center and Department of Pathology
University of California, Los Angeles, School of Medicine
Los Angeles, California 90024

The purpose of this article is to review our current (mid-1985) understanding of the molecular biology of the myb gene family. Two avian acute leukemia viruses, avian myeloblastosis virus (AMV) and the E26 virus, contain myb-related oncogenes. As is the case for other retroviral oncogenes, normal cellular DNA contains a closely related, highly conserved genetic precursor, c-myb (or proto-myb). This proto-oncogene also appears to be activated in several malignancies which are not caused by acutely transforming retroviruses containing myb. The molecular mechanisms by which c-myb may be rendered oncogenic, by viral transduction or by other means, will be a focus of this review. The general biology of retroviruses will not be discussed in detail since the subject has recently been extensively reviewed[1].

I. THE ONCOGENE OF AMV

A. Transformation by AMV

Avian myeloblastosis virus (AMV) is a replication defective retrovirus which causes acute myelomonocytic leukemia following injection into chicken embryos or newly hatched chicks[2]. AMV transforms immature avian myeloid precursors and mature macrophages, but no other cell type in vitro[3-6a]. Transfection of a cloned AMV proviral DNA has recently been reported to cause fibroblast transformation, but the role of myb in this process remains unknown[6b]. The bone marrow target cells for AMV transformation appear to differ from those of the myc viruses (MC29, CMII, OK10, and MH2) and the erb virus (AEV) by cell surface markers, functional assays, and velocity sedimentation[7,8]. A temperature-sensitive mutant of AMV exists which has a greatly decreased transformation capacity at the non-permissive temperature in vitro and does not cause leukemia in chickens[9]. Cells previously transformed in vitro with this ts-AMV display a partial morphological conversion into macrophage-like cells when shifted to the non-permissive temperature. Cells transformed with wild-type AMV can also be induced to differentiate into apparently mature macrophages by phorbal myristate acetate (PMA), a tumor promoting agent[10,11].

B. AMV Oncogene Structure and Transcription.

The myb oncogene was first discovered as a transduced genetic element of cellular origin which is present in AMV (v-myb^{AMV}) but not in its helper viruses, the myeloblastosis-associated viruses (MAV-1 and MAV-2)[12,13]. Molecular cloning of the AMV and MAV proviruses from the DNA of virally transformed leukemic myeloblasts and subsequent restriction enzyme mapping and heteroduplex analyses indicated that transduced cellular sequences had replaced the env gene during the genesis of AMV[13-16]. However, the gag and pol genes appeared to be largeley intact. These results were supported by direct oligonucleotide mapping of viral RNAs and by the observation that "non-producer" leukemic cells harboring only the AMV provirus produce virus particles, albeit non-infectious ones[17]. These non-infectious particles contain protein products of the gag and pol genes, but not those of the env gene.

AMV thus appeared to have a genetic structure similar to that of the Bryan strain of Rous sarcoma virus which expresses src as a subgenomic mRNA, but lacks the env gene[18]. Analysis of viral RNA species in AMV transformed myeloblasts demonstrated that a 2 kilobase (kb) subgenomic mRNA as well as the 7 kb genomic viral RNA both contain myb-specific sequences[19,20]. This 2 kb subgenomic mRNA species was also shown to contain sequences related to the U5 region of the viral long terminal repeat (LTR), suggesting that this mRNA is generated by the splicing of 5' LTR sequences to 3' myb-specific sequences, as is the case for the env ans src mRNAs of Rous sarcoma virus[21]. In order to determine the precise structure of the v-myb[AMV] oncogene, the nucleotide sequence of the transduced region of the AMV provirus was determined[22,23]. Comparison of this sequence with that of the Prague C strain of Rous sarcoma virus[24] revealed that transduced sequences (amv) provide coding sequences for the pol gene as well as the myb gene of AMV. These sequences of cellular origin had replaced a short 3' terminal region (36 codons) of the pol gene and nearly the entire env gene, leaving only the eleven C-terminal env codons intact (Figure 1). These transduced sequences are predicted to provide 27 codons which constitute an abnormal C-terminus for the AMV reverse transcriptase, offering a possible explanation for its reported lack of functional activity[17]. (Note: The well-studied "AMV reverse transcriptase" thus appears to actually be the product of its MAV helper viruses.)

Downstream of the termination codon of the transduced C-terminus of the AMV reverse transcriptase, a single long open reading frame extends through the remaining 371 codons of the inserted cellular sequences and across the 3' cellular-viral recombination site through the 11 in-frame terminal env codons. The first initiation codon in this transduced open reading frame is preceded by what appear to be consensus transcriptional and translation control sequences[23]. Thus, the product of v-myb[AMV]

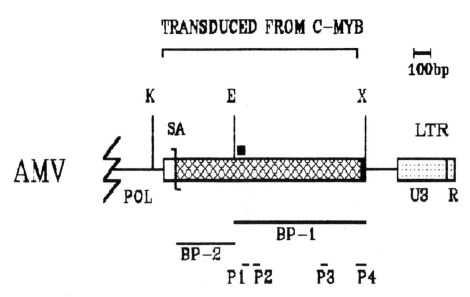

Figure 1. The Structure of v-myb^AMV. The 3' portion of the AMV genome which contains the transduced cellular sequences is shown. Symbols are as follows: open box--transduced sequences encoding pol C-terminus; hatched box--transduced sequences encoding internal p48myb residues; black box--env sequences encoding p48myb C-terminus; stippled box--viral LTR; small black square-initial AUG within the transduced sequences. SA denotes the splice acceptor site for generating the myb-specific 2 kb viral mRNA. K, E, and X denote the positions where KpnI, EcoRI and XbaI restriction endonuclease sites occur within proviral DNA. Shown below are the relative sizes and locations of synthetic immunogens used to raise anti-myb antibodies (see text for details).

was initially predicted to be a protein of 30,000 molecular weight (MW) initiating within the transduced cellular sequences. However, the AMV oncogene product was subsequently identified as an unglycosylated 48,000 MW protein[25,26] inconsistent with these initial predictions.

This gave rise to an alternate model in which the v-myb^AMV product has its N-terminus encoded by a short viral sequence upstream of the splice junction of the AMV subgenomic mRNA[25-27]. S1 nuclease mapping of this 2 kb mRNA identified a splice acceptor site immediately following the altered pol termination codon within the transduced sequences of cellular origin[28].

By analogy with the splice donor site used to generate the Rous sarcoma virus subgenomic mRNAs[21], the first six codons of the gag gene are predicted to be joined in-frame to the entire long myb-specific open reading frame at this splice acceptor site. This would result in translation of a myb-encoded protein of the observed size.

These S1 mapping studies also showed that the homologous splice acceptor site is used in generating c-myb mRNA[28]. This proved that the 5' recombination event which generated AMV occured within a c-myb intron and therefore must have been at the DNA rather than the RNA level. In contrast, the 3' recombination event was shown to have occured within an exon of c-myb.

Sequencing of part of the AMV provirus also revealed that its LTR contains a U3 region unlike that of any known retrovirus, while its R and U5 regions are nearly identical to those of RSV[22-24]. The role of these presumed transcriptional control sequences in the unique pathogenesis of AMV remains to be determined. Both DNA restriction mapping and RNA oligonucleotide mapping have shown that MAV-1 and MAV-2 appear to share this unusual transcriptional control region[13,17,34].

C. AMV oncogene product and possible functions.

The identification of the product of the AMV oncogene proved difficult for two reasons. First, sera from leukemic chickens do not immunoprecipitate the v-myb[AMV] gene product. Presumably, this is because AMV can only induce leukemia in relatively immunoincompetent hatchling birds and is rapidly fatal[2]. Secondly, since the AMV oncogene product does not contain large segments encoded by viral structural genes, antisera raised against viral components do not immunoprecipitate any novel fusion proteins such as those encoded by the MC29 and Fujinami sarcoma viruses[17,29]. Analysis of the products of in vitro translation of AMV RNA were ambiguous in identifying a myb-encoded gene product[30,31].

Two strategies were eventually successful in identifying the product of v-myb[AMV]. Both methods used knowledge of the nucleic acid sequence in order to produce immunological reagents specific for myb-encoded proteins. In one case, rabbits were immunized with four distinct synthetic peptides predicted from the v-myb[AMV] DNA sequence[25]. Three of these four antisera (anti-P1, P2, and P4; see Figure 1) specifically immunoprecipitated a 48,000 MW metabolically-radiolabelled protein, p48[myb], from a clonal AMV-transformed "nonproducer" cell line and from polyclonal AMV-induced peripheral blood leukemic myeloblasts. This protein was not present in uninfected chicken tissues or in cells infected only with helper virus. p48[myb] is non-glycosylated[25], exists in several forms separable by isoelectric point[11,32] and is phosphorylated at low levels on serine and threonine[32].

The same 48,000 MW protein was independently identified in the same AMV transformed cell line by a rabbit antiserum raised against a bacterial fusion protein whose myb portion (BP-1 in Figure 1) was encoded by the v-myb[AMV] sequence downstream of the first internal AUG[26]. Immunoprecipitation of the products of in vitro translation of AMV RNA also identified a 34,000 MW protein in addition to p48[myb]. This may represent initiation of translation at the "cryptic" first internal AUG discussed above, however, this 34,000 MW protein was not observed in vivo.

Recently, a rabbit antiserum raised against a bacterial fusion protein containing the v-myb[AMV] coding sequences upstream from this first internal AUG (BP-2 in Figure 1) has also been shown to immunoprecipitate p48[myb32a]. This proves that the sequence upstream of this first AUG within v-myb[AMV] is indeed protein coding and implies that translation must begin in a spliced leader sequence.

The protein product of the oncogene of AMV differs structurally in three ways from p75[c-myb], its 75,000 MW normal cellular homolog[26]. Firstly, it has N- and C-terminal residues of viral origin. The presence of six gag-encoded N-terminal amino acids in p48[myb], which are encoded by the spliced viral mRNA leader, has been documented by tryptic peptide mapping[33]. The presence of eleven in-frame env-encoded C-terminal amino acids has been shown by nucleic acid sequencing[22,23] and by immunologic cross-reactivity of anti-p48[myb] C-terminal peptide antiserum with the gp37[env] protein of MAV-1 (but not, interestingly, of MAV-2)[34]. Secondly, coding sequences for both the N- and C-termini of p75[c-myb] have been deleted during the genesis of AMV[22,26,33]. Thirdly, point mutations predict the presence of eleven altered amino acids in p48[myb] relative to the homologous region of p75[c-myb] [22].

A mutant of AMV which is temperature-sensitive for the initiation and maintenance of transformation has been isolated[9]. Cells transformed by this virus exhibit a 5- to 10-fold decrease in the amount of p48[myb] when shifted to the non-permissive temperature[35], offering the first genetic evidence that p48[myb] is indeed the cause of transformation by AMV. This decrease in p48[myb] is apparently due to a specific reduction in the level of subgenomic v-myb[AMV] mRNA. The lesion in this ts-mutant thus appears to perturb the regulation of viral RNA splicing or stability rather than p48[myb] structural sequences.

Because the predicted sequence of p48[myb] bears no strong homolgy to any other published protein sequence, the initial steps taken to identify its probable functions have largely focused on its intracellular location. p48[myb] has been identified as a nuclear protein in AMV-transformed cells both by immunofluorescence and by subcellular fractionation and immunoprecipitation[36,37].

PMA-induced terminal differentiation of an AMV-transformed cell line into macrophages does not appear to alter the intracellular level of p48[myb] [11]. Surprisingly, however, the p48[myb] in these differentiated cells was mostly found in the cytoplasm rather than the nucleus[37]. The physiological significance of this latter finding remains unclear, since myeloblasts transformed by temperature-sensitive mutants of the closely related E26 virus do not show an altered intracellular distribution of their myb-encoded nuclear protein during terminal differentiation at the non-permissive temperature[38].

More refined ultrastructural studies and biochemical fractionation of AMV-transformed myeloblasts have revealed that substantial fractions of p48[myb] are present in the insoluble nuclear matrix (64%) and in the readily soluble nucleoplasm (29%), but little if any p48[myb] is specifically associated with chromatin (7%)[39]. Consistent with a nuclear matrix localization, immunofluorescent analysis of cycling cells has revealed that p48[myb]-specific staining is homogeneously nuclear during interphase with the exception of nucleolar centers; is nuclear, but excluded from the condensed chromosomes during metaphase; and is diffusely cytoplasmic during telophase.

In addition to its definition as a structural entity, the nuclear matrix is also a functional site where DNA replication and active gene transcription are believed to occur[40]. Perturbations of either of these basic nuclear functions can easily be envisaged to result in cellular transformation. Interestingly, association with the nuclear matrix has also been observed for the products of the myc oncogene of MC29 and related viruses[41] and for the product of the E1A transforming gene of adenovirus[42].

The nature of DNA association with the nuclear matrix is unknown, but it is likely to involve protein-DNA interactions. Recent experiments have shown that immunoaffinity purified p48[myb] can bind to DNA in vitro[38] as can native p48[myb] from nucleoplasmic extracts[43]. Similar results have also been obtained with products of the myc-related genes[41,44], however, the specificity and functional significance of such in vitro DNA binding remains unknown.

Some similarity has been noted between the predicted p48[myb] amino acid sequence and (i) a DNA-binding domain common to numerous proteins including bacteriophage lambda repressor[27]; (ii) the products of the myc and adeno-virus E1A genes[97]. The functional significance of these proposed distant relationships is unclear.

The goal of future studies of p48myb will be to establish the physiological significance of its DNA-binding properties and to determine its role, if any, in the processes of DNA replication and transcription. The short half-life (~30 minutes) of p48myb in vivo[32] is similar to that of the myc and E1A-encoded nuclear transforming proteins[44,45] and is consistent with a regulatory role for these proteins. However, although p48myb can be expressed in the nuclei of normal fibroblasts[37], it does not appear capable of transforming these cells.

II. THE ONCOGENE OF E26 VIRUS

A. Transformation by E26 virus.

The replication defective E26 acute leukemia virus contains an additional putative oncogene (ets) in addition to v-myb[E26]. In contrast to AMV, it causes a leukemia in chickens in which erythroid cells predominate, but in which myeloid cells are also present[47-50]. This leukemic phenotype appears to be independent of the helper virus but may result from the production of specific growth factors[50]. E26 transforms myeloid as well as erythroid bone marrow target cells in vitro[50-52]. Furthermore, either erythroid or myeloid E26-transformed cells can be selectively grown out of leukemic peripheral blood or in vitro transformed bone marrow by using appropriate growth factors[50,52]. The factor required for outgrowth of E26-transformed myeloid cells, cMGF, has been purified to apparent homogeneity, consists of two glycoproteins of 23,000 and 27,000 MW, and is active in the picomolar range[53]. Studies of E26 transformation of early embryonic tissues have suggested that unlike AMV or AEV, this virus can transform uncommitted bipotential erythroid-myeloid stem cells[52]. In further contrast to AMV, the E26 virus has also been reported to transform fibroblasts in vitro [51,54]. These E26-transformed fibroblasts are similar to myc virus-transformed fibroblasts in that they exhibit altered growth characteristics in vitro, but do not cause tumors in nude mice.

Four temperature-sensitive mutants of E26 virus have recently been isolated[55]. Myeloid cells transformed by these viruses stop growing and differentiate into macrophage-like cells when shifted to the non-permissive temperature (42°C). They also lose their responsiveness to cMGF and secrete a cMGF-like factor. However, transformation of erythroblasts and fibroblasts is unaffected by temperature shift and the three mutants tested retained their leukemogenicity in chickens (Note: The chicken basal temperature is

41.5°C.). The molecular lesions in these interesting mutants remain to be determined.

B. E26 virus oncogene structure and transcription.

The E26 virus was initially shown to bear myb-related sequences by nucleic acid hybridization[12,56]. Oligonucleotide mapping and molecular cloning of viral DNA has confirmed this and has further established the presence of transduced sequences (ets) apparently unrelated to c-myb[57,58]. The nucleotide sequence of the E26 virus predicts a single long open reading frame which joins 272 viral gag-specific codons, 283 transduced myb-specific codons, and 491 transduced ets-specific codons[58,59]. The myb-specific sequences of E26 (v-myb^{E26}) are an internal subset of the c-myb exons transduced by AMV. v-myb^{E26} lacks 106 bp present at the 5' end of v-myb^{AMV}, including the AMV splice acceptor site, and also lacks 240 bp present at the 3' end of v-myb^{AMV}. Both the 5' and 3' recombination events which generated v-myb^{E26} from c-myb occurred within exons. v-myb^{E26} differs by only a single nucleotide and predicted codon from the homologous c-myb sequences and does not share any common point mutations with v-myb^{AMV} relative to c-myb.

Transduction of the myb and ets sequences has resulted in deletion of the entire pol gene and substantial portions of gag and env as well. Although the usual viral splice donor site in gag which is used to generate subgenomic env mRNA has been preserved, the E26 provirus transcribes a single, presumably unspliced genome-length 5.7 kb mRNA[33,58]. The E26 virus contains LTR sequences which are closely related to those of the Rous sarcoma and MH2 viruses and appear unrelated to the unique U3 sequences present in AMV and its MAV helper viruses[59]. The biological role of these differing transcriptional control elements between E26 and AMV remains to be determined.

The role of ets-specific sequences in transformation by the E26 virus is also unclear at present. The predicted ets-encoded protein sequences bears a significant homology to the protein sequence deduced for the products of the CDC4 and CDC36 genes in yeast, mutations of which alter the cell cycle[59a]. This suggests that ets may be more than an idle passenger in the E26 virus, although no acutely transforming retrovirus bearing only ets sequences has yet been described. In this regard, mutants of E26 which lack nearly the entire ets coding region transform myeloid bone marrow targets in vitro, but do not appear to cause leukemia in vivo [59b].

C. E26 virus oncogene product and possible functions.

The product of the E26 virus oncogene, p135gag-myb-ets, was first identified by immunoprecipitation using antisera directed against gag-encoded viral proteins[56,60]. This protein is present in both erythroid and myeloid E26-transformed cells[50]. Comparative tryptic peptide mapping has confirmed the presence of gag-specific amino acid sequences[33,60]. The presence of myb-specific amino acid sequences in p135gag-myb-ets has also been established by immunological cross-reactivity and by peptide mapping[25,33,38].

The subcellular location of p135gag-myb-ets appears to be similar to that of p48myb described above. Immunofluorescence and subcellular fractionation have identified this protein in the nuclei of E26-transformed myeloblasts[36-38] and a substantial fraction is tightly bound to the nuclear matrix[38a]. The common myb-encoded domains in p48myb and p135gag-myb-ets are likely to determine the nucleotropism of these proteins because p75c-myb is also a nuclear protein. Furthermore, this nucleotropism is likely to be due to a carrier mediated process rather than passive diffusion and "trapping", since p135gag-myb-ets is large enough to be excluded by the nuclear membrane pore complex.

Affinity purified p135gag-myb-ets binds DNA in vitro and a correlation was established between this DNA-binding activity and the transforming capacity of several temperature-sensitive E26 virus mutants[38]. The oncogene products of these mutant viruses either lacked any apparent DNA-binding in vitro or lost this activity at the non-permissive temperature. Although the nature of the molecular lesions in these mutants are unknown, they are hypothesized to be in the v-myb[E26] sequence, since only myeloblasts and not erythroblasts or fibroblasts are temperature sensitive for transformation[55]. Interestingly, the mutant p135gag-myb-ets proteins remain in the nuclei of tsE26-transformed myeloblasts following shift to the non-permissive temperature, despite the terminal differentiation of these cells into macrophages.

D. The role of growth factors in E26 transformation.

E26-transformed myeloblasts are dependent upon cMGF for proliferation in vitro[60], but this requirement can be abrogated by superinfection with avian retroviruses containing src-related oncogenes (src, fps, yes, ros, erbB and mht/mil)[60a]. Such src-superinfected E26-transformed cells then appear to produce their own cMGF-like factor. Viruses containing myb or myc (in the absence of mht/mil) cannot substitute for those containing src-related oncogenes in inducing this supposed autocrine growth stimulation. Interestingly, the intracellular level of p135gag-myb-ets appears to be increased by cMGF in E26-transformed myeloblasts, whereas levels of helper virus proteins and of the oncogene products of cells transformed by AEV and MC29 appear to be unaffected by this factor[60].

Two recent findings appear to support a linkage between src-related onco-genes and growth factor independence of transformed myeloid cells. First, the c-fms gene product, which is a cell-surface tyrosine kinase related to src, is closely related and possibly identical to the receptor for murine CSF-1 (also known as G-CSF), a macrophage growth factor[61]. The receptor for the presumably related avian cMGF is also likely to be a src-related tyrosine kinase. Secondly, the src-related oncogene of the Abelson murine leukemia virus (abl) can malignantly transform myeloid cells and mast cells from growth factor dependence to growth factor independence[62,63]. However, in this case, transformation does not appear to occur via an autocrine mechanism.

These results suggest that myeloid transformation by E26 and possibly AMV may produce growth factor-dependent clones which can then progress to growth factor-independence by subsequent alterations in the genes for myeloid growth factors or their receptors. However, the continuous production of myb appears likely to be required since the src-containing viruses themselves do not transform myeloid cells, even when pp60[src] is expressed at high levels[64]. In addition, progression to growth factor independence may not be required for E26-induced leukemogenesis, since freshly isolated peripheral blood leukemic cells are growth factor dependent[50].

III. THE NORMAL c-myb GENE

A. Structure of the c-myb gene.

A single-copy normal cellular gene closely related to the myb oncogenes of AMV and E26 is present in the genome of widely divergent vertebrate species including man [12,65]. A more distantly related gene has recently been identified in Drosophila as well, but not thus far in yeast[66]. The evolutionary conservation of the c-myb gene implies that it serves an essen-tial function in metazoan species. A comparison of the normal c-myb gene with the partially transduced viral myb genes may reveal how the latter cause leukemia.

The 9 kb region of the chicken c-myb gene from which the oncogenes of AMV and E26 arose has been cloned[67-71] and the regions of v-myb homology have been sequenced[22]. These analyses reveal that the v-myb coding sequence of AMV has arisen by precise splicing of six c-myb introns. At least one additional intron is present in c-myb both 5' and 3' to the transduced v-myb[AMV] coding sequences[28,28a,69]. Both the size of the chicken c-myb gene product and the sequences at the 5' and 3' flanking splice sites imply that additional c-myb coding exons are also present both 5' and 3' to the region homologous to v-myb[AMV].

The human c-myb locus has also been cloned and mapped with restriction endonucleases[70,72]. The v-myb[AMV] homologous sequences are distributed in the expected order over approximately 6 kb and contain at least four introns. Hybridization of human c-myb mRNA with cloned human genomic DNA flanking the region of v-myb homology indicates that the entire c-myb transcription unit may exceed 30 kb[72]. The single copy human c-myb gene is located on chromosome 6q22-24[73-75].

The organization of the murine c-myb gene appears to be similar to the human c-myb gene[76]. Comparison of cloned genomic DNA[76] with cDNA clones[76,77] and mRNA reveals that the murine c-myb transcription unit appears to encompass approximately 45 kb and that its 5' end is likely to lie within 8 kb of the v-myb[AMV] homologous region[76]. The murine c-myb gene has been mapped to chromosome 10[78].

A gene which is at least partially homologous to c-myb has also been cloned from Drosophila melanogaster[66]. This single copy gene is present at position 13E-F on the X chromosome. DNA sequencing has revealed a 375 nucleotide domain which is 67% identical to the homologous coding region of the chicken c-myb gene. This conserved region corresponds to the most 5' coding sequences of v-myb[AMV] and is predicted to encode a protein domain of 125 amino acids which is 73% identical to that of the chicken (see below). Interestingly, at least two of the introns present in this region of chicken c-myb are absent in Drosophila c-myb.

    B. Transcription of c-myb.

Transcripts of the c-myb gene ranging in size from 3.4 to 4.5 kb have been detected in diverse species. In the chicken a 4 kb c-myb RNA has been identified primarily in hematopoietic tissues, particularly those which contain a large proportion of immature cells[69,79-83]. Such transcripts appear to be present in cells of the lymphoid, erythroid, and myeloid lineages. The variable presence of hematopoietic elements in frehsly isolated "non-hematopoietic" tissues makes the interpretation of low levels of c-myb expression difficult. However, c-myb expression has recently been reported in cultured chicken embryonic fibroblasts[84].

Levels of expression of chicken c-myb do not appear to correlate with susceptibility to transformation by AMV. Mature macrophages express little if any c-myb[80,81], whereas embryonic yolk sac myeloid precursors express high levels of c-myb[83], yet both cell types appear to be targets for transformation by AMV[6,6a]. The yolk sac cells which express c-myb comprise only about 5% of the hematopoietic cells in this tissue and their levels of c-myb RNA appears to excede that of v-myb expression in AMV or

E26-transformed cells[83]. These cells have been identified primarily as M-CFC, the committed progenitor for the macrophage lineage. As they differentiate to the promonocyte stage there is an abrupt decrease in c-myb expression of over 100-fold.

In several cell types, c-myb expression appears to be cell cycle dependent[84]. Steady state levels of c-myb mRNA are specifically increased during the late G1 or early S phase of the cell cycle in the Marek Disease Virus-transformed MSB-1 chicken T lymphoma cell line, in normal chicken embryo fibroblasts, and in B lymphocytes of the Bursa of Fabricius. In these cell types, regulation of c-myb expression occurs via post-transcriptional mechanisms and steady state levels of c-myb mRNA can be stabilized by pretreatment of cells with cycloheximide. In contrast, chicken thymocytes which contain a much higher overall level of c-myb mRNA do not exhibit cell cycle or cycloheximide-inducible variation in its expression. These studies suggest that c-myb may serve both a general function during the cell cycle and a tissue specific function in thymocytes. The thymus is an unusual organ in that its lymphocytes undergo rapid turnover, with most cells apparently destined to die before reaching the peripheral tissues. The high, cell cycle-independent levels of c-myb in this tissue may be involved in its unusual cellular replication and differentiation.

Human c-myb transcripts of 3.4 to 4.5 kb have also been detected in human hematopoietic cells and transformed cell lines of the lymphoid, erythroid, and myeloid lineages[85,87]. The most mature cells in these lineages do not appear to express c-myb and its expression can be dramatically reduced in the HL60 promyelocytic leukemia cell line by cheimcally induced differentiation[85]. A similar decrease in c-myb expression has been observed in the human ML-1 myeloblastic leukemia cell line following treatment with PMA and this decreased expression appears to occur rapidly, prior to the decrease in DNA synthesis which accompanies differentiation[88]. Transcription of c-myb has also been observed in human breast, colon, and small cell lung carcinomas and derived cell lines[87,89,90]. The small cell lung carcinomas are particularly interesting since c-myb transcription has only been detected in the more malignant variant cell form and appears to yield a smaller 2 kb as well as a presumably normal 4 kb c-myb mRNA[90]. These variant cells also display an amplification and increased expression of c-myc[91].

Feline c-myb is expressed in high levels as a 4.5 kb mRNA in bone marrow, thymus and spleen[92]. In addition, fetal kidneys and early gestational liver and brain are rich in c-myb transcripts, again suggesting that c-myb function may not be limited to hematopoietic tissues.

Murine c-myb is abundantly expressed as a 4 kb transcript in thymus and bone marrow, to a lesser extent in fetal liver, and barely if at all in adult liver, spleen, lymph nodes, and brain[93]. c-myb expression decreases at least 10-fold in cells of the T-lymphocyte lineage as they progress from immature cortical thymocytes to mature, resting peripheral T cells. However, no decrease in c-myb expression was observed during age-dependent thymic involution. The lymphoid organs of lpr/lpr mice, which exhibit an autoimmune-lymphoproliferative syndrome, contain increased levels of c-myb mRNA, as do those of humans with a similar disorder[94]. In studies similar to those of human HL60 and ML-1 differentiation described above, the WEHI-3B murine myeloid leukemia cell line showed decreased expression of both c-myb and c-myc during G-CSF-induced differentiation into monocytes, while c-fos expression increased markedly[95]. However, in this case, c-myb mRNA levels remained high until the later stages of differentiation. Increased c-myb expression has recently been observed in quiescent murine 3T3 cells following stimulation with growth factors[96], again suggesting that myb may have more than one function and may be involved in cell replication in general.

Drosophila c-myb is expressed in early embryos as a predominant 3.8 kb mRNA and a much less abundant 3.0 kb mRNA[66]. Preliminary work also indicates that myb-related transcripts are expressed at roughly equal levels at all major stages of Drosophila development.

C. Product of the c-myb gene and its possible function.

The product of the chicken c-myb gene is a 75,000 MW protein, p75[c-myb], identified by immunoprecipitation from hematopoietic tissues and cell lines with antisera directed against either BP-1 or BP-2 (see Figure 1)[26,32a]. The partial homology of p75[c-myb] to p48[myb] of AMV and to p135[gag-myb-ets] of E26 has been shown by tryptic peptide mapping[26,33]. Like p48[myb] and p135[gag-myb-ets], p75[c-myb] is a nuclear protein[26,32a]. A cytoplasmid, hematopoietic-specific 110,000 MW protein previously identified using anti-myb peptide antibodies[25,27,36] is not recognized by antisera directed against either BP-1 or BP-2 and does not appear to be a product of the c-myb gene.

Nuclear proteins of 75,000 and 79,000 MW have recently been identified in murine and human hematopoietic tissues and cell lines using affinity purified anti-BP-2 antibodies[32a]. Like the viral p48[myb] and p135[gag-myb-ets], a substantial fraction of the candidate human p79[c-myb] is present in the insoluble nuclear matrix. These murine and human proteins appear likely to represent authentic c-myb products because the protein domain against which these antibodies were raised is very highly conserved from Drosophila to man (see below).

Sequencing of a partial 2.8 kb murine c-myb cDNA clone has revealed an open reading frame of at least 1944 nucleotides which is predicted to encode a 71,000 MW protein of 636 amino acids[77]. The disposition of this coding region within the entire 4 kb mRNA is not yet known. The predicted protein has a high alpha-helical content, a basic region toward the N-terminus of the protein, and an overall globular configuration. The deduced amino acid sequence predicts an imperfect threefold tandem repeat of 52 residues near the N-terminus of the protein beginning at residue 38. The first copy of this repeated sequence, first identified in v-myb[AMV] [97], has been largely deleted during the generation of AMV and E26.

Comparison of the amino acid sequence predicted from this murine cDNA with that from the chicken genomic coding sequences corresponding to v-myb[AMV] reveals an 82% overall identity beginning with an initial match of 129 out of 130 residues[77] (see Figure 2). The BP-2 antigen used to raise anti-myb antibodies which recognize murine p75 and human p79, as well as chicken p75[c-myb], contains the first 115 of these 129 identical amino acids[32a]. This same region is also highly conserved in the predicted protein product of Drosophila c-myb[66], but a second region which is highly conserved between mouse and chicken c-myb products is not present within the identified Drosophila sequences (Figure 2).

Analysis of this murine c-myb cDNA clone has allowed the orientation of the chicken c-myb regions transduced by AMV and E26 relative to the normal c-myb coding sequences[77]. The murine c-myb domain which is homologous to v-myb[AMV] is preceded by at least 71 amino acids and followed by 200 amino acids (Figure 3). This would leave approximately 2 kb of presumptive untranslated mRNA.

The function of the c-myb gene product is currently unknown. Its nuclear location, short half-life, and apparent cell-cycle dependent expression suggest that it may play an important role in controlling normal cell division. The cell cycle dependence of c-myb expression in some tissues stands in contrast to the expression of c-myc which increases during G0 to G1 shifts[98], but appears constant in continuously cycling cells[99,100]. Although formerly believed to be specific to hematopoietic cells, c-myb expression now appears likely to play a more general role in dividing cells.

IV. ONCOGENIC ACTIVATION OF c-myb

A. Retroviral transduction.

AMV and E26 have independently transduced a nearly identiccal coding region of c-myb to form dominantly acting oncogenes which are rapidly leukemogenic[22,23,59]. The common feature of these transduction events is trun-

cation of the c-myb coding region at both ends with retention of a specific
internal domain. Because of the location of the 5' and 3' recombination
sites, both of these viral oncogenes produce fusion proteins with the structure x-myb-y. The AMV oncogene product p48myb has only six N-terminal
and 11 C-terminal non-myb virally-encoded residues, whereas the E26 oncogene
product p135gag-myb-ets contains large non-myb N- and C-terminal domains.
These differing v-myb oncogene product structures suggest that the deletion
of particular c-myb regions may be essential for c-myb activation.

In addition to c-myb truncation, the retroviral myb oncogenes both contain
point mutations within v-myb coding sequences[22,23,59]. Thus, p48myb is predicted to have eleven amino acid differences and p135gag-myb-ets is predicted
to have a single amino acid difference relative to the homologous region of
p75c-myb. However, the single mutant codon in v-myb[E26] is not altered in
v-myb[AMV], suggesting that these mutations may not be important for c-myb
activation. Nevertheless, it is possible that activating mutations exist
in AMV which are compensated for in E26 by the presence of ets sequences.

An additional difference between normal c-myb and its derived viral oncogenes is that the latter are driven by strong, retroviral transcriptional
promoters. Levels of c-myb in some normal cells which are in excess of those
of v-myb in AMV transformed cells[83] argue that high levels of myb-related
transcripts alone are not sufficient for transformation. The cell cycle
dependence of c-myb expression in some cell types[84] suggests that temporally
aberrant expression of viral myb genes may be important for transformation.
However, AMV does not appear to transform fibroblasts despite nuclear expression of p48myb driven by a retroviral LTR[37].

The relevance of these potential modes of c-myb activation can be addressed
experimentally by the construction of retroviruses expressing c-myb, either
in toto or with appropriate alterations. The recent cloning of c-myb cDNAs
should allow an early answer to these questions[77,101].

B. Mutagenesis by Retroviral Insertion.

The non-acutely transforming, non-defective retroviruses which do not
carry transduced oncogenes can also cause malignancies. In at least some
cases, they appear to do so by acting as insertional mutagens which alter the
transcription and/or structure of proto-oncogenes[102,103,107]. Presumably,
this mode of oncogenesis is the form fruste from which the acutely transforming viruses occasionally arise.

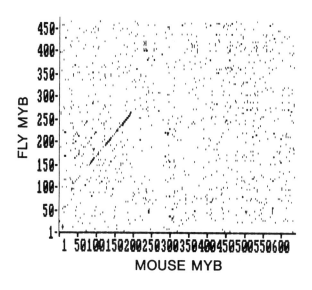

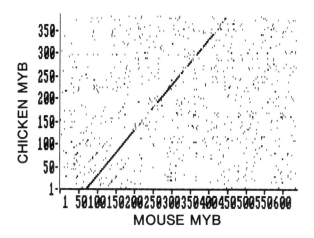

Figure 2. Evolutionary Conservation of c-myb Coding Domains. The protein sequence predicted from a presumed full-length murine c-myb cDNA[77] has been compared to that of: (left panel) the protein segment predicted from the partial sequence of Drosophila c-myb [66]; or (right panel) the protein segment predicted from the sequence of chicken c-myb regions which are homologous to v-myb[AMV] [22,23]. Protein sequences were compared two residues at a time. Dots indicate the positions of identical dipeptides.

A distinct subgroup of murine hematopoietic tumors induced by Abelson murine leukemia virus (A-MuLV) have been found to contain rearrangements within the c-myb locus and to express altered myb-containing mRNAs[104]. These tumors do not contain integrated A-MuLV proviruses, but the rearranged c-myb loci of at least four independently derived tumors contain internally deleted Moloney murine leukemia (M-MuLV) helper proviruses[105]. These proviruses are inserted within a 1.5 kb stretch of cellular DNA at the 5' end of the v-myb-related sequences. Recent studies have shown that the 5' viral LTR is used to generate an aberrant transcript which splices into a c-myb splice acceptor site homologous to that of v-myb[AMV] [106]. This would appear to result in a 5' truncation of the c-myb coding region similar to that of AMV and E26. Interestingly, these presumably myb-induced tumors are myeloid rather than lymphoid, as previously thought.

This mode of activation of c-myb by 5' retroviral integration, aberrant splicing and proto-oncogene truncation is very similar to the mechanism recently described for avian leukosis virus activation of c-erbB[107]. In the case of c-erbB activation, defective transforming viruses containing erbB arise at a high frequency[108], suggesting that murine myb viruses could similarly arise from tumors with M-MuLV perturbation of c-myb.

Additionaly murine hematopoietic tumors have recently been discovered in which retroviral insertion into the c-myb locus has occurred in the 3' region of the v-myb homologous sequences[106,109]. In at least one such tumor, the integration site is very near the location corresponding to the point in chicken c-myb at which the 3' recombination with E26 virus occurred[106].

Thus, alterations of c-myb by retroviral insertion appear to mimic the viral truncation of c-myb coding sequences in AMV and E26 (Figure 3). These studies suggest that either 5' or 3' truncation may be sufficient to convert c-myb into a transforming gene. However, it is unknown if the observed insertional mutagenesis of c-myb is itself sufficient for oncogenesis.

C. Gene amplification and chromosome translocation.

Amplification of the human c-myb gene has been observed in primary cultures and three cell lines derived from a single case of acute myelogenous leukemia (AML)[86]. Accompanying cytogenetic abnormalities were observed in the region 6q22-24 where c-myb is normally located. In addition, two cell lines independently drived from a single adenocarcinoma of the colon also exhibited c-myb amplification[89]. In this case, the amplified copies of c-myb are carried on an anomalous marker chromosome which is characteristic of both colon carcinoma cell lines. In both of these tumors, amplification of c-myb correlated with increased expression of apparently normal 4 kb c-myb mRNA. The role of these amplifications in the genesis of these two malignancies is unclear, but the presence of amplified c-myb in the primary AML cultures and the presence of an apparently identical myb-containing marker

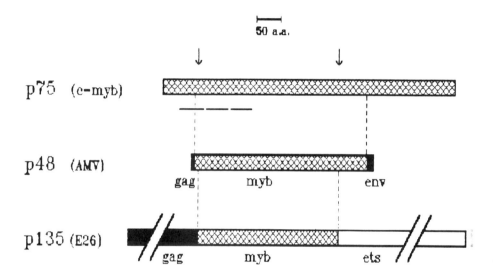

Figure 3. The Structures of myb-encoded Proteins. The predicted relationships of murine p75[c-myb], AMV p48[myb], and E26 p135[gag-myb-ets] are diagrammed [22,23,59,77]. Symbols: hatched boxes--myb-encoded domains; black boxes--domains encoded by segments of viral replicative genes; open box--ets-encoded domain. The horizontal black bars indicate the location of the predicted imperfect three-fold tandem repeat within p75[c-myb]. The broken vertical lines demarcate homologous myb-encoded domains. The vertical arrows indicate approximate points of disruption of murine c-myb coding sequences by MuLV insertions.

chromosome in two independently derived colon cell lines suggests that these phenomena are not artifacts of selection in tissue culture.

Furthermore, deletions of the distal half of chromosome 6 near the region where c-myb is located have been consistently observed in acute lymphocytic leukemia, ovarian carcinoma and melanoma[110]. However, a specific demonstration of myb translocation has not yet been reported in these tumors.

V. SUMMARY

The highly conserved, single copy c-myb gene has been independently transduced by two avian acute leukemia viruses, AMV and E26. This gene has also undergone insertional mutagenesis by non-acutely transforming murine leukemia viruses in a number of hematopoetic tumors. The common denominator of these retroviral activations of c-myb appears to be truncation of the normal coding region at either or both ends. The role of point mutations in myb-induced leukemogenesis is currently unknown.

The products of the c-myb gene and its altered viral counterparts are nuclear proteins, a large fraction of which are associated with the nuclear matrix. In addition, the myb gene products have short half-lives and bind DNA in vitro. These features suggest that myb may act by regulating DNA replication or transcription. Consistent with this notion, the expression of c-myb is cell cycle dependent in several cell types. However, the abundant expression of c-myb in the thymus is not similarly regulated and may serve a different function.

The expression of c-myb appears not to be limited to hematopoietic tissues as previously thought and the nature of the hematopoietic specificity of transformation by v-myb is not currently understood. Nevertheless, hematopoietic growth factors and their receptors appear to play an important role in such transformation.

Two new experimental systems for studying myb have recently been described. First, the discovery of a myb-related gene in Drosophila should allow the application of powerful classical and molecular genetic approaches. The functional similarity of this distantly related gene to the much more closely related avian and mammalian myb genes is unknown. Second, recent studies of murine myb in normal and abnormal hematopoiesis offers several advantages relative to the avian system, such as in-bred animal strains, a wealth of specific cell-surface markers, and cloned hematopoietic growth factor and receptor genes. Isolation or construction of an acutely transforming murine myb retrovirus may thus be very useful. Several obvious goals for future research will be to define the function of myb proteins within the nucleus, to understand the regulation of myb expression during the cell cycle, to establish which molecular alterations are essential for converting c-myb into a transforming gene, and the determine the role of myb in human malignancies.

VI. ACKNOWLEDGMENTS

We thank our many fellow mybologists for providing materials and discussions used in assembling this review. In particular, we thank Mike Bishop, David Boettiger, Mike Dvorak, Tom Gonda, James Ihle, Giovanella and Carlo Moscovici, Mike Nunn, Bernard Perbal, Grace Shen-Ong, Diana Sheiness, and Craig Thompson for sharing results with us prior to publication. Work in the authors' laboratory was supported by USPHS Research Grant CA-10197. J.S.L. is a Fellow of the Leukemia Society of America, Inc.

VII. REFERENCES

1. Weiss, R., Teich, N., Varmus, H. and Coffin, J., eds. (1982) RNA Tumor Viruses, Cold Spring Harbor Laboratory, Cold Spring Harbor, New York.

2. Beard, J. W. (1980) in Viral Oncology, Klein, G., ed., Raven Press, New York, pp. 55-87.

3. Baluda, M. A. and Goetz, I. E. (1961) Virol. 15, 185-197.

4. Moscovici, C., Gazzolo, L. and Moscovici, M. G. (1975) Virol. 68, 173-181.

5. Beug, H., von Kirchbach, A., Doderlein, G., Conscience, J.-F. and Graf, T. (1979) Cell 18, 375-390.

6. Durban, E. M. and Boettiger, D. (1981) J. Virol. 37, 488-492.

6a. Boettiger, D. and Durban, E. (1984) J. Virol. 49, 841-847.

6b. Soret, J., Kryceve-Martinerie, C., Crochet, J. and Perbal, B. (1985) J. Virol. 55, 193-205.

7. Gazzolo, L., Moscovici, C., Moscovici, M. G. and Samarut, J. (1979) Cell 16, 627-638.

8. Graf, T., von Krichbach, A. and Beug, H. (1981) Exper. Cell Res. 131, 331-343.

9. Moscovici, M. G. and Moscovici, C. (1983) Proc. Natl. Acad. Sci. USA 80, 1421-1425.

10. Pessano, S., Gazzolo, L. and Moscovici, C. (1979) Microbiologica 2, 379-392.

11. Symonds, G., Klempnauer, K.-H., Evan, G. I. and Bishop, J. M. (1984) Mol. Cell. Biol. 4, 2587-2593.

12. Roussel, M., Saule, S., Lagrou, C., Rommens, C., Beug, H., Graf, T. and Stehelin, D. (1979) Nature 281, 452-455.

13. Souza, L. M., Strommer, J. N., Hillyard, R. L., Komaromy, M. C. and Baluda, M. A. (1980) Proc. Natl. Acad. Sci. USA 77, 5177-5181.

94

14. Souza, L. M., Komaromy, M. C. and Baluda, M. A. (1980) Proc. Natl. Acad. Sci. USA 77, 3004-3008.
15. Souza, L. M. and Baluda, M. A. (1980) J. Virol. 36, 317-324.
16. Souza, L. M., Briskin, M. J., Hillyard, R. L. and Baluda, M. A. (1980) J. Virol. 36, 325-336.
17. Duesberg, P. H., Bister, K. and Moscovici, C. (1980) Proc. Natl. Acad. Sci. USA 77, 5120-5124.
18. Wang, L.-H., Duesberg, P. H., Kawai, S. and Hanafusa, H. (1975) Proc. Natl. Acad. Sci. USA 73, 447-451.
19. Chen, J. H., Hayward, W. S. and Moscovici, C. (1981) Virol. 110, 128-136.
20. Gonda, T. J., Sheiness, D. K., Fanshier, L., Bishop, J. M., Moscovici, C. and Moscovici, M. G. (1981) Cell 23, 279-290.
21. Hackett, P. B., Swanstrom, R., Varmus, H. E. and Bishop, J. M. (1982) J. Virol. 41, 527-534.
22. Klempnauer, K.-H., Gonda, T. J. and Bishop, J. M. (1982) Cell 31, 453-463.
23. Rushlow, K. E., Lautenberger, J. A., Papas, T. K., Baluda, M. A., Perbal, B., Chirikjian, J. G. and Reddy, E. P. (1982) Science 216, 1421-1423.
23a. Rushlow, K. E., Lautenberger, J. A., Reddy, E. P., Souza, L. M., Baluda, M. A., Chirikjian, J. G. and Papas, T. S. (1982) J. Virol. 42, 840-846.
24. Schwartz, D. E., Tizard, R. and Gilbert, W. (1983) Cell 32, 853-869.
25. Boyle, W. J., Lipsick, J. S., Reddy, E. P. and Baluda, M. A. (1983) Proc. Natl. Acad. Sci. USA 80, 2834-2838.
26. Klempnauer, K.-H., Ramsay, G., Bishop, J. M., Moscovici, M. G., Moscovici, C., McGrath, J. P. and Levinson, A. D. (1983) Cell 33, 345-355.
27. Lipsick, J. S., Boyle, W. J., Lampert, M. A. and Baluda, M. A. (1984) in Cancer Cells 2/Oncogenes and Viral Genes, Vande Woude et al., eds., Cold Spring Harbor Laboratory, Cold Spring Harbor, New York, pp. 143-151.
28. Klempnauer, K.-H. and Bishop, J. M. (1983) J. Virol. 48, 565-572.
28a. Dvorak, M., unpublished.
29. Silva, R. F. and Baluda, M. A. (1980) J. Virol. 35, 766-774.
30. Anderson, S. M. and Chen, J. H. (1981) J. Virol. 40, 107-117.
31. Wright, S. E., Harmon, S. A., Smith, D. P., Hayes, J. K., Robertson, P. A. and Wayne, A. W. (1984) Intervirol. 21, 17-24.

32. Ong, J. and Baluda, M. A., unpublished.

32a. Boyle, W. J., Lipsick, J. S. and Baluda, M. A., unpublished.

33. Klempnauer, K.-H. and Bishop, J. M. (1984) J. Virol. 50, 280-283.

34. Perbal, B., Lipsick, J., Svoboda, J., Silva, R. F. and Baluda, M. A. (1985) J. Virol. 56, in press.

35. Moscovici, M. G., Klempnauer, K.-H., Symonds, G., Bishop, J. M. and Moscovici, C., unpublished.

36. Boyle, W. J., Lampert, M. A., Lipsick, J. S. and Baluda, M. A. (1984) Proc. Natl. Acad. Sci. USA 81, 4265-4269.

37. Klempnauer, K.-H., Symonds, G., Evan, G. I. and Bishop, J. M. (1984) Cell 37, 537-547.

38. Moelling, K., Pfaff, E., Beug, H., Beimling, P., Bunte, T., Schaller, H. E. and Graf, T. (1985) Cell 40, 983-990.

38a. Boyle, W. J., unpublished.

39. Boyle, W. J., Lampert, M. A., Li, A. C. and Baluda, M. A. (1985) Mol. Cell. Biol., in press.

40. Shaper, J. H., Pardoll, D. M., Kauffman, S. H., Barrack, E. R., Vogelstein, B. and Coffey, D. S. (1979) Adv. Enz. Regul. 17, 213-248.

41. Eisenman, R. N., Tachibana, C. Y., Abrams, H. D. and Hann, S. R. (1985) Mol. Cell. Biol. 5, 114-126.

42. Feldman, L. T. and Nevins, J. R. (1983) Mol. Cell Biol. 3, 829-838.

43. Lampert, M. A., Boyle, W. J. and Baluda, M. A., unpublished.

44. Donner, P., Greiser-Wilke, I. and Moelling, K. (1982) Nature 296, 262-266.

45. Eisenman, R. N., Linial, M., Groudine, M., Shaikh, R., Brown, S. and Neiman, P. E. (1979) Cold Spring Harbor Symp. Quant. Biol. 44, 1235-1247.

46. Spindler, K. R. and Berk, A. J. (1984) J. Virol. 52, 706-710.

47. Ivanov, X., Mladenov, Z., Nedyalkov, S. and Todorov, T. G. (1962) Bulgarian Acad. Sci. Bull. Inst. Pathol. Comp. Anim. Domest. 9, 5-36.

48. Nedyalkov, S., Bozhkov, S. and Todorov, T. G. (1975) Acta. Vet. Brno. 44, 765-768.

49. Moscovici, C., Samarut, J., Gazzolo, L. and Moscovici, M. G. (1981) Virol. 113, 765-768.

50. Radke, K., Beug, H., Kornfeld, S. and Graf, T. (1982) Cell 31, 643-653.

51. Graf, T., Oker-Blom, N., Todorov, T. G. and Beug, H. (1979) Virol. 99, 431-436.

52. Moscovici, M. G., Jurdic, P., Samarut, J., Gazzolo, L., Mura, C. V. and Moscovici, C. (1983) Virol. 129, 65-78.

53. Leutz, A., Beug, H. and Graf, T. (1984) EMBO J. 3, 3191-3197.

54. Palmieri, S., Kahn, P. and Graf, T. (1984) Cell 39, 579-588.

55. Beug, H., Leutz, A., Kahn, P. and Graf, T. (1984) Cell 39, 579-588.

56. Bister, K., Nunn, M., Moscovici, C., Perbal, B., Baluda, M. A. and Duesberg, P. H. (1982) Proc. Natl. Acad. Sci. USA 79, 3677-3681.

57. LePrince, D., Gegonne, A., Coll, J., de Taisne, C., Schneeberger, A., Lagrou, C. and Stehelin (1983) Nature 306, 395-397.

58. Nunn, M. F., Seeburg, P. H., Moscovici, C. and Duesberg, P. H. (1983) Nature 306, 391-395.

59. Nunn, M., Wehier, H., Bullock, P. and Duesberg, P. (1984) Virol. 139, 330-339.

59a. Peterson, T. A., Yochem, J., Byers, B., Nunn, M. F., Duesberg, P. H., Doolittle, R. F. and Reed, S. F. (1984) Nature 309, 556-558.

59b. Nunn, M. F. and Hunter, T., unpublished.

60. Beug, H., Hayman, M. J. and Graf, T. (1982) EMBO J. 1, 1069-1073.

60a. Adkins, B., Leutz, A. and Graf, T. (1984) Cell 39, 439-445.

61. Scherr, C. J., Rettermier, C. W., Sacca., R., Roussel, M. F., Look, A. T. and Stanley, E. R. (1985) Cell 41, 665-676.

62. Cook, W. D., Metcalf, D., Nicola, N. A., Burgess, A. W. and Walker, F. (1985) Cell 41, 677-683.

63. Pierce, J. H., Di Fiore, P. P., Aaronson, S. A., Potter, M., Pumphrey, J., Scott, A. and Ihle, J. N. (1985) Cell 41, 685-693.

64. Lipsick, L., Brugge, J. S. and Boettiger, D. (1984) Mol. Cell. Biol. 4, 1420-1424.

65. Bergmann, D. G., Souza, L. M. and Baluda, M. A. (1981) J. Virol. 40, 450-455.

66. Katzen, A. L., Kornberg, T. B. and Bishop, J. M. (1985) Cell 41, 449-456.

67. Perbal, B. and Baluda, M. A. (1982) J. Virol. 41, 250-257.

68. Perbal, B. and Baluda, M. A. (1982) J. Virol. 44, 586-594.

69. Gonda, T. J. and Bishop, J. M. (1983) J. Virol. 46, 212-220.

70. LePrince, D., Saule, S., de Taisne, C., Gegonne, A., Begue, A., Righi, M. and Stehelin, D. (1983) EMBO J. 2, 1073-1078.

71. Perbal, B., Cline, J. M., Hillyard, R. L. and Baluda, M. A. (1983) J. Virol. 45, 925-940.

72. Franchini, G., Wong-Staal, F., Baluda, M. A., Lengel, C. and Tronick, S. R. (1983) Proc. Natl. Acad. Sci. USA 80, 7385-7389.

73. Dalla-Favera, R., Franchini, G., Matrinotti, S., Wong-Staal, F., Gallo, R. C. and Croce, C. M. (1982) Proc. Natl. Acad. Sci. USA 79, 4714-4717.

74. Harper, M., Franchini, G., Love, J., Simon, M. I., Gallo, R. C. and Wong-Staal, F. (1983) Nature 304, 169-171.

75. Zabel, B. U., Naylor, S. L., Grzeschik, K.-H. and Sakaguchi, A. Y. (1984) Somat. Cell. Molec. Genet. 10, 105-108.

76. Castle, S. and Sheiness, D., unpublished.

77. Gonda, T. J., Gough, N. M., Dunn, A. R. and ed Blaquiere, J. (1985) EMBO J., in press.

78. Sakaguchi, A. Y., Lalley, P. A., Zabel, B. U., Ellis, R. W., Scolnick, E. M. and Naylor, S. L. (1984) Proc. Natl. Acad. Sci. USA 81, 525-529.

79. Chen, J. H. (1980) J. Virol. 36, 162-170.

80. Gonda, T. J., Sheiness, D. K. and Bishop, J. M. (1982) Mol. Cell. Biol. 2, 617-624.

81. Coll, J., Saule, S., Martin, P., Raes, M. B., Lagrou, C., Graf, T., Beug, H., Simon, I. E. and Stehelin, D. (1983) Exper. Cell Res. 149, 151-162.

82. Duprey, S. P. and Boettiger, D. (1985) Proc. Natl. Acad. Sci. USA, in press.

83. Thompson, C. B., Challoner, P. B., Neiman, P. E. and Groudine, M., unpublished.

84. Westin, E. H., Gallo, R. C., Arya, S. K., Eva, A., Souza, L. M., Baluda, M. A., Aaronson, S. A. and Wong-Staal, F. (1982) Proc. Natl. Acad. Sci. USA 79, 2194-2198.

85. Pellici, P.-G., Lanfrancone, L., Brathwaite, M. D., Wolman, S. and Dalla-Favera, R. (1984) Science 224, 1117-1121.

86. Slamon, D. J., deKernion, J. B., Verma, I. M. and Cline, M. J. (1984) Science 224, 256-262.

87. Craig, R. W. and Bloch, A. (1984) Cancer Res. 44, 442-446.

88. Alitalo, K., Winqvist, R., Lin, C. C., de la Chapelle, A., Schwab, M. and Bishop, J. M. (1984) Proc. Natl. Acad. Sci. USA 81, 4534-4538.

89. Griffin, C. A. and Baylin, S. B. (1985) Cancer Res. 45, 272-275.

90. Little, C. D., Nau, M. M., Carney, D. A., Gazdar, A. F. and Minna, J. D. (1983) Nature 306, 194-196.

91. Busch, M. P., Devi, B. G., Soe, L. H., Perbal, B., Baluda, M. A. and Roy-Burman, P. (1983) Hematol. Oncol. 1, 61-75.

92. Sheiness, D. and Gardiner, M. (1984) Mol. Cell. Biol. 4, 1206-1212.

93. Mountz, J. D., Steinberg, A. D., Klinman, D. M., Smith, H. R. and Mushinski, J. F. (1984) Science 226, 1087-1089.

94. Gonda, T. J. and Metcalf, D. (1984) Nature 310, 249-251.

95. Greenberg, M. E. and Ziff, E. B. (1984) Nature 311, 433-438.

96. Ralston, R. and Bishop, J. M. (1983) Nature 306, 803-806.

97. Kelly, K., Cochran, B. H., Stiles, C. D. and Leder, P. (1983) Cell 35, 603-610.

98. Thompson, C. B., Challoner, P. B., Neiman, P. E. and Groudine, M. (1985) Nature 314, 363-366.

99. Hann, S. R., Thompson, C. B. and Eisenman, R. N. (1985) Nature 314, 366-369.

100. Gerondakis, S. and Bishop, J. M., personal communication.

101. Hayward, W. S., Neel, B. G. and Astrin, S. M. (1981) Nature 209, 475-479.

102. Payne, G. S., Bishop, J. M. and Varmus, H. E. (1982) Nature 295, 209-217.

103. Mushinski, J. F., Potter, M., Bauer, S. R. and Reddy, E. P. (1983) Science 220, 795-798.

104. Shen-Ong, G. L. C., Potter, M., Mushinski, J. F., Lavu, S. and Reddy, E. P. (1984) Science 226, 1077-1080.

105. Shen-Ong, G. L. C., unpublished.

106. Nilsen, T. W., Maroney, P. A., Goodwin, R. G., Rottman, F. M., Crittenden, L. B., Raines, M. A. and Kung, H.-J. (1985) Cell 41, 719-726.

107. Miles, B. D. and Robinson, H. L. (1985) J. Virol. 54, 295-303.

108. Ihle, J. N. and Weinstein, Y., unpublished.

109. Mitelman, F. and Levan, G. (1981) Hereditas 95, 79-139.

6

Structure and Mechanism of Activation of the <u>myb</u> Oncogene

Dan Rosson and E. Premkumar Reddy

Department of Molecular Oncology
Roche Institute of Molecular Biology
Nutley, NJ   07110

I. INTRODUCTION

The myb oncogene was first identified as the transforming gene of Avian myeloblastosis virus (AMV) which causes myeloblastic leukemia in chickens and transforms myelomonocytic hematopoietic cells in culture[1,2]. Like other acute transforming viruses, AMV is replication defective having arisen by recombination between its non-defective helper virus and host cellular sequences. The latter sequences which constitute the myb oncogene are responsible for the oncogenic potential of this virus. However, unlike most other acute transforming viruses, AMV does not induce morphological transformation of cultured fibroblasts suggesting that only a restricted cell population is the target of its transforming gene product[1,2]. A more recently isolated avian virus, E26, also contains the myb oncogene in addition to a second oncogene ets. E26 virus causes erythroblastosis and a low level of concomitant myeloblastosis in chickens[3,4,5].

The normal cellular counterpart of this oncogene (c-myb) is highly conserved and is present in all vertebrates as well as some invertebrate species examined[6,7]. The function of the myb gene product has not been identified but appears to be restricted to a set of immature hematopoietic cells of the myeloid and T lymphoid series[8,9,10]. Levels of myb expression appear to be high in thymic lymphocytes from young mice with active thymuses. Activity decreases in thymuses of older mice whose thymuses have undergone involution. Similarly, studies on a collection of fresh and cultured human cells revealed that the expression of the myb gene is limited only to immature myeloid and T lymphoid cells and not to mature cells of the same lineage[9]. Thus the function of the normal myb gene appears to be associated with the maturation process of hematopoietic cells of this lineage. This is corroborated further by the restricted ability of AMV to transform a limited set of lymphoid cells in vitro and in vivo[1,2].

Proteins encoded by the myb gene of both AMV and E26 are located in the nucleus of the transformed cells[11]. Similarly, the c-myb encoded protein also appears to be localized in the nucleus of normal myeloid cells[12]. Studies with purified v-myb proteins also indicated that these proteins have an associated DNA-binding activity[13]. Furthermore, v-myb proteins encoded by temperature-sensitive mutant of E26 lost their DNA-binding capability when shifted to non-permissive temperatures suggesting that this activity is essential for the transforming function of the virus. These results, taken together, suggest a role for the myb gene in the control and/or differentiation of hematopoietic cells of the myeloid and T lymphoid series.

II. RESULTS AND DISCUSSION

A. Structural organization of Avian Myeloblastosis virus and a comparison of v-myb and c-myb encoded messenger RNAs.

The stucture of the AMV provirus is shown in Figure 1[14]. The complete nucleotide sequence of the transforming gene of this virus has been determined[15,16]. Recently, we have cloned the reverse transcript of the subgenomic messenger RNA encoded by this virus genome and determined the nucleotide sequence of this cDNA clone. The results of these studies indicate that AMV transforming gene is synthesized via a spliced messenger RNA in which the leader sequence, derived from the 5' terminus of the genomic RNA, is spliced to the body of the v-myb encoded sequences. Protein synthesized by this spliced mRNA would contain six amino acids derived from the gag gene of the helper virus and 371 amino acids derived from the v-myb sequences. The open reading frame of the v-myb region extends into the viral sequences at the 3' end, terminating in the envelope portion of the viral gene. Thus, the last 11 amino acids at the carboxy terminal end of the transforming protein are derived from the 3' end of the viral envelope gene. The structure of this subgenomic mRNA is schematically shown in Figure 1.

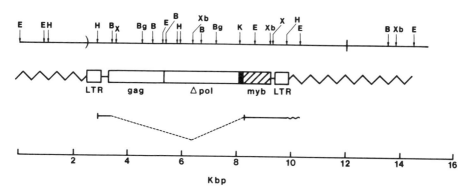

Figure 1. Summary of the major structural features of AMV proviral genome described by Souza et al.[14]. Restriction map of the entire DNA clone is shown at the top. B, BamHI; E, EcoR1; H, HindIII; K, KpnI; X, XhoI; Xb, XbaI. Flanking host cellular sequences are represented by wavy lines, and the large terminal repeats (LTRs) are indicated as rectangles. The portion of the cell-derived transforming gene (v-myb) is indicated by the hatched box. The botton portion shows the structure of the spliced subgenomic mRNA that codes for the transforming protein.

102

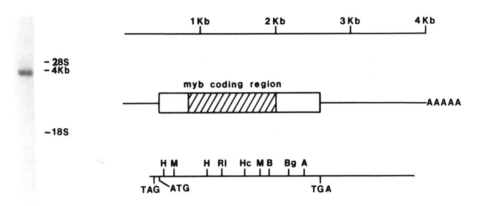

Figure 2. Molecular cloning of c-myb cDNA. Poly(A)-RNA was isolated from chicken thymus and analyzed by hybridization to ^{32}P-labeled v-myb probe which revealed the presence of a 4.0 Kbp message (left). The cDNA library was constructed from this RNA using the λ gt10 vector system. The restriction map of one of the cDNA clones which was 3.6 Kbp long and contained the entire coding sequence is shown. Restriction sites shown are: A, AhaIII; B, BalI; Bg, BglII; H, HaeII; Hc, HincII, M, MstII; RI, EcoRI.

To compare the structure of v-myb encoded sequences with the c-myb gene product, we undertook to cDNA cloning of its mRNA. The c-myb genome is functionally active in several lymphoid organs including the thymus coding for an mRNA species which is 4.0 kb long (Fig. 2). A c-myb cDNA clone was obtained using this RNA whose restriction map in shown in Figure 2. Figure 3 shows the nucleotide sequence of the coding region of this cDNA clone. The longest open reading frame in this sequence extends from nucleotide

Figure 3. Nucleotide sequence of the coding region of the c-myb cDNA clone. The amino acid sequence predicted for the proto-oncogene product is shown below the nucleotide sequence. Pertinent restriction enzyme sites as well as the v-myb homologous sequences are shown. The two terminator codons in frame with the reading frame are indicated by ***. Small arrows pointing upwards denote the nucleotide differences between c-myb and v-myb (AMV) that have resulted in amino acid change.

```
TTCGGCGGGC CGTAGCGGGC CATCTGCACG CGGAGCTCCG GGCATCCAG CACGGCCCCG TCC
***                                          50         100
```

LEFT BLOCK:

```
ATG GCG TCC ATC GCG TCC CGT TTG TCG GCG AAA CGG TCG AGG ACG AAT GCG
MET Ala Ser Ile Ala Ser Arg Leu Ser Ala Lys Arg Ser Arg Thr Asn Ala
                                                  Hae II         150

AAC CCG CGG CTC CTC GGC ACT TCG CGC GGC GGA CGC CCT GGA CCC CCA AGC
Asn Pro Arg Leu Leu Gly Thr Ser Arg Gly Gly Arg Pro Gly Pro Pro Ser
                                      200

CCG GCA GGG GGC ATG GGC GGC GGG CGC CTC CCC CGT CCT CTT CCC CCA GCG
Pro Ala Ala Ala Arg MET Ala Arg Gly Leu Pro Arg Pro Leu Pro Pro Ala
                  250

GCC GCC AGG ACG CCC AGA CCC AGA TAC AGC AGC AGC GAT GAC
Ala Ala Arg Thr Pro Arg Pro Arg Tyr Ser Ser Ser Asp Asp
                        300

GAT GAA GAT GTT GAG GTG ATG GAC CAC TAC GAT GGC CTG CTT CCT AAG
Asp Glu Asp Val Glu Val MET Asp His Tyr Asp Gly Leu Leu Pro Lys
              350

GCT GGG GCA CGT CAC CTA GGG GAA CGT GAA GAG GAG AAA
Ala Gly Ala Arg His Leu Gly Glu Arg Glu Glu Glu Lys
      400

CTG AAG AAA GTG GTG GAA CAG GTC ATT GGC ATT GCC AGT
Leu Lys Lys Val Val Glu Gln Val Ile Gly Ile Ala Ser
                              start AMV homology

TTC TTC CCT AAT CGG ACA GAT GTT CAG CAC CGG TGG CAG
Phe Phe Pro Asn Arg Thr Asp Val Gln His Arg Trp Gln
      500                      start E26 homology

AAC CCA GAA CTT ATC AAA GGT CCA GAA GAG GAT GAA ATA
Asn Pro Glu Leu Ile Lys Gly Pro Glu Glu Asp Glu Ile
Asn Pro Glu Leu Ile Lys Gly Pro Glu Glu Asp Glu Ile    (500)

GAA CTC GTG CAG AAA TAC GGT GTC CCA AAG GCT AAG CAT TTG
Glu Leu Val Gln Lys Tyr Gly Val Pro Lys Ala Lys His Leu
Glu Leu Val Gln Lys Tyr Gly Val Pro Lys Ala Lys His Leu   Hae II

AAG GGA ATT GGA TGC AGG AGG AGA GAA GAG ATT GCA CAT CAT
Lys Gly Ile Gly Cys Arg Arg Arg Glu Glu Ile Ala His His
                              650              Eco RI

GAA GTG GTG CTG AGC AGC AAC TGG TGG ATT GCA GAT ATT GCA
Glu Val Val Leu Ser Ser Asn Trp Trp Ile Ala Asp Ile Ala
                                          700

CAC CCA GGA ATC CTG GGA AAC ACC AGA TAC CTG CTG GAG ATT
His Pro Gly Ile Leu Gly Asn Thr Arg Tyr Leu Leu Glu Ile
                                          750

ACT GAT GCT TAC GTC CTG AAA TAC GGT TGG AAT CAC CGC TGG
Thr Asp Ala Tyr Val Leu Lys Tyr Gly Trp Asn His Arg Trp
                                      800      Hae II

AAG GAG ATT GGA ATT GGA TGC AGC AAG ATC AAG AAT ATG
Lys Glu Ile Gly Ile Gly Cys Ser Lys Ile Lys Asn MET
                              850

GAA GTG GTG AAA ACC TCC TGG TGG TCC AAA GCC TTT GGC GTC
Glu Val Val Lys Thr Ser Trp Trp Ser Lys Ala Phe Gly Val
                          900

CAC CCA GGC TTC CAG TAC AGC AGC AGC AGT GGC TTC TTA CAC
His Pro Gly Phe Gln Tyr Ser Ser Ser Ser Gly Phe Leu His
              950

GAA GTG TTC CAG AAG AGC ATG GGC AGT GGC GGC CCG CAG CAA
Glu Val Phe Gln Lys Ser MET Gly Ser Gly Gly Pro Gln Gln
                      1000

GGC TTC CAG AAG AGC ATC GGT GTA CCG CAG CTG ATT GCT GCT
Gly Phe Gln Lys Ser Ile Gly Val Pro Gln Leu Ile Ala Ala
              1050

ATT GCT AAT ATT GTC GAT GTT CCT CCA GCT GCT ATA CGA TTA GAG
Ile Ala Asn Ile Val Asp Val Pro Pro Ala Ala Ile Arg Leu Glu

GTA AAT ATT ATT GAC GAA CCT GAA AAA GAA GAC CGA AAG ATT AAG
Val Asn Ile Ile Asp Glu Pro Glu Lys Glu Asp Arg Lys Ile Lys
1140

AAT GAT GAA GAC CCA GAA AAT AAG GAA ATA CAC
Asn Asp Glu Asp Pro Glu Asn Lys Glu Ile His
```

RIGHT BLOCK:

```
             Sal I
ATG TCG ACT GAG AAT CTG AAA GGG CAG GCA TTA CCA ACA CAG AAC CAC
MET Ser Thr Glu Asn Leu Lys Gly Gln Ala Leu Pro Thr Gln Asn His
1200                                              1250

ACA GCA AAC TAC CCC GGC TGG CAC AGC ACC GTT GCT GAC AAT ACC AGG ACC
Thr Ala Asn Tyr Pro Gly Trp His Ser Thr Val Ala Asp Asn Thr Arg Thr

AGT GGT GAC AAT GCA CCT GTT TCC TGT GTT GGG GAG CAT CAC CAC TGT CCA
Ser Gly Asp Asn Ala Pro Val Ser Cys Val Gly Glu His His His Cys Pro
                                          end E26 homology        1300

TCT CCA CCA GTG GAT CAT GGT TGC TTA CCT GAG GAA AGT GCG TCC GCA CGG
Ser Pro Pro Val Asp His Gly Cys Leu Pro Glu Glu Ser Ala Ser Pro Ala Arg
                                                          1350

TGC ATG GTT ATT CAC CAG AAC ATC CTG GAT AAT GTT AAG AAT CTC AAT GAA
Cys MET Val Ile His Gln Asn Ile Leu Asp Asn Val Lys Asn Leu Asn Glu
                                            1400

TTT GCA GAA ACA CTC CAG TTA TTA AAC TCG TTC TCC AAT AAT
Phe Ala Glu Thr Leu Gln Leu Leu Asn Ser Phe Ser Asn Asn
                      1450

GAG AAT CTG GAC AAC CCT GCA CTA ACC TCC ACC CCA GTG TGT GGC CAC
Glu Asn Leu Asp Asn Pro Ala Leu Thr Ser Thr Pro Val Cys Gly His
                      1500

AAG ATG TCT GTT GAC GTT TTC ACT TTC AAA ACT CAG AAG
Lys MET Ser Val Asp Val Phe Thr Phe Lys Thr Gln Lys
                          end AMV homology

GAA AAC CAC GTT AGA ACT CCT AAG AGG ATC ATA TTA TTA GAG AGC TCT
Glu Asn His Val Arg Thr Pro Lys Arg Ile Ile Leu Leu Glu Ser Ser
              1650

CCA CGA ACA ACA CCT CCA TTC AAA AAC GCA CTT AAA CTT GCA CTT GAA ATC AAA TAT
Pro Arg Thr Thr Pro Pro Phe Lys Asn Ala Leu Lys Leu Ala Leu Glu Ile Lys Tyr
      1700                                                    Bgl II

GGT CCT TTG ATG ATG ATG CTG CCT CAA GGA ACT CAT CAT GTA GAT CTG CAG
Gly Pro Leu MET MET MET Leu Pro Gln Gly Thr His His Val Asp Leu Gln
                  1750

GAC GTT ATC AAG CAG GAG TCG CTG GAA TCT AAA GCA GTG GTG GCA GGG GAA CTA CAT GAA
Asp Val Ile Lys Gln Glu Ser Leu Glu Ser Lys Ala Val Val Ala Gly Glu Leu His Glu
      1800

AGT GGA ATC CCC CTT TTG AAA AAA ATC ATT TGC TCA AAA GTG GTG GGG GAA AAC CTG AAC ACT
Ser Gly Ile Pro Leu Leu Lys Lys Ile Ile Cys Ser Lys Val Val Gly Glu Asn Leu Asn Thr
1850

AAA GCT GGA AAT TTT TTA TTA TGC TCA AAT TTT ACA CAT CTT CAC AGC AGC
Lys Ala Gly Asn Phe Phe Leu Cys Ser Asn Phe Thr His Leu His Ser Ser
                                                          1950

CAG CTC ATT ACA CAT GCC ATG AAG AGA AAT GAA GAT GTG CCA AAT CTT CTT ACC AGC
Gln Leu Ile Thr His Ala MET Lys Arg Asn Glu Asp Val Pro Asn Leu Leu Thr Ser
                                              2000

TCC ATT TTA TTA GCC CCG GGC TCG GAA GTG GCT CCA GGG AGT GGT CTG CTG AAC AAT GCT
Ser Ile Leu Leu Ala Pro Gly Ser Glu Val Ala Pro Gly Ser Gly Leu Leu Asn Asn Ala
                                          2100

GGC TTC CAG AAG AGC CAC CAC AGG CTG TGC CGG CCA CAT CTG CAG CAT CTG CTG AAC AAT GCT
Gly Phe Gln Lys Ser His His Arg Leu Cys Arg Pro His Leu Gln His Leu Leu Asn Asn Ala
                                      2100

TGG GGG TCG AAG TGC TCT GTG CCA GCT AAC ACC CTG TAC ATG CAG CAG ATG CTG ACT GAC CAG
Trp Gly Ser Lys Cys Ser Val Pro Ala Ser Pro Lys Thr MET Gln Gln MET Leu Thr Asp Gln
                                                          2150

GCA GGA CGC GCC AAG TAC GCC GGC TTC CCA GCG GGC TTC TTC TAC ACT TTG ATG TGAAAGGGGCC
Ala Gly Arg Ala Lys Tyr Ala Gly Phe Pro Ala Gly Phe Phe Tyr Thr Leu MET ***
Ala Arg Lys Tyr Ala Gly Phe Pro Ala Ala Phe Ala Leu Thr Asp Gln
                  2200

GATGGACTTC TCCGGAGAAG CATTATGGTT GGCAAACACT TCTCGTTC
```

position 13 to 2160 and contains an initiator codon, ATG, at position 63-65 and a terminator codon at position 2161-2163. Such an open reading frame could code for a polypeptide of 699 amino acids with an estimated molecular mass of 77 kd. This is in agreement with the estimated size of 75 kd for the c-myb encoded protein (16). This open reading frame is preceded by approximately 500 bp of non-coding sequences at the 5' end and followed by a stretch of 1400 bp of non-coding sequences at the 3' end.

Analysis of the predicted c-myb amino acid sequence by a dot-matrix program reveals a structure of three tandem repeats that extend for amino acid positions 96 to 147, 148 to 199 and 200 to 250. The first two repeats are more homologous to each other than to the third repeat. The role of these repeats is unknown. However, since this protein is localized in the nucleus and known to bind DNA[12,13], it is possible that these repeats are involved in one of these two properties. A comparison of these sequences with those of mouse c-myb[20] and Drosophila c-myb[7] encoded proteins shows this region is the best conserved region between the three species. Thus, it is probable that this region codes for a critical function of normal cellular myb protein.

A comparison of the cDNA sequence with that of the v-myb sequences of AMV and E26 reveals that the two genes are homologous from nucleotide position 450 to 1560 in AMV and position 478 to 1341 in E26. These comparisons suggest features that may be required for retroviral activation of this proto-oncogene. In both cases similar stretches of amino and carboxy terminal sequences have been deleted. Thus, the normal c-myb protein contains an additional stretch of 142 and 150 amino acids at the amino terminal end and 192 and 272 amino acids at the carboxy terminal end compared to AMV and E26 encoded proteins, respectively. The observation that the myb gene has undergone deletions in both the amino and carboxy terminal ends in similar locations in the two viruses suggests that such alterations are essential for the activation of the gene's oncogenic potential. Additional support is provided for the hypothesis by two murine model systems.

B. Activation of myb gene in murine ABPL tumors.

A second model system, which allows us to examine the activation of the myb locus more carefully, is the ABPL tumor system where rearrangements in this locus have been observed[10,17,18]. These tumors arose in BALB/c mice following the injection of pristane and Abelson murine leukemia virus along with its helper, Moloney murine leukemia virus[19]. In the presence of pristane, which induces intraperitonial granulomatous tissue, the virus rapidly induces a variety of lymphoid neoplasms, predominantly of the pre-B cell series, which have been termed as ABLS tumors. Two other classes of tumors that are induced at a much lower frequency by this virus are plasmacytomas (ABPC tumors) and a morphological subset of tumors that appear to be myeloid and have been termed as ABPL tumors. Later studies indicated that these ABPLs do not produce the Abelson virus nor do they contain the integrated proviral genome[8]. Instead, all the ABPL tumors examined were found to have undergone rearrangements in the myb locus resulting in the synthesis of abnormal messenger RNA transcripts[8]. Molecular cloning and structural comparison of the normal and rearranged c-myb DNA sequences revealed that the rearrangements in all ABPL tumors were due to the integration of Mo-MuLV genome into a 1.5 Kpb stretch of cellular DNA immediately upstream to the v-myb related sequences[17,18]. A detailed characterization of the mouse c-myb coding exons revealed that this integration occurs in intron sequences that lie between the third and fourth coding exons[20]. This has been shown to result in the initiation of transcription immediately downstream to the viral integration site which results in the synthesis of mRNAs that lack the 5' coding sequences. This results in an analogous deletion of amino terminal amino acids in the myb gene product of ABPL tumors as is produced in the two viral myb genes. The fate of the DNA sequences toward the 3' end of the myb gene is not known but preliminary analysis of the aberrant myb RNAs from one of the ABPL tumors suggests the possibility of alterations at this end also. These results lend additional strength to the hypothesis that amino and/or carboxy terminal deletions in the myb locus are essential for the oncogenic activation of this gene.

A third example of myb activation is seen in some of the myeloid leukemias induced by Cas-Br Mo-MuLV in NSF mice. The nature of the myb rearrangements in one of these cell lines (NSF-60) has been studied in detail by molecular cloning and nucleotide sequence analysis[21]. These results demonstrate that, as in the case of ABPL tumors, the rearrangements are due to the integration of the proviral genome in the c-myb locus of this cell line. However, unlike the case of ABPL tumors, the integration occurs toward the 3' end of the myb locus resulting in the premature termination of the rearranged myb gene transcription. This results in the synthesis of a truncated mRNA which lacks the entire 3' half of the normal coding sequences. The myb coding sequences in this aberrant mRNA terminate at a point corresponding to nucleotide 1425 in the c-myb sequences presented in Figure 2. As can

106

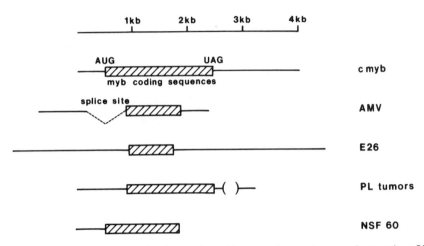

Figure 4. Comparison of the myb-coding region of normal c-myb mRNA (chicken) with activated forms of myb mRNAs in the AMV and E26 viruses and ABPL and NSF60 tumor cells. The boxes represent myb coding sequences. The parentheses in PL tumor RNA indicate rearrangements toward the 3' end which have not yet been precisely defined.

be seen this point lies close to the site of deletion observed in AMV and E26 viruses. This would result in the synthesis of a myb protein that would contain a carboxy terminal deletion similar to that synthesized in AMV or E26 virus-transformed cells. This is schematically shown in Figure 4.

III. SUMMARY AND CONCLUSIONS

The results summarized in this review show that the normal chicken myb gene codes for a protein of 77 kd which appears to play an important role in the control and/or differentiation of hematopoietic cells of myeloid and T lymphoid series. The activation of this gene has been observed in chicken and murine systems. In the avian system, this has been achieved by trans-duction of the myb oncogene into a retrovirus. Such a tranduction resulted in the deletion of coding sequences from both the 5' and 3' ends of the gene. Initiation and terminator codons in helper viral sequences have been substi-tuted for the analogous sequences in the proto-oncogene. Deletion of simi-lar stretches of sequence in both the viruses suggested the possibility that these deletions may play an important role in the activation of this gene.

The availability of the murine model system allowed us to examine this question further. In the ABPL tumor system, the activation of the myb locus occurred as a result of viral integration in a region immediately upstream to the v-myb related sequences. In NSF-60 cell line, the activation is due to the viral integration toward the 3' end of the gene. In both cases the viral integration results in the synthesis of aberrant mRNAs that have suffered deletions similar to those observed in the avian system. In all instances this results in the synthesis of truncated proteins which appear to mediate the transforming function. The availability of chicken and mouse c-myb cDNA clones makes it possible to test this hypothesis directly by construction of retroviruses containing various deletion mutations.

IV. REFERENCES

1. Baluda, M. A. and Goetz, I. E. (1961) J. Virol. 15, 185-199.
2. Moscovici, C. (1975) Curr. Top. Microbiol. Immunol. 71, 79-96.
3. Moscovici, C., Samarut, J., Gazzolo, L. and Moscovici, M. G. (1981) Virology 118, 765-768.
4. Graf, T., Olser-Blom, N., Todorov, T. G. and Beug, H. (1979) Virology 99, 643-653.
5. Nunn, M. F., Seebert, B. H., Moscovici, C., Duesberg, P. H. (1983) Nature (London) 306, 391-395.
6. Franchini, G., Wong-Staal, F., Baluda, M. A., Lengel, C. and Tronick, S. A. (1983) Proc. Natl. Acad. Sci. USA 80, 7385-7389.
7. Katzen, A. L., Kornberg, T. B. and Bishop, J. M. (1985) Cell 41, 449-456.
8. Westin, E. H., Gallo, R. C., Arya, S. K., Eva, A., Souza, L. M., Baluda, M. A., Aaronson, S. A., Wong-Staal, F. (1982) Proc. Natl. Acad. Sci. USA 79, 2194-2198.
9. Sheiness, D. and Gardinier, M. (1984) Mol. Cell. Biol. 4, 1206-1212.
10. Mushinski, J. F., Potter, M., Bauer, S. R. and Reddy, E. P. (1983) Science 220, 795-798.
11. Klempnauer, K. H., Symonds, G., Evans, G. I. and Bishop, J. M. (1984) Cell 37, 537-547.
12. Boyle, W. J., Lampert, M. A., Lipsick, J. S. and Baluda, M. A. (1984) Proc. Natl. Acad. Sci. USA 81, 4265-4269.
13. Moelling, K., Pfaff, E., Beug, H., Beimling, P., Bunte, T., Schaller, H. and Graf, T. (1985) Cell 40, 983-990.
14. Souza, L. M., Briskin, R., Hillyard, R. and Baluda, M. (1980) J. Virol. 36, 325-330.

15. Rushlow, E. K., Lautenberger, J. A., Papas, T. S., Baluda, M. A., Perbal, B., Chirikjian, J. G. and Reddy, E. P. (1982) Science 216, 1421-1423.

16. Klempnauer, K. H., Ramsey, G., Bishop, J., Moscovici, M., Moscovici, C., McGrath, J. and Levinson, A. (1983) Cell 33, 345-355.

17. Shen-Ong, G., Potter, M., Mushinski, J., Lavu, S. and Reddy, E. P. (1984) Science 226, 1077-1080.

18. Lavu, S., Mushinski, J. F., Shen-Ong, G. L. C., Potter, M. and Reddy, E. P. (1985). Growth Factors and Transformation, p. 301-306. Cold Spring Harbor Laboratory, Cold Spring Harbor, NY.

19. Potter, M., Reddy, E. P. and Wivel, N. A. (1978) Natl. Cancer Inst. Monogr. 48, 311.

20. Lavu, S. and Reddy, E. P. (1985) EMBO Journal (communicated).

21. Weinstein, Y., Ihle, J. N., Lavu, S. and Reddy, E. P. (1985) Proc. Natl. Acad. Sci. USA (communicated)

7

Viral myc Genes and their Cellular Homologs

Takis S. Papas, James A. Lautenberger, Nancy C. Kan,
Dennis K. Watson, Rebecca Van Beneden, Miltos Psallidopoulos,
Robert J. Fisher, Shigeyoshi Fujiwara, Kenneth Samuel,
Christos Flordellis, Ren-Ping Zhou, Peter Duesberg,
Arun Seth[+] and Richard Ascione

Laboratory of Molecular Oncology, National Cancer
Institute, Frederick, Maryland 21701

[*]Department of Molecular Biology, University of California,
Berkeley, California 94740

[+]LBI-Basic Research Program, NCI-Frederick Cancer Research
Facility, Frederick, Maryland 21701

Research supported in part by contract no. NO1-CO-23909
with Litton Bionetics, Inc.

I. INTRODUCTION

Our laboratory has been heavily committed toward studies identifying and understanding the acute avian leukemia virus transforming genes, responsible for the malignant transformation of normal cells in vitro, and neoplastic disease in the animal. These retroviral transforming genes have been termed viral onc-genes (v-onc), and DNA sequences homologous to them have been iden- tified in a wide-variety of normal eukaryotic non-transformed cells ranging from yeast to man[1]. We have also felt it mandatory to include within the scope of our research investigations on viral transforming genes, stu- dies on their normal cellular counterparts, the cellular onc-genes (c-onc). The molecular characterization and precise structure of these genes, particu- larly of the acute transforming viruses and their cellular homologs, have been greatly facilitated by the methods of recombinant genetic cloning and gene transfection techniques; these techniques have been very valuable and served as powerful probes in unraveling the intracacies involved in the manifestation of malignancy at the cellular level[2]. More importantly, evidence has accumulated in laboratories like ours[3] and our colleagues[4] which stressed the value of retroviral oncogene research and the utility of employing acute transforming retroviruses as model systems, for studying the induction of malignancy in a variety of vertebrate systems. In particular it is now widely accepted that this category of retroviruses, capable of efficiently inducing tumors rapidly and in large numbers, arose by incorpo- rating a portion of the host cellular genome by transduction[5] and that these captured cellular onc-gene sequences are quite limited in number and highly conserved amongst eukaryotic and especially vertebrate genomes[6]. This high degree of onc gene conservation implies an essentiality of func- tion which may be critical to the cell's growth and regulation and thus may be common to many eukaryotic cell types. In spite of the general acceptance of the host origin of retroviral genes and that the action of the altered cellular oncogenes may in fact experimentally cause certain kinds of neo- plastic disease in animals; the precise oncogenetic events leading to these malignant changes is not at all clearly understood.

Our laboratory having been the first to clone and determine the nucleotide sequence of the MC29 avian acute transforming viruses gene, now known as v- myc, has attempted to compare and characterize this transforming gene a variety of other such genetic relatives obtained from the MC29 family of viruses. We have, in addition, attempted to molecularly compare these transforming genes to their normal cellular onc-gene counterparts, the c-myc genes; examining their expressed transcripts as well, using a variety of animal cells and tissue[7]. Our expectation is that since myc has been linked with a number of different avian leukemias, as well as associated in certain cellular proliferative events, such systematic, molecular comparisons may reveal recognizable domains(s) common to these onc-genes or perhaps susceptible to activation by specific mutagenic alteration(s) or chromosomal rearrangement. Ultimately, it is hoped that such studies can be utilized to design specific immunologic reagents able to locate and characterize protein(s) encoded by the normal and altered myc-genes, elucidating their subcellular location and functional role(s) in the process.

II. Comparison of the nucleotide and deduced protein sequences of cellular and viral myc genes. The sequence of the human and chicken[8] cellular myc genes as well as those of the avian acute transforming retroviruses MC29 [9], MH2 [10], and OK10 [11] have been reported. Recently, the sequence of the rainbow trout cellular myc gene has been established[12] in this laboratory (Fig. 1).

Figure 1. Pairwise comparison of the trout sequence with that of the chicken and human indicated a high degree of homology at both the level of nucleotide and deduced amino acid sequence. In order to obtain a consistent alignment between the trout, chicken, and human sequences, the deduced amino acid sequences were compared by the computer program of Murata et al.[13]. The results of this comparison is shown in Fig. 2. The structure of the myc genes deduced from the sequences are depicted in Fig. 3. For all three sequences, the region homologous to the MC29 v-myc gene are organized in two exons. Studies of the structure of myc messages from chicken and human cells indicate that there also is an exon located 5' from the major exons with homology to MC29 v-myc.

Figure 2. Comparison of the deduced protein sequences of the rainbow trout (TR-MYC), human (HU-MYC), and chicken (CH-MYC) cellular myc genes with the myc genes of avian retroviruses MC29 (MC-MYC), MH2 (MH-MYC), and OK10 (OK-MYC). The amino acids are abbreviated by the standard one letter code[14]. While the amino-terminal end of the cellular myc proteins have not been established, position 1 is assigned to the first initiation codon in the second exon. Dashes represent deletions inserted by the three protein alignment program of Murata et al.[13]. The matrix of pairwise amino acid comparisons used was that of MacLachlan[15] and the gap penalty used was 8. Asterisks represent identity between human myc

Figure 1

```
                                                                                                              -3182
                                                                                                              CTGCAGT
CH-MYC

        -3172      -3162      -3152      -3142      -3132      -3122      -3112      -3102      -3092      -3082      -3072
CH-MYC  TAGTTTCTCT GCATATAATT ATATTGCAGC ACAGGATTAT GATTTTCAAC CCTAGGTGTA CTGGAGTAAT TTTGAAGTAT TTCTGCTGCT TCCAGCTGAA TTTCGATGGC

        -3062      -3052      -3042      -3032      -3022      -3012      -3002      -2992      -2982      -2972      -2962
CH-MYC  TTTTACAGCT CTGAGAGCAT TACTGTGTAT TGGGTCATTC TGATACTGTT CTTAAATGAG TAAAAGAACC ATAGAATGGT TTGAGTTGGA AGGGACCTTC AAAGGTCATC

        -2952      -2942      -2932      -2922      -2912      -2902      -2892      -2882      -2872      -2862      -2852
CH-MYC  TAGTCCAACA TCCCTGCAAT GAGCTGGGAC ATCTACAGCT TGATCAGAGC CCTGTAGAGC CTGGCTTTGA GTGTCTCCAG GGATGGGGCA TCCACCACCT CTCTGGGCAA

        -2842      -2832      -2822      -2812      -2802      -2792      -2782      -2772      -2762      -2752      -2742
CH-MYC  CCCGTTCCAG TGCCTCACTG CCCTTATTTT AAAAAAAACA TCTTCCTAAT ATCCAGTCTA AATCTCCCCT GTCCTACTTT GAAACCATTT CCCCATGTCC TATCACAAGA

        -2732      -2722      -2712      -2702      -2692      -2682      -2672      -2662      -2652      -2642      -2632
CH-MYC  AACCCTCCTA AAGAGTCTGT CTCCTTCTTT CTGGTAGCAT CCCTACGAAC TTTCACACTG GGTCAATTCA GATCCTGCCC CTTTCTGGCA GAATCCTTCA GCCACGCTAT

        -2622      -2612      -2602      -2592      -2582      -2572      -2562      -2552      -2542      -2532      -2522
CH-MYC  TTCCAGTCAC ACCAGCAAAG TCCACTACAG ACACAGCGTT GTAGCATTCA AGAACAGCAC GATGTATTTT AAGCCACCTA GGAGCAAGAG CAAACCCAAT GCTTAAAATT

        -2512      -2502      -2492      -2482      -2472      -2462      -2452      -2442      -2432      -2422      -2412
CH-MYC  GGGACTGCTC AGCACTCCCC GTTTCTGATC CCCTCTTCTT GTTTTCATGA ATCCGTCCCT CTTTGCTACC CAACAGCGGC AGAAAGGGCT GCGAACTGCA CTCGGAGCGG

        -2402      -2392      -2382      -2372      -2362      -2352      -2342      -2332      -2322      -2312      -2302
CH-MYC  AATTTGGCTG CAAACATTCC GCTGCTCAGC GGAAATGGGC GATTTCCACT TAAAAAAAAA AAGGGGGGGG GGGGATTTTT TTTTTTTTT TTTCATTATT TTTTCGCCG

        -2292      -2282      -2272      -2262      -2252      -2242      -2232      -2222      -2212      -2202      -2192
HU-MYC                     C CCCGGGTTCCC AAAGCAGAGG GCGTGGGGGA AAAGAAAAAA GATCCTCTCT CGCTAATCTC CGCCCACCGG CCCTTTATAA TGGCAGGGTC
CH-MYC  GGAGGGGTTC GTGCAGGTGC CGGGCCGGGG CTGCGCGCTG CATCCCGCGG GCGCTATCGG GCGCCGGGAG AGGGCGCGAT GGCCCACCAG TAGCGTTGGC CGTGGGAAAG
```

Start of human exon 1

```
        -2182      -2172      -2162      -2152      -2142      -2132      -2122      -2112      -2102      -2092      -2082
HU-MYC  TGGACGGCTG AGGACCCCCG AGCTGTGCTG CTCGCGGCCG CCACCGCCGG GCCCCGGCCG TCCCTGGCTC CCCTCCTGCC TCAGAGAAGG CAGGGCTTCT CAGAGGCTTG
CH-MYC  CCGGGCCGCC CCCAGCGCCG GGGAACCGCA ACGGGGGGAT GGATGGGGAA GGGGGTGCGG GGGTCCTCCC GCCCGGCGAT CCGTGTTCCT CCCCGAGCTT CTACGCTTAG

        -2072      -2062      -2052      -2042      -2032      -2022      -2012      -2002      -1992      -1982      -1972
HU-MYC  GCGGGAAAAA GAACGGAGGG AGGGATCGCG CTGAGTATAA AAGCCGGTTT TCGGGGCTTT ATCTAACTCG CTGTAGTAAT TCCAGCGAGA GGCAGAGGGA GCGAGCGGGC
CH-MYC  AAATGATACA AATACTTATA AGTCCGTTTG GTGTGCGTGT GTGTGTGGGG AGGAGGGGGG GGGAGGGGGG AGGGGGTGAA GAAATAAATG CGAAATAAAT AAGAAATGCA

        -1962      -1952      -1942      -1932      -1922      -1912      -1902      -1892      -1882      -1872      -1862
HU-MYC  GGCCGGCTAG GGTGGAAGAG CCGGGCGAGC AGAGCTGCGC TGCGGGCGTC CTGGGAAGGG AGATCCGGAG CGAATAGGGG GCTTCGCCTC TGGCCCAGCC CTCCCGCTGA
CH-MYC  TGAGAAAATAG GAATGATATA TATGTATATA TCTTAGCGGG GTGCCCGCAG GTGCGGGTAT TGCAGCGGGA GGGGCGCAGA TAGCGGTCCC GCGGGGCCGG GAAGACGCGA

        -1852      -1842      -1832      -1822      -1812      -1802      -1792      -1782      -1772      -1762      -1752
HU-MYC  TCCCCCAGCC AGCGGTCCGC AACCCTTGCC GCATCCACGA AACTTTGCCC ATAGCAGCGG GCGGGCACTT TGCACTGGAA CTTACAACAC CCGAGCAAGG ACGCGACTCT
CH-MYC  TGCGGGAGCG CCCGTCGGGT CTCGGCTCCG CGCACCTCCG GGGATGGGTA ACGGGGAAGG GGTGACCCCG GGGTGGGGAA GGAGCCGCTG GGTGAGGGGC TGCGGAGCGA

        -1742      -1732      -1722      -1712      -1702      -1692      -1682      -1672      -1662      -1652      -1642
HU-MYC  CTCGACGCGG GGAGGCTATT CTGCCCATTT GGGGACACTT CCCCGCCGCT GCCAGGACCC GCTTCTCTGA AAGGCTCTCC TTGCAGCTGC TTAGACGCTG GATTTTTTTC
CH-MYC  GCGGGGGGAG CCCGGGGGTC CCCGGGGGTC ACCTTGCAGC CGCTCCCCCC GCAGCCTCCT CCTCCCGTTT AATCCTCCGG GATAACGAAG CAGCGACACG GGCGGGGGTG
```

End of human exon 1

```
        -1632      -1622      -1612      -1602      -1592      -1582      -1572      -1562      -1552      -1542      -1532
HU-MYC  GGGTAGTGGA AAACCAGGATA AGCACCGAAG TCCACTTGCC TTTTAATTTA TTTTTTTATC ACTTTAATGC TGAAGATGAGT CGAATGCCTA AATAGGGTGT CTTTTCTCCC
CH-MYC  CGCCAGGCTAC GGACGCTCCT TTGTGCCGGT AGGGTAGCCG GCAACCGCCC CGCCCGCAGC CGCGTTACGG GTGGACACGG AGCGTGAACC TCCCCTGCCG CCGTCGGGGG

        -1522      -1512      -1502      -1492      -1482      -1472      -1462      -1452      -1442      -1432      -1422
HU-MYC  ATTCCTGCGC TATTGACACT TTTCTCAGAG TAGTTATGGT AACTGGGGCT GGGGTGGGGG GTAATCCAGA ACTGGATCGG GGTAAAGTGA CTTGTCAAGA TGGGAAGAGA
CH-MYC  GCAGCGGGAG GAGGGGGAGC GGAGAGCGAA GAGGGAAGGA GGGAGGGGGG AAGGCAGCGA GGAGGGAAGC AGCCAGGAAG GCCCTTTTCA TCCCCGCTCG TATTTTTTTT

        -1412      -1402      -1392      -1382      -1372      -1362      -1352      -1342      -1332      -1322      -1312
HU-MYC  GAAGGCAGAG GGAAAAACGG AATGTTTTTT AAGACTACCC TTTCGAGATT TCTGCCTTAT GAATATATTC ACGCTGACTC CCGGCCGGTC GGACATTCCT GCTTTATTGT
CH-MYC  TTTTTTTTAC TATGTTTACT TCCGACCTCT CCTTGTAGTA AGAGAAAAAA AACCAACCGC TGCTCCGCAT CGCCTCTCCC CGGCCCCTCT CCCTCCCTCC CTCCCTCCCG

        -1302      -1292      -1282      -1272      -1262      -1252      -1242      -1232      -1222      -1212      -1202
HU-MYC  GTTAATTGCT CTCTGGGTTT TGGGGGGCTG GGGGTTGCTT TGCGGTGGGC AGAAAGCCCC TTGCATCCTG AGCTCCTTGG AGTAGGGGCC GCATATCGCC TGTGTGAGCC
CH-MYC  CCCGCCCAGC TCCGGCTCCG AGTACTCGGG GGGGGGCACG GAGCCCCTCG GCCGCCCCCT CGCCGGCCGC CCTCCCGCGT CACGGAGCCC GCGCGGAANC GGGGGCGAGC

        -1192      -1182      -1172      -1162      -1152      -1142      -1132      -1122      -1112      -1102      -1092
HU-MYC  AGATCGCTCC GCAGCCGCTG ACTTGTCCCC GTCTCCGGGA GGGCATTTAA ATTTCGGCTC ACCGCATTTC TGACAGCCGG AGACGGACAC TGCGGCGCGT CCCGCCCGCC
CH-MYC  GGGAGGGACA TGAAGCGGCG ACGCGCACCG CGAGAGCGCG CACTCGCGGG GCCCCGCCGT GCCGCTCGTG CTCCCGCCCC CGCTGCATCT CCCGCCCGCC CCGCTGCCGG

        -1082      -1072      -1062      -1052      -1042      -1032      -1022      -1012      -1002       -992       -982
HU-MYC  TGTCCCCGCG GCGATTCCAA CCCGCCCTGA TCCTTTTAAG AAGTTGGCAT TTGGCTTTTT AAAAAGCAAT AATACAATTT AAAACCTGGG TCTCTAGAGG TGTTAGGACG
CH-MYC  GCTTTAAGAG CAGCAAAGCA ACTTAACTTC TATTGTACGC GACGGAGCGC GCGCGGCCGC CTTGGACCGT ACAATCTGCC GCACGCCGGG AAGGCGAGCC CTCTCCGCTG

         -972       -962       -952       -942       -932       -922       -912       -902       -892       -882       -872
HU-MYC  TGGTGTTGGG TAGGCGCAGG CAGGGGGAAA GGGAAGGCAG GATGTGTCCG ATTCTCCTGG AATCGTTGAC TTGGAAAAAC CAGGGCGAAT CTCCGCACCC AGCCCTGACT
CH-MYC  TATTTTTTTT TCATCGTGG TGGGAGGAAG CGATCTACGT TCTCCCGCG TTTGGCTCC CTTTTTTCCC CCGTCTTCTC CGGCGGTTCT TTTTATATTT TTATCTCCAA

         -862       -852       -842       -832       -822       -812       -802       -792       -782       -772       -762
HU-MYC  CCCCTGCCGC GGCCGCCCTC GGGTGTCCTC GCGCCCGAGA TGCCGGAGGAA CTGCGAGGAG CGGGGCTCTG GGCGGTTCCA GAACAGCTGC TACCCTTGGT GGGGTGGCTC
CH-MYC  TTTCCTGATT TTGTTGTTCC CCGCACCGCC CGCAATTATT GCCTCGCTCC GTCTCGCAGC CGGCGCGTTG GAGGAGCCGG TGAGTGGGGC GGCTCCGGTT TACCCATCAC

         -752       -742       -732       -722       -712       -702       -692       -682       -672       -662       -652
HU-MYC  CGGGGGAGGT ATCCGACGGG GGTCTCTGGC GCAGTTGCAT CTCCGTATTG AGTGCAGAGG GAGGTGCCCC TATTATTATT GGACACCCCC CTTGTATTTA TGGAGGGGTG
CH-MYC  TCGATCCACC GCGGTCGGGC TGACAGCGCG GGGCCGCGGG ACCGCCGGTG CCTCCCGGGG GACGCGGCGC TGCTCCGGGC ACGGCGCGCT CCATCCTTCT CGGCTGCTCT

         -642       -632       -622       -612       -602       -592       -582       -572       -562       -552       -542
HU-MYC  TTAAAGCCCG CGGCTGAGCT CGCCACTCCA GCCGGCGAGA GAAAGAAGAA AAGCTGGCAA AAGGAGTGTT GGACGGGGGC GGTACTGGGA GTGGGGACGG GGGCGGTGGA
CH-MYC  GGCTTGGATA TATAATTCTA TTTTTTGGAG GGGGGGGGGG GGTGGGGGAG GGCAAGAAGC ATTTGCTTCT CCGCGTACGC ACGGCAGGTT ATGCTTATTG CACATATATA

         -532       -522       -512       -502       -492       -482       -472       -462       -452       -442       -432
HU-MYC  GAGGGAAGGT TGGGAGGGGC TGCGGTGATCG GCGGGGGTAG GAGAGCGGCT AGGGCGCGAG TGGGAACAGC CGCAGCGGAG GGGCCCCGGC GCGGAGCGGG GTTCACGCAG
CH-MYC  CGTATATATA TGTGCGTGTG TGGATATATA TGTATATATG ATAAATTTGG CAAAGTTTGC CCAGCTCCGT GCAGCGGCAG GTGGTGGCT GGGGAGCAGC CCGGCTCTGC
MC-MYC  ---------  ---------  ---------  ---------  ---------  ---------  ---------  [CGCAGCGGAG] GGGCCCCGGC GCGGAGCGGG GTTCACGCAG
```

v-myc/chicken c-myc homology

```
         -422       -412       -402       -392       -382       -372       -362       -352       -342       -332       -322
HU-MYC  CCGCTCAGCGC CCAGGCGCCT CTCAGCCTCC CTTCAGGGTG GCGCAAAACT TTGTGCCTTG GATTTTGGCA AATTGTTTTC CTCACCGCCA CCTCCGCGGG CTTCTTAAGG
CH-MYC  GCTGGAGCAT ACCGGCCCTT CTCGCCCGGT TCCCGGTGCC GGAGCTGGGC ACCGGCTGAG CGCGGCGGCT GCGGGAGCTG TGCCCGAGCG GAGCCCCTCC GGAGAGTCGC
MC-MYC  ---------  ---------  ---------  ---------  ---------  ---------  ---------  ---------  ---------  ---------  ---------

         -312       -302       -292       -282       -272       -262       -252       -242       -232       -222       -212
HU-MYC  GCGCCAGGCG CGATTTCGAT TCCTCTGCCG CTGCGGGGCC GACTCCCGGG CTTTGCGCTC CGGGCGCCCG GGGGAGCGGG GGCTCGGCGG GCACCAAGCC GCTGGTTCAC
CH-MYC  GGGGAGAGCG CTCCGGGCGT CCCCGGGCGC TGACCCCTCG ATGGAGGGGG TCGCGACTCC CGGTCGCCCC GCTGAGCTGG GGAGGGGGTG AGGCGGGGGG CTCACGGAGG
MC-MYC  ---------  ---------  ---------  ---------  ---------  ---------  ---------  ---------  ---------  ---------  ---------
```

```
            -202       -192       -182       -172       -162       -152       -142       -132       -122       -112       -102
HU-MYC  TAAGTGCGTC TCCGAGATAG CAGGGGACTG TCCAAAGGGG GTGAAAGGGT GCTCCCTTTA TTCCCCCACC AAGACCACCC AGCCGCTTTA GGGGATAGCT CTGCAAGGGG
CH-MYC  GTCGTGCTTT TTATTATTAT TATTATTTTA TTATTATTAT TAGTTTATAT ATATATATAT ATATATAAAT CAATCTGACG GCGCGGGGTG CCGGGAGGGA GCGCTGCGTG
MC-MYC  ---------- ---------- ---------- ---------- ---------- ---------- ---------- ----T----- ---------- ---------- ----------
MH-MYC                                          '''''  '''''-G' '''''''''' '''''''''' '''''''''' '''''''''' '''''''''' ''''''''''

            -92        -82        -72        -62        -52        -42        -32        -21        -11        -1
HU-MYC  AGAGGTTCGG GACTGTGGCG CGCACTGCGC GCTGCGCCAG GTTTCCGCAC CAAGACCCCT TTAACTCAAG ACTGCC---- -----TCCCG CTTTGTGTGC CCCGCTCCAG
CH-MYC  CCGAGGGTCG ATCTCCCCCG CTATAGGGGC CGGGGGGAGC GGAGCCTCGC GGCCCCGAGC GCGGCTCACC CGGCCC---- -----CCCCG TGTCCCCCTC CCGCCCGCAG
MC-MYC  ---------- ---------- ---------- ---------- ---------- ---------- ---------- ---------- ---------- ---------- ----------
MH-MYC  ''''''''''  '''''T''''  '''''''''' '''G C'''' '''''''''' '''''''''' '''''''''' '''''CCCC CCCCG''''' '''''''''' '''''''''
OK-MYC  Start of          Initiation     '''''''''' '''''''''' '''''''''' '''''''''' '''''''''' '''''''''' '''''''''' '''''''''
        exon 2            codon

TR-MYC  --- --- --- --- --- --- --- --- --- AAT TCA AGT TTG GCG AGT AAA AAC TAC GAC TAC GAC TAT GAT TCT ATC CAG CCA TAT TTT TAT GTT  66
                                              **  *   ** ** *  *    *  * ** *** ** *** * **  *  *   *** ** *** *** **
HU-MYC  CAG CCT CCC GCG ACG ATG CCC CTC AAC GTT AGC TTC ACC AAC AGG AAC TAT GAC CTC GAC TAT GAC TTC GAC TTC TAC TGC  90
          *    * ** **  ** **  ** *   *** ** *  * ** *** * *   *** ** ** * *  *** **  ** **  ** *** * ** ** *** **
CH-MYC  GCA GCA GCC GCC GCG ATG CCG CTC AGC GCC AGC CTC CCC AGC AAG TAC TAC GAT TAC GAC TAC GAC TCG GTG CAG CCC TAC TTC TAC TTC  90
MC-MYC  ''' ''' ''' ''' ''' ''' ''' ''' ''' ''' ''' ''' ''' ''' ''' ''' ''' ''' ''' ''' ''' ''' ''' ''' ''' ''' ''' ''' '''
MH-MYC  ''' ''' ''' ''' ''' ''' ''' '''  ''T' '''
OK-MYC  ''' ''' ''' ''' ''' ''' ''' '''

                                                                                                                  box 1
TR-MYC  GAC AAC GAA GAT GAG GAT TTC TAT --- --- --- CAC CAG CAG CCA GGA CAG CTT CAG CCA GCT CCA GAC GAG GAC ATC TGG AAG AAA  147
          *    *** *   ** *** *   ***                **  *** *** * *  ** *  *** ** ** *** **  ** *** *** *** *** *** ***
HU-MYC  GAC --- GAG GAG GAG AAC TTC TAC CAG --- --- CAG CAG CAG AGC CAG CAG CTG CAG CCC GCG CCC AGC GAG GAT GAT ATC TGG AAG AAA  171
          **    *** ***  *** *  *** ***         ** *** ** *** ** ** *** **  ** ** **  ** *** *** *** *** *** *** *** ***
CH-MYC  GAG GAG GAG GAG GAG AAC TTC TAC CTG GCG GCG CAG CAG CGG GGC AGC GAG GAG CTG CAG CCT GCC GCC TCC GAG GAC ATC TGG AAG AAG  180
MC-MYC  ''' ''' ''' ''' ''' ''' ''' ''' ''' ''' ''' ''' ''' ''' ''' ''' ''' ''' ''' ''' ''' ''' ''' ''' ''' ''' ''' '''
MH-MYC  ''' ''' ''' ''' ''' ''' ''' TC' ''' ''' ''' A''' ''' ''' ''' ''A '''
OK-MYC  ''' ''' ''' ''' ''' ''' ''' ''' ''' ''' ''' ''' ''' '''

TR-MYC  TTT GAG TTG CTC CAC ACT CCT CCT CTC TCC CCG AGC CGA CCA TCA --- CTG --- --- --- TCT AGT ATT --- --- --- --- TTC CCA ---  210
          **  *** *** *** **  **  ** ** ** *** *** *** *** ***    **                              ***  *
HU-MYC  TTC GAG CTG CTG CCC ACC GCC CCG CTG TCC CCT AGC CGC CGC TCC GGG CTC TGC TCG CCC TCC TAC GTT GCG GTC ACA CCC TTC TCC CTT  261
          ***  *** *** ** *** * ** *** ** *** *** *** ***    *** *  *   *    *                          *** *
CH-MYC  TTT GAG CTC CTG CCC ACG CCC CCC CTC TCG CCC AGC CGC CGC TCC AGC CTG GCC GCC GCC TCC TGC --- --- --- --- --- TTC CCT ---  252
MC-MYC  ''' ''' ''' ''' ''' ''' ''' ''' ''' ''' ''' ''T' ''' ''' ''' ''' ''' ''' ''' ''' ''' ''' ''' ''' ''' ''' ''' '''
MH-MYC  ''' ''' ''' ''' ''' ''' ''' ''' G''' ''' ''' ''' ''' ''' T' ''' ''' ''' ''A '''
OK-MYC  ''' ''' ''' ''' ''' ''' ''' ''' G''' ''' ''' ''' ''' ''' ''' ''' ''' '''

TR-MYC  --- --- --- --- --- --- --- --- --- TCG ACT GCT GAC CAA CTA GAA ATG GTG ACC GAG TTT CTC GGG GAC GAC GTT GTA AAC  267
                                                **  ** *** *** *** *** *** *** ***  *   ** ** *  *** ***
HU-MYC  CGG GGA GAC AAC GAC GGC GGT GGC GGG AGC TTC TCC ACG GCC GAC CAG CTG GAG ATG GTG ACC GAG CTG CTG GGA GAC GAC ATG GTG AAC  351
                                                *** *** *** *** *** *** *** *** *** *** *** *** ** *** *** *** ***
CH-MYC  --- --- --- --- --- --- --- --- --- TCC ACC GCC GAC CAG CTG GAG ATG GTG ACG GAG CTC CTG GGG GGG GAC ATG GTC AAC  309
MC-MYC  ''' ''' ''' ''' ''' ''' ''' ''' ''' ''' ''' ''' ''' ''' ''' ''' ''' ''' ''' ''' ''' ''' ''' ''' ''' ''' '''
MH-MYC  ''' ''' ''' ''' ''' ''' ''' ''' ''' ''' ''' ''' ''' ''' ''' ''' ''' ''' 'G'' '''
OK-MYC  ''' ''' ''' ''' ''' ''' ''' ''' ''' ''' ''' ''' ''' ''' ''' ''' ''' '''

                                            box 2
TR-MYC  CAG AGT TTC ATC TGC GAT GCC GAC TAC TCC CAA ACC TTC CTC AAG TCA ATC ATC ATT CAG GAC TGT ATG TGG AGC GGC TTC TCT GCC ACA  357
          *** *** *** *** *** *  ** *** *** ***  *   ** ** ** ** *** *** *** *** *** *** *** *** *** *** *** ** *** **
HU-MYC  CAG AGT TTC ATC TGC GAC CCG GAC --- GAC GAG ACC TTC ATC AAA AAC ATC ATC ATC CAG GAC TGT ATG TGG AGC GGC TTC TCG GCC GCC  438
          *** *** *** *** *** *   *** ***     *** **  ** ** ** *** *** *** *** *** *** *** *** *** *** *** *** ** *** **
CH-MYC  CAG AGC TTC ATC TGC GAC CCG GAC --- GAC GAA TCC TTC GTC AAA TCC ATC ATC ATC GAC GAC TGC ATG TGG AGC GGC TTC TCC GCC GCC  396
MC-MYC  ''' ''' ''' ''C' ''' ''' ''' ''' ''' ''' ''' ''' ''' ''' ''' ''' ''' ''' ''' ''' ''' ''' ''' ''' ''' ''' ''' '''
MH-MYC  ''' ''' ''' ''' ''' ''' ''' ''' ''' ''' ''' ''' ''' ''' ''' ''' 'G'' ''' '''
OK-MYC  ''' ''' ''' ''' ''' ''' ''' ''' ''' ''' ''' ''' ''' ''' ''' ''' ''' '''

TR-MYC  GCC AAG TTA GAG AAA GTG GTG TCT GAA AGA CTC GCA TCG CTC CAG ACT GCT AGG AAA GAT --- --- --- --- --- --- --- --- ---  417
          *** *** *  ** ** **  ** ** *  *   **  * ** *** ** *** ** ***
HU-MYC  GCC AAG CTC ------------- GTC TCA GAG AAG CTG GCC TCC TAC CAG GCT GCG CGC AAA GAC --- --- --- --- --- --- --- --- ---  489
          *** *** **             **  ** *** *** ** *** ** *** *** ** *  *** *** ***
CH-MYC  GCC AAG CTG GAG AAG GTG GTG TCG GAG AAG CTC GCC ACC TAC CAA GCC TCC CGC GAG GGG GGC CCC GCC GCC GCC GTC TCC CGA CCC GGC  486
MC-MYC  ''' ''' ''' ''' ''' ''' ''' ''' ''' ''' ''' ''' ''' ''' ''' ''' ''' ''A'' ''' ''' '''
MH-MYC  ''' ''' ''' ''' ''' ''' ''' ''' ''' ''' ''' ''' ''' ''' ''' ''' ''' '''
OK-MYC  ''' ''' ''' ''' ''' ''' ''' ''' ''' ''' ''' ''' ''' ''' ''' ''' ''' '''

TR-MYC  --- --- --- TCA GCC GTT GGC GAC AAC GCA GAG TGT CCT ACT --- --- CGG TTG AAC GCA AAC TAC TTG CAG GAT CCG AAT ACT TCC GCG  492
                      **  *   *   ** ** *  *** ** *  **               **  * *** *** **  ** ** *** ***
HU-MYC  --- --- --- AGC GGC AGC CCG AAC CCC GCC CGC GGC CAC AGC GTC TGC TCC ACC TCC AGC TTG TAC CTG CAG GAT --- --- CTG AGC GCC  564
                      **  *** ***  ** **  * *** *  *** *  ** * *** ** *  *** *** **               ***  *  ***
CH-MYC  CCG CCG CCC TCG GCG GCG CCT CCT CCT GGC GGC TCC GCC --- --- --- GCC TCG GCC GGC CTC TAC CTG CAC --- --- CTG GGA GCC  564
MC-MYC  ''' ''' ''' ''' ''' ''' ''' ''' ''' ''' ''' ''' ''' ''' ''' ''' ''' ''' ''' '''
MH-MYC  ''' ''' ''' ''' ''' ''' ''' ''' ''' ''' ''' ''' ''' ''' ''' ''' ''' '''
OK-MYC  ''' ''' ''' ''' ''' ''' ''' ''' ''' ''' ''' ''' ''' ''' ''' ''' ''' '''

TR-MYC  TCA GAA TGC ATT GGT CCG AAT ACT TCC GCG TCA GAA TGC ATT GGT CCC TCA GTG GTC TTC CCC TAC CCA ATA ACT GAG ACT --- --- CCC  576
          *                          **  *** *** ** *** *  ** *** *** ***  *   ** ** *   **  *   *** ***
HU-MYC  GCC --- --- --- --- --- --- --- --- --- GCC TCA GAG TGC ATC GAC CCC TCG GTG GTC TTC CCC TAC CCT CTC AGC AGC AGC TCG --- CCC  630
          **                                      ***  *  *** *** **  ** *** *** ** *** ** *** ** *** ** *** *** *** ***
CH-MYC  GCG --- --- --- --- --- --- --- --- --- GCC GCC GAC TGC ATC GAC CCC TCG GTG GTC TTC CCC TAC CCG TC AGC GAG CGC GCC --- CCG  627
MC-MYC  ''' ''' ''' '''
MH-MYC  ''' ''' ''' '''                               'G' ''' 'G' T''' ''' ''' 'G' '''  'G' '' AG' ''' 'G' ---
OK-MYC  ''' ''' ''' '''

TR-MYC  AAA --- --- --- --- --- --- --- --- --- --- --- --- --- --- --- --- --- --- --- --- --- --- --- --- CCA AGT AAG GTG GCA  594
          **
HU-MYC  AAG TCC TGC GCC TCG CAA GAC TCC AGC GCC TTC TCT CCG TCC TCG GAT TCT CTG CTC TCC TCG ACG GAG TCC TCC CTC CAG GGC AGC CCC  720
CH-MYC  CGG GCC GCC --- --- --- --- --- --- --- --- --- --- --- --- --- --- --- --- --- --- --- --- --- --- CCC CCC GCC AAC  651
MC-MYC  ''' ''' '''
MH-MYC  --- --- ---                                                                                          ''' ''' 'GG'
OK-MYC  ''' ''' ---
```

Fig. 1 (continued)

End of exon 2 — Start of exon 3

```
TR-MYC CCA CCC ACG GAT TTG GCA TTG GAC ACC CCA CCC AAC AGT GGT AGC AGC AGC AGT GGT AGT GAC GAT GAT GAT GAG GAG GAA 684
       ••• •   • •       •   •     •   • ••  •• ••  •••            ••• •• •                        ••  ••  •• • •
HU-MYC GAG CCC CTG GTG CTC CAT GAG GAG ACA CCG CCC --- --- --- ACC ACC AGC AGC --- --- --- GAC TCT GAG --- --- --- GAG GAA CAA 783
       •      •                 •   •• •• •• •••            ••  •• ••• •••            •   •      •• ••• •••
CH-MYC CCC GCG GCT CTG CTG GGG GTC GAC ACG CCC --- --- --- ACG ACC AGC AGC --- --- --- GAC TCG GAA --- --- --- GAA GAA CAA 714
MC-MYC ''' ''' ''' ''' ''' '''                  ''' '''       ''' ''' '''                  ''' '''          ''' ''' '''
MH-MYC ''' ''' ''' ''' ''' ''' ''' G'' ''' '''           ''' GT' G'' G''            ''' 'G' ''' ''G
OK-MYC ''' ''' ''' ''' ''' '''

TR-MYC GAT GAT GAG GAC GAG GAG ATA GAT GTC GTT ACT GTG --- GAG AAG AGG CAA GCT GTG --- AAG CGG TGC GAC CCC AGC ACG --- --- --- 762
       ••  •• ••  •••   •• ••  •• • ••• •• ••• •• •••      ••  ••• ••• •• •••      ••  •• • •  •  •   •     •
HU-MYC --- --- GAA GAT GAG GAA GAT ATC GAT GTT TCT GTG --- GAG AAG AGG CAG GCT CCT GGC AAG GTG TCA GGA TCT GGA TCA CCT --- 861
       •••    ••• ••• •• • •• •• ••  •• ••• ••  •••       •   •• ••• •• •••      ••  •• • •   •   •••
CH-MYC --- --- GAA GAT GAG GAG GAA ATC GAT GTC GTT ACA TTA GCT GAA GAG AAC GAG TCT GAA --- TCC AGC ACA GAG TCC AGC ACA GAA GCA 795
MC-MYC --- --- ''' ''' ''' ''' ''' ''' ''' ''' ''' ''' ''' ''' ''' ''' ''' ''' ''' ''' ''' ''' G'' ''' '''
MH-MYC ''' ''' ''' ''' ''' ''' ''' ''' ''' '''
OK-MYC ''' ''' ''' ''' ''' '''

TR-MYC TCA GAG --- --- --- --- ACC AGA CAT CAC AGT CCC CTT GTG CTG AAG AGG TGC CAT GTC TCC ACC CAC CAG CAC AAC TAC GCC GCC CAC 840
       •   •                  •  •• •   •• •• •• •• •  •• •• ••• ••• •• •• • •• •• ••• •• ••• ••• •• • •
HU-MYC TCT GCT GGA GGC CAC AGC AAA CCT CCT CAC AGC CCA CTG GTC CTC AAG AGG TGC CAC GTC TCC ACC CAC CAG CAC AAC TAC GCT GCT CCT 951
       ••  •        •          •• •• • •• ••  • •    •• •• ••• •• •• •
CH-MYC TCA GAG GAG CAC TGT --- AAG CCC CAC CAC AGT CCG CTG GTC CTC AAG CGG TGT CAC GTC AAC ATC CAC CAA CAC AAC TAC GCT GCT CCT 882
MC-MYC ''' ''' ''' ''' ''' ''' ''' ''' ''' ''' ''' ''' ''' ''' ''' ''' ''' ''' ''' ''' ''' ''' G'' ''' '''
MH-MYC ''' ''' ''' ''' ''' ''' ''' ''' ''' '''
OK-MYC ''' ''' ''' ''' ''' '''

TR-MYC CCC TCC ACA CGG CAC GAC CAG CCA GCT GTC AAA AGG CTG AGG CTG GAG AAC AGC AGC CGG GTC CTC AAG CAG ATC AGC AGC AAC CGC 930
       ••• ••  •• • ••    •• • •• •   •• •• ••• •• •• • •                  ••  •• • •••  ••  • •   ••• •• ••• •• • •••
HU-MYC CCC TCC ACT CGG AAG GAC TAT CCT GCT GCC AAG AGG GTC AAG TTG GAC --- --- AGT GTC AGA GTC CTG AGA CAG ATC AGC AAC AAC CGA 1035
       ••• ••  •• • ••  •• • •   •• • •• •• ••• •• •• • •           •••     ••  ••  • • ••  ••  • •   •   •• ••• •• • •••
CH-MYC CCC TCC ACC AAG GTG GAA TAC CCA GCC GCC AAG AGG CTA AAG TTG GAC --- --- AGT GTC GTC CTC AAA CAG ATC AGC AAC AAC CGA 966
MC-MYC ''' ''' ''' ''' ''' ''' ''' ''' ''' ''' ''' ''' ''' ''' ''' ''' ''' ''' ''' ''' ''' ''' G'' ''' '''
MH-MYC ''' ''' ''' ''' ''' ''' ''' ''' ''' '''
OK-MYC ''' ''' ''' ''' ''' '''

TR-MYC AAA CTG TCA AGT CCC CGG ACA TCG GAC ACG GAG GAC TAC GAC AAA AGA ACT CAT AAT GTA CTG GAG CGC CAG CGG CTG GAG CTC 1020
       ••• •• •  •   •   •  • •   •• •• • •••  •• •• • ••  •• •• ••• •• • •  •• •• • ••• •• ••• ••• •• •• • ••• ••• ••• ••
HU-MYC AAA TGC ACC AGC CCC AGG TCC TCG GAC ACC GAG GAA AAT GTC AAG AGG CGA ACA CAC AAC GTC TTG GAG CGC CAG CGG CGG AAC GAG CTG 1125
       ••• •• • ••  •   •  • •   •• •• • ••• •• • •••  •• ••  •• ••  •• • ••  •• ••• •• • •• ••• ••• ••• ••• •   •• •• • ••
CH-MYC AAA TGC TCC AGT CCC CGC ACG TCA GAC TCA GAG GAC AAC GAC AGG CGA ACG CAC AAC GTC TTG GAG CGC CAG CGA GGG AAT GAG CTG 1056
MC-MYC ''' ''' ''' ''' ''' ''' ''' 'T' ''' ''' ''' ''' ''' ''' ''' ''' ''' ''' ''' ''' ''' ''' G'' ''' '''
MH-MYC ''' ''' ''' ''' ''' ''' ''' 'T' ''' '''
OK-MYC ''' ''' ''' ''' ''' ''' ''' 'T'

TR-MYC AAG CTG GAC TTT TTT GCT CTA CGG GAT GAG ATA CCG GAT GTG GCC AAC AAT GAG AAG GCA GCC AAA GTG GTC ATC CTA AAG AAG GCT ACA 1110
       •• • •• •   •• •• ••• •• • ••  •• ••  •• •• •   ••• •• •• ••• •••  •• ••• •• • •  •• •• •••  •• •• ••• •• ••• ••• ••
HU-MYC AAA CGG AGC TTT TTT GCC CTG CGT GAC CAG ATC CCG GAG TTG GAA AAT AAT GAA AAG GCC CCC AAG GTA GTT ATC CTT AAA AAA GCC ACA 1215
       ••• ••  •  •• •• ••• •• • •• • ••  •• •• ••  •• •   •  •• ••• •• • •• ••• ••• ••• ••  •• •• •••  •• •• ••• •• ••• ••
CH-MYC AAG CTG AGC TTC TTT GCC CTG CGT GAC ATA CCC GCG GCC AAC AAC GAG GCG CCC AAG GTT GTC ATC CTG AAA AAC GCC ACG 1146
MC-MYC ''' ''' C'' ''' ''' ''' ''' 'G' ''' ''' ''' ''' ''' ''' ''' ''' ''' ''' ''' ''' ''' ''' 'G' ''' '''
MH-MYC ''' ''' ''' ''' ''' '''
OK-MYC ''' ''' ''' ''' ''' '''

TR-MYC GAG TGC ATT TAC AGC ATG CAG ACA GAT GAG CAG AGA CTA GTC AAC CTC AAA GAG CAA CTA AGG AGG AAA AGT GAA CAT TTG AAC AG AAG 1200
       ••• •• • •  •• • •••       •  • •• •• •• •  •• • •• •• •• • ••  • •  • •• •• ••• •• • •• •• ••• •• ••• •• • •• ••• ••
HU-MYC GCA TAC ATC CTG TCC GTC CAA GCA GAG GAG CAA AAG CTC ATT TCT GAA GAG GAC TTG TTG CGG AAA CGA CGA GAA CAG TTG AAA CAC AAA 1305
       ••  •• • •   •  • •  •  • •• • •   •• •• •• •••    •  • •• •• ••• ••• ••  •• ••  •• ••• ••  •• •• • •• •• ••• •• • •• ••
CH-MYC GAG TAC GTT CTG TCT ATC CAA TCG GAC GAG CAC AGA CTA ATC GCA GAG AAG AGG CTT GTG AGG CGG AGG AGA CAG CTG AAA GAC AAA C 1236
MC-MYC ''' ''' ''' ''' ''' C'' ''' ''' ''' ''' 'A' ''G ''' ''' ''' ''' ''' ''' ''' ''' ''' ''' ''' ''' '''
MH-MYC ''' ''' ''' ''' ''' '''
OK-MYC ''' ''' ''' ''' ''' '''
```

Termination   Start of
codon   noncoding region

```
TR-MYC CTG GCA CAA CTG CAG --- --- --- --- ---
       •• • •   •• •• ••
HU-MYC CTT GAA GAG CTA CGG AAC TCT TGT GCG TAA GGAAAAGTAA GGAAAACGAT TCCTTCTAAC AGAAATGTCC TGAGCAATCA CCTATGAACT TGTTTCAAAT
CH-MYC CTT GAG CAG CTA AGG AAC TCT CGT GCA TAG GAACTCTTGG ACATCACTTA GAATACCCCA AACTAGACTG AAACTATGAT AAAATATTGG TGTTTCTAAT
MC-MYC ''' ''' ''' ''' ''' ''' ''' ''' ''' ''' ''''''''''
MH-MYC ''' ''' ''' ''' ''' '''
OK-MYC ''' ''' ''' ''' ''' '''
```

```
         1345        1355        1365        1375        1385        1395        1405
HU-MYC
         1276        1286        1296        1306        1316        1326        1336
CH-MYC

         1415        1425        1435        1445        1455        1465        1475        1485        1495        1505        1515
HU-MYC GCATGATCAA ATGCAACCTC ACAACCTTGG CTGAGTCTTG AGACTGAAAG ATTTAGCCAT AATGTAAACT GCCTCAAATT GGACTTTGGG CATAAAAGAA CTTTTTTATG
         1346        1356        1366        1376        1386        1396        1406        1416        1426        1436        1446
CH-MYC ATCACTCATG AACTACATCA GTCCATTGAG TATGGAACTA TTGCACTGC ATGCTGTGCG ACTTAACTTG AGACTACACA ACCTTGGCCG AATCTCCGAA CGGTTTGGCC
MC-MYC '''''''''' '''''''''' '''''''''' '''''''''' '''''''''' '''''''''' '''''''''' '''''''''' '''''''''' '''''''''' ''''''''''
OK-MYC

         1525        1535        1545        1555        1565        1575        1585        1595        1605        1615        1625
HU-MYC CTTACCATCT TTTTTTTTTC TTTAACAGAT TTGTATTTAA GAATTGTTTT TAAAAAATTT TAAGATTTAC ACAATGTTTC TCTGTAAATA TTGCCATTAA ATGTAAATAA
         1456        1466        1476        1486        1496        1506        1516        1526        1536        1546        1556
CH-MYC AGAACCTCAA AACTGCCTCA TAATTGATAC TTTGGGCATA AGGGATGATG GGACATTCTT CATGCTTGGG GATGAACTCT TCAACTTTTT TTCTTTTAAA ATTTTGTATT
MC-MYC '''''''''' '''''''''' '''''''''' '''''''''' '''''''''' '''''''''' '''''''''' '''''''''' '''''''''' '''''''''' ''''''''''
OK-MYC
```

Polyadenylation signal   Poly A addition site

```
         1635        1645        1655        1665        1675        1683
HU-MYC CTTTAATAAA ACGTTTATAG CAGTTACACA GAATTTCAAT CTAGTATAT AGTACCTA
         1566        1576        1586        1596        1606        1616        1626        1636        1646        1656        1666
CH-MYC TAAGGCATTT TTTCTTAGCG AGAATTCCAA ATAGAGTTGT CCCCAGATTG CTGTATATAT TTACACATCT TCTTGCCATG TAAATACCTT TAATAAAGTC TTTATAGAAA
MC-MYC '''''''''''
```
Polyadenylation signal

```
         1676        1686        1696        1706        1716        1726        1736        1746        1756   1761
CH-MYC AATGTGCAAC ATTAATACAC AGCAGTTGTG GGAACTGGAT TTATACTTGT CTTGAACTTG TGTGCCATAA CATTTCACAG TTTTGTTTTT TATTT
```
Poly A addition site

Figure 2

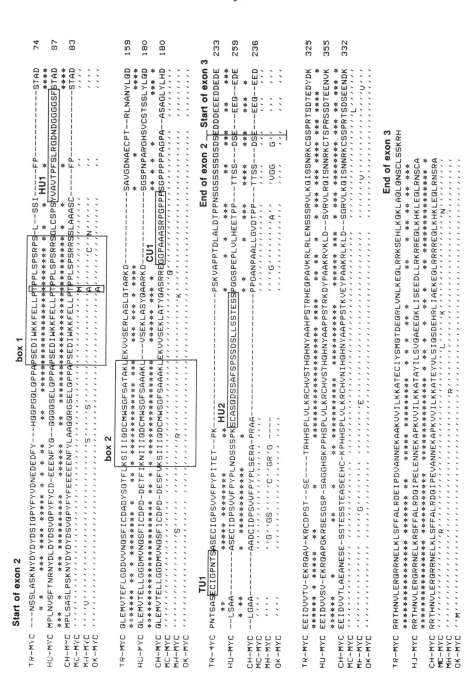

Figure 2 (con't)...and trout or chicken myc amino acid sequences. Apostrophes represent identity of a viral residue with the corresponding chicken residue. The position (number 61 in chicken) where each of the viral sequences differs from the chicken progenitor is highlighted. Also indicated are the division between the second and third exons as well as myc boxes 1 and 2. These represent the area of high homology with the N-myc gene. TU1, HU1, HU2, and CU1 represent the major species specific unique sequences that possibly arose through insertion events.

The degree of homology between the three sequences using this alignment procedure is presented in Table 1. Overall, the third exon is more highly conserved as indicated by the greater percent homology and the lower number of gaps that are required in this region for optimal alignment. However, several segments of the second exon are very highly conserved among the three organisms including the two regions that have been shown to be homologous to N-myc. It should be noted, however, that several other regions as long as these myc boxes are also highly conserved. These include the region between the myc boxes as well as the central portion of the third exon. It is of interest to note that in the first coding exon all three of the sequences

Table 1. Degree of myc homology myc between three cellular genes.

	Triple Matches	Trout vs Chicken	Trout vs Human	Chicken vs Human
Amino Acid				
total gene	55	64	62	68
exon 2	52	60	58	64
exon 3	58	70	66	73
box 1	93	94	94	96
box 2	89	95	89	95
Nucleic Acid				
total gene	53	62	60	70
exon 2	49	58	55	67
exon 3	58	67	66	74
box 1	70	74	77	81
box 2	81	85	83	92

Table 1. The percent homology was determined from alignment of the three sequences as described in the legend to Fig. 2. The ratio used was the number of matches over the average number of non-gap residues in the region examined. If the constraint of having a consistent alignment between the three sequences is removed, it is likely that somewhat higher percent matches could be obtained for the pairwise comparisons.

Viral and Cellular *myc* Genes

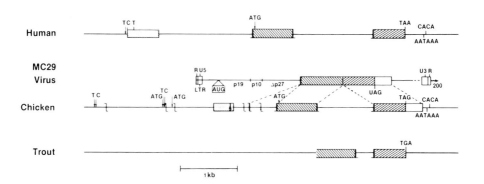

Figure 3. Summary of the major features of the structure of the human (Hu-c-myc), chicken (C-p-myc), trout (Ft-c-myc), and MC29 myc genes. The hatched regions represent the second and third exons while the dotted regions represent the first exon. The potential regulatory sites shown are: T, TTATA box; C, capping site; AATAAA, polyadenylation signal; CACA, poly A addition site; (2) and (5) represent donor and acceptor signals.

have inserted regions that are unique to themselves (cf. Fig. 2). There are two such regions in the human sequences (HU1 and HU2) while the chicken and trout each have a single region (CU1 and TU1, respectively). Other than these insertion events and other smaller insertions and deletions, the second and third exons seem to have evolved by the gradual acceptance of point mutations. The human and chicken sequences are somewhat more similar to each other than each of these sequences to one another. This observation is consistent with a phylogenetic model in which birds and mammals share a common lineage that diverged from the lineage that has lead to modern fish.

The highlights of the structural comparisons are diagrammatically represented in Fig. 3 and can be summarized as follows: (i) MC29 is a defective virus because it lacks the entire polymerase (pol) gene, part of the gag gene, and 71 amino acids from the amino terminus of the envelope (env) gene. Instead of these retroviral genetic elements, the MC29 genome contains the cell-derived myc sequence. (ii) An open reading frame is observed extending form the first ATG intitiation codon located at the 5' end of the gag gene into the myc sequence. This open reading frame is designated as the hatched area in Fig. 1. (iii) Nucleotide sequence comparison of MC29 and cellular myc genes reveals a stretch of 12 nucleotides shared by the virus and the chicken cell genomes, but not shared by the human proto-myc gene. A perfect consensus donor-acceptor splice signal is located at the 3' border of the 12 nucleotide region. This splice signal has probably functioned in linking up the 12-nucleotide sequence with the 5' end of the second exon of chicken protomyc whenever the MC29 virus originated. Thus, the 5' end of this 12-mer defines the 5' recombination point between the helper virus and chicken proto-myc gene. (iv) Human, chicken and trout proto-myc genes contain at least two coding exons interrupted by introns of: human, 1.38 kb; chicken, 0.97 kb; and trout, 0.27 kb - decreasing in size from human to fish. This reduction is consistent with the correlation of smaller sized introns in primative organisms[12]. These exons are clearly defined by consensus donor-accpetor splice signals and by the absence of introns in the v-myc sequence. (v) The two exons in the chicken and human proto-myc genes share a common reading frame which is terminated by a conserved translation termination signal: TAG in v-myc, and TGA in fish proto-myc. (vi) Using the following approaches we have been able to demonstrate that mRNA from normal cells may be generated from proto-myc sequences: (a) by direct examination of the nucleotide sequence of cloned myc genes consensus transcriptional signals were detected; (b) by hybridization studies using mRNA extracted from appropriate cells a major proto-myc mRNA species of 2.5 kb and minor species up to 4 kb were detected; and (c) by comparison of myc-related sequences isolated from genomic DNA libraries and by identifying proto-myc mRNAs from cDNA libraries. (vii) The fish, chicken and human proto-myc genes are distinctive cellular eukaryotic genes, possessing all the characteristic signals of a eukaryotic gene. These genes are transcriptionally active, generating mRNA approximately similar in size (~2.5kb). When one examines the cellular myc sequence for open reading frames (ORF's), several additional, potential coding domains can be found in both chicken and human myc genes (Fig. 4).

CHICKEN MYC PROTEIN TERMINATION CODONS

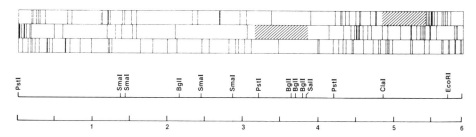

HUMAN MYC PROTEIN TERMINATION CODONS

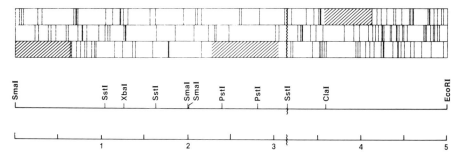

Figure 4. Open reading frames of the (top) chicken and (bottom) human myc genes. Diagrammatic representation of the position of protein translation termination codons in each possible reading frame. Cross hatched areas define the position and frame of the myc gene exons. Several restriction sites are presented to aid comparison with Figure 4 and 5. The symbol (⅔) at the Sst I represents a discontinuity in sequence for the second human myc intron.

III. Identification and characterization of the c-myc product of chicken
      and human.

There have been two general approaches in our laboratory to identify and characterize the myc gene products in chicken and human. The first makes use of synthetic peptides corresponding to amino acid sequences deduced from the DNA sequence of <u>myc</u> and the use of these peptides to prepare peptide specific antibodies. The second approach utilizes <u>E. coli</u> expression vectors to synthesize the cloned <u>myc</u> product and to purify the bacterially expressed protein as antigen for specific antibody production. These techniques have led to the identification and characterization of the normal chicken <u>myc</u> protein and tentative identification of protein(s) in certain human tumor cells such as: COLO 320, HL60, and several Burkitt lymphoma lines.

A. <u>Identification of c-myc protein from chicken.</u> Synthetic peptides derived from the proto-<u>myc</u> sequence of the chicken was used to identify and characterize the normal <u>myc</u> protein in Chicken Embryo Fibroblasts (CEF). The <u>myc</u> proteins of Q8 quail cells and CEF were labeled with $[^{35}S]$-methionine and were immunoprecipitated with the appropriate antibodies of synthetic peptides derived form the predicted amino acid sequences (cf. Fig. 2). Figure 5 represents the results from a typical experiment.

Large-scale immunoprecipitation of cell extracts has allowed isolation of p110 from nonproducer Q8 cells and p55 from chicken embryo fibroblasts. The overlapping tryptic peptide fingerpring patterns generated from p110 and p55 polypeptides suggest that the two proteins have a common origin (Fig. 6A and B). These results offer the first conclusive evidence that defines p55 as the chicken proto-myc gene product. These findings were further supported by mixing experiments depicted in Fig. 7, confirming a systematic pattern of overlapping tryptic peptides.

B. <u>The human myc proteins.</u> The human <u>myc</u> proteins in tumor cells have been isolated from a variety of cells such as: COLO 320, HL60 and several Burkitt lymphoma cells lines. The proteins thus far identified have a nuclear location and molecular weights of 58,000 to 66,000[16]. All of these studies are subject to the criticism that the <u>myc</u> protein identified by immunological criteria, have not been confirmed to be <u>myc</u> by amino acid sequence analysis - the ultimate test.

We modified our earlier procedure to include an immunoaffinity purification method in order to make efficient use of the limited supply of peptide specific, polyclonal antibody. Instead of linking the antibody to sepharose, we made use of the ability of protein A-sepharose to bind IgG. This enabled us to isolate <u>myc</u> from biosynthetically labeled cells in sufficient quantity for amino acid sequence analysis. For an antibody directed against a <u>myc</u> peptide, we selected an amino acid sequence from the second exon of <u>myc</u>. The sequence portion of <u>myc</u> used is hydrophilic and did not contain

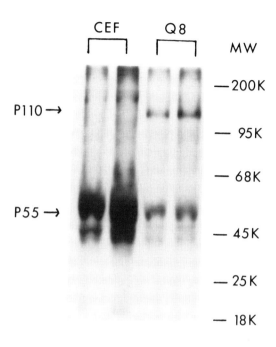

Figure 5. Immunoprecipitation of chicken p55 and MC29 p110. MC29 transformed quail cells (Q8) and chicken embryonic fibroblasts (CEF) were labelled with [^{35}S]-methionine and [^{35}S]-cysteine for 1 hour. The cells were lysed and treated with anti-myc (second exon) sera, and the resulting immunocomplexes were analyzed on SDS-polyacrylamide gels.

any common protease sites. The second exon anti-peptide antibody was affinity purified on sepharose columns to which its corresponding peptide had been linked. The purified anti-peptide antibody had a titer of 10^6 on ELISA assay.

The data in Table 2 summarizes the purification of myc by immunological methods. The nuclei were isolated from ^{3}H-arginine labeled COLO 320 cells. The nuclei were extracted in RIPA buffer (see text of Table 2) and the extract treated with the peptide specific antibody and protein A sepharose. After extensive washing, the myc protein was eluted from the immunoprecipitate by addition of excess peptide. Some 70% of the myc protein was specifically eluted with peptide, while 23% of ^{3}H-arginine remained

122

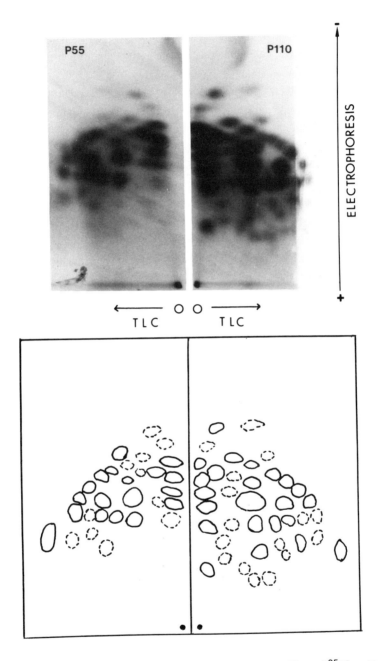

Figure 6. Tryptic peptide analysis of p110 and p55. [^{35}S]-methionine (left panel) and [^{35}S]-cysteine (right panel) labelled p110 and p55, isolated from preparative gels, were digested with trypsin to completion; the resulting tryptic peptides were separated on TLC plates by electrophoresis and chromotography.

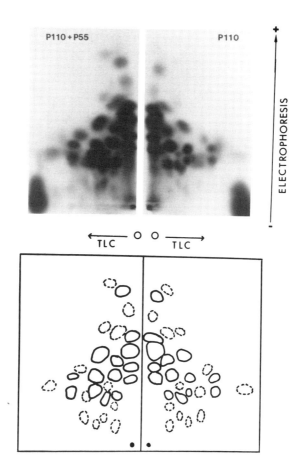

Figure 7. Reconstitution experiment of tryptic peptide analysis using a mixture of p110 and p55 comparing to p110 digests. Conditions were as in Fig. 6.

associated with the protein A sepharose. The ^{3}H-_myc_ protein was ethanol pre-cipitated to remove salts and to prepare the sample for amino acid sequence analysis. We recovered 54% of the ^{3}H-_myc_ protein by this method. To be sure we had a homogeneous protein, we analyzed the isolated protein by SDS-gel electrophoresis followed by fluorography. The x-ray film was

Table 2. Purification of Hu-c-myc Protein from COLO 320 Cells

	$[^3H]$-Arginine (counts/min)	$\%[^3H]$-Arginine
Immunoprecipitate from nuclear extract (6 x 10^7) cells	1.26 x 10^6	100
Hu-c-<u>myc</u> eluted with peptide	8.87 x 10^5	70
Arginine not released with peptide (SDS-solubilized residue)	2.88 x 10^5	22
		% Recovery
Hu-c-<u>myc</u> recovered by ethanol precipitation	4.82 x 10^5	54

Table 2.   COLO 320 cells (6x10^7) were incubated 1 hour with RPMI medium
μ deficient in arginine.   The cells were given 5 mCi ^3H-arginine (360
μCi/ml) and the incubation continued for 4 hours. The cells were collected
by centrifugation and washed 2 times with Phosphate buffered saline (PBS).
The cells were lysed in 3ml of a buffer (containing: 0.14 M NaCl, 1.5 mM
$MgCl_2$, 10 mM Tris-Cl pH 8.6, 0.5% NP40, 1mM each of TLCK, TPCK and PMSF
and 0.06 ml of aprotinin) kept at 0-4 C. The mixture was underlayed with
12 ml of lysis buffer containing 24% sucrose and 1% NP40, incubated 10
minutes at 0°C, and centrifuged at top speed in the Sorvall RT6000 for 20
minutes. The pellet (crude nuclei) was resuspended in 1 ml RIPA buffer
(0.050 M Tris-Cl pH 7.5, 0.15 M NaCl, 0.1% SDS, Triton X-100, 0.5% sodium
deoxycholate, 1.0 mM PMSF and 0.06 ml of aprotinin) sonicated 1 minute,
diluted to 8 ml with RIPA and then centrifuged at 40,000 RPM for 20 minutes.
The supernatant fluid was incubated at 0°C with 1 ml of protein A-sepaharose.
The protein A-sepharose was removed by centrifugation, and the supernatant
fluid incubated with the <u>myc</u> antibody overnight at 0°C. The <u>myc</u> protein
and its antibody were collected by binding to protein A-sepharose.   The
protein A-<u>myc</u> complex was washed 5 times with RIPA buffer, twice in PBS
containing 0.05% SDS and the <u>myc</u> protein was eluted using PBS containing
0.1% SDS and 200μg/ml of <u>myc</u> peptide. The eluted <u>myc</u> protein was dried
overnight, dissolved in 0.1 ml of HPLC grade water and 0.9 ml of ethanol
was added. The sample was stored at -20°C overnight and the <u>myc</u> precipitate
was collected by centrifugation for further analysis.

exposed for 1 or 7 days. As can be observed in Figure 8, as little as 1,000 cpm of the ^{3}H-arginine labeled myc could be visualized after 1 day exposure. Longer exposure times and larger samples reveal that the immuno-affinity purified myc is sufficiently homogeneous for amino acid sequence analysis.

IV. Myc containing acute leukemia viruses. The myc containing viruses possess a wide spectrum of oncogenicity causing leukemias and solid tumors in chickens and transform specific hematopoeitic cells and fibroblasts in tissue culture. This characteristic is unlike the narrow spectrum of myb containing viruses; such as AMV and E26, which cause only leukemias in animals and transforms only specific hematopoeitic cells in tissue culture (Table 3).

Immunoaffinity Purified *myc*: Peptide Specific Elution [³H]Arginine

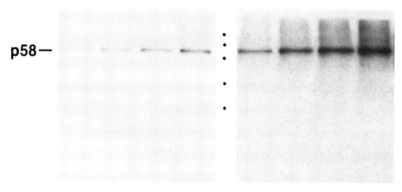

p58—

Exposure

1 Day   7 Days

Figure 8. SDS-gel electrophoresis of ^{3}H-arginine labeled myc. The ethanol precipitated, immunoaffinity purified myc was applied to SDS PAGE. After electrophoresis, the gels were fixed, impregnated with fluors and xray films were exposed for 1 or 7 days. The lanes contain 0.5×10^4, 2×10^4 and 3×10^4 CPM of the ^{3}H-arginine labeled myc. The dots represent molecular weight markers of 90,000, 68,000 43,000 and 25,000 daltons.

Thus far, the DNA sequences of the three avian transforming retroviruses, MC29, MH2 and OK10, containing the v-<u>myc</u> oncogene (cf. Fig. 1), as well as the sequence of the chicken proto-<u>myc</u> (cf. Fig. 1)[4] have been presented. Careful examination of their predicted amino acid sequences (cf. Fig. 2) reveal that there is a unique codon site, where as a result of adjacent mutations, none of the three viral sequences codes for the amino acid res idue that is encoded by the cellular proto-<u>myc</u> gene. This observation is highlighted at position 61 numbered from the first ATG in chicken exon 2 (Fig. 9). Position 61 and its neighbors are seen to be conserved among the proto-<u>myc</u> genes from chicken, human, mouse, and fish[17].

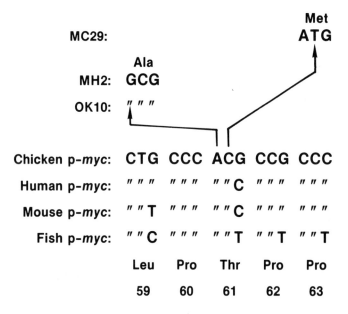

Figure 9. Sequence of a segment of the <u>myc</u> gene from avian retroviruses and animal cells. The references for the sequences are given in the text. Except where noted, the viral sequences are identical to the chicken p-<u>myc</u> sequence for the segment shown. The codons are numbered from the first init- iation codon in the second exon of chicken.

Due to the relatively low number of amino acid differences noted between the viral and chicken myc sequences, it is rather unlikely that this occurrence is by chance alone. Counting from the first ATG in exon 2, the chicken proto-myc locus codes for 416 amino acid residues. The number of amino acid substitutions between viral and chicken proto-myc is 7, 27, and 2 for MC29 [9], MH2 [10], and OK10 [11], respectively. We calculate that there would be only one chance in 458 that all three viral sequences contain an amino acid substitution at a common position if these substitutions were to have occurred randomly. We suggest, therefore, as a possible explanation of this observation that substitutions at position 61 might lead to an increase in the oncogenic potential of the virus and thus would confer a growth-advantage upon the cells so transformed. We are currently evaluating this hypothesis by altering viral v-myc and animal proto-myc genes by site specific mutagenesis to thereby determine if such substitutions, at position 61, indeed modulate oncogenic potential.

The occurence of substitutions at a common location in the viral and myc genes may be analogous to the observation made in many laboratories, that codon 12 of a ras gene is altered in viruses containing ras sequences and in tumor DNA which upon transfection is capable of transforming NIH 3T3 cells (see ref. 18 for review). While each of the three viruses containing the ras gene differ from the normal sequences by a G to A transition in the first position of codon 12, the mutations in transforming tumor DNA occur in either the first or second position. For example, the first position of codon 12 of the c-Ha-ras 1 allele of rat is altered in Harvey murine sarcoma virus and Rasheed rat sarcoma virus while the second position in this codon is altered in rat mammary carcinomas induced by nitrosomethylurea. Similarly, the human c-Ki-ras 2 allele was found to be altered in the first position in a human lung carcinoma cell line and in the second position in a human colon carcinoma cell line.

V. MH2 virus contains dual genes myc and mht.

A. Molecular Structure of MH2. We have molecularly cloned the MH2 provirus and determined its exact genetic structure by nucleotide sequence analysis shown in Figure 10.

128

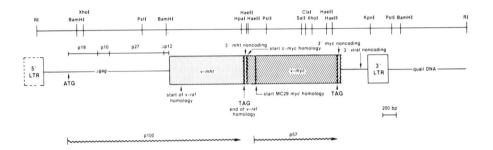

Figure 10. Genetic structure of MH2 proviral genome. A restriction enzyme map of the 6.5-kb Eco RI-resistant quail DNA fragment that includes the MH2 provirus is shown above the genetic map of MH2 proviral genome. Dashed lines represent sequences not present in the 6.5-kb Eco RI fragment; boxes between the 5' and 3' LTRs represent cell-derived sequences: solid lines between the two LTRs represent viral sequences. p100 and p57 represent the δgag-mht hybrid protein and the myc-containing protein in MH2-transformed cells, respectively.

Unexpectedly, this analysis revealed an MH2-specific sequence of 1.2 kb, termed mht, which is totally unrelated to the myc sequence[19]. The nucleotide sequence of MH2 viral genome indicates that the gag region and the mht gene form an open reading frame starting in the gag and terminating at a TAG stop codon near the 3' end of mht. This open reading frame contains 894 amino acids capable of accounting for a 100K dalton protein. This prediction is in accordance with a p100 sized gag-mht fusion protein observed in MH2-transformed cells[20].

By nucleotide sequence comparison one observes that the myc sequence of MH2 has 182 nucleotides not found in the MC29 viral myc sequence, but present in the cellular proto-myc gene flanking the first major coding exon. This region consists of the 3' end of the intron preceeding the first of the two major exons and contains an RNA splice acceptor site found in the chicken cell. Thus, the myc sequence of the MH2 genome includes the cellular splice acceptor site which can be used to generate the 2.6 kb subgenomic mRNA[21]. This spliced subgenomic RNA species is subsequently translated into a 57K dalton protein, the myc-containing protein detectable in MH2-transformed cells[22]. In addition, the myc sequence of MH2 differs from the of

Table 3. Oncogenic properties of myc containing avian acute leukemia viruses.

Virus Strain	Neoplastic growth induced in vivo			Cell types transformed in vitro	Viral onc sequences
	Sarcoma	Carcinoma	Acute leukemia		
	(Fibrosarcoma=F) (Hepatocytoma=H)	(Renal adenocarcinoma=RC) (Carcinoma=C)	(Myelocytomatosis=M) (Erythroblastosis=E) (Myeloblastosis=My)	(Fibroblastic=f) (Epitheloid=ep) (Myeloid=m) (Erythroid=e)	
MC29-subgroup					
MC29	F, H	C, RC	M, E	f, ep, m, e	myc
MH2	F, H	C, RC	M, E	f, ep, m, e	myc, mht
OK10	F, H	C, RC	M, E	f, ep, m, e	myc
CMII	F, H	C, RC	M, E	f, ep, m, e	myc

MC29 in 33 substitutions out of 419 amino acids, and a deletion of 4 amino acids in the MH2 myc sequence.

B. v-mht Homology to v-raf. When the mht sequence of MH2 was compared with the onc-specific raf sequence of murine sarcoma virus (MSV) 3611, a striking homology was observed (Fig. 11). Notably, the sequence homology between the two onc-genes is 80 percent. Most of the observed nucleotides changes are third base substitutions. The raf sequence of MSV 3611 differs from the mht sequence of MH2 by having 19 amino acid substitutions and one inserted proline. The bulk of these amino acid changes occurs at the 3' half of the respective onc-genes. Significantly, the homology between these two oncogenes at the deduced amino acid level is 94 percent. This region of homology is flanked on both sides by MH2- and MSV 3611-specific sequences, with essentially no homology between the two viruses. As shown in Figure 11, at the 5' side, the homology begins 174 bp 3' the gag-mht junction in MH2. Thus, the first 58 amino acids of mht preceding the start of homology with raf are MH2-specific[23]. At the 3' side, the two sequences share a common termination codon at position 1186 and diverge beyond this point. It is concluded from these studies that the MH2 virus has two non-structural genes with oncogenic potential.

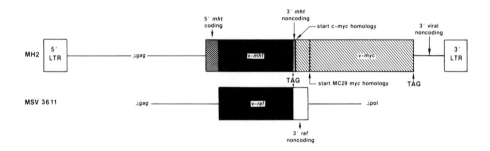

Figure 11. Comparison of the genetic maps of v-mht and v-raf genes. The MH2 proviral genome is shown above the v-raf gene of MSV 3611. Boxes at both ends of MH2 represent long terminal repeats (LTR); boxes between the LTR's represent cell-derived sequences; and lines represent viral sequences. Solid areas indicate the highly homologous regions of v-mht and v-raf genes.

C. Mutagenesis of Avian Carcinoma Virus MH2. To test whether each of the two potential onc genes of MH2 can transform fibroblasts independently of the other, we have prepared deletions mutants of mht and myc as well as frame shift mutants of MH2.

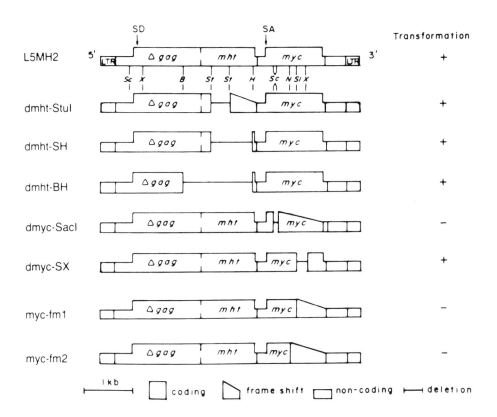

Figure 12. Genomes of MH2 proviruses used to test for the effects of mht and myc mutation of fibroblast transformation. The plasmid clones containing wild type L5MH2, a 456 nucleotide mht deletion, d mht-StuI, a 923 nucleotide mht deletion, d mht-SH, a 1396 nucleotide Δ gag-mht deletion, d mht-BH, a 128 nucleotide myc deletion, d myc-SacI, a 165 nucleotide myc deletion, d myc-SX, and two myc frameshift mutations, myc-fm 1 and myc-fm 2, are shown and their abilities to transform fibroblasts are indicated. The location of restriciton enzyme sites of the 4.4 kb MH2 provirus is indicated on the map of L5MH2. SD and SA are splice donors and splice acceptors. Sc is the restriction enzyme SacI, X is XhoI, B is BglII, St is StuI, H is HpaI, N is NotI, Sl is SalI.

The MH2 clone used for site-specific mutagenesis was derived from a MH2 provirus cloned in a prokaryotic pBR325 plasmid vector. The nucleotide sequence of this provirus has been determined previously[19]. We have utilized this clone and have created several deletion or frameshift mutants in both the myc and/or mht oncogenes. The details of these constructions have been presented elsewhere[24]. A diagram of each of these constructs are shown in Figure 12.

Biological activity of the mutant MH2 provirus. About 7 μg of the plasmids carrying wild type, mht or myc mutations of MH2 provirus were each transfected as Ca-precipitates[25] into chick or quail embryo fibroblasts together with 1 μg proviral DNA of avian myeloblastosis associated virus (MAV-1) cloned in lambda phage[26] as helper virus. Two days after transfection cells were transferred at a dilution of 1:4. Transformed focal areas were detected 5 to 7 days later in cultures infected with L5MH2, d mht-StuI, d mhtSH, d mht-BH, and d myc-XS but not with d myc-Sac I and the two myc frameshift mutants fm-1 and 2. Virus from growth media of cultures transfected with L5MH2, d mht-Stu I, d myc-SX and myc fml 1 was assayed physically by hybridizing RNA of purified virus "dot-blotted" on nitrocellulose paper with ^{32}P labeled DNA probes. These included a Taq resistant mht DNA fragment cloned in pBR322, a 443 nucleotide StuI-resistant mht segment in Fig. 12, and a 10 kb Bam H1-resistant fragment of a chicken proto-myc[27]. Virus from all four cultures tested was positive for mht and myc. As expected, virus from the culture infected with d mht-StuI was negative with the Stu 1-resistant mht probe[29]. We conclude that L5MH2, all the transforming mutants, and the non-transforming mutants tested for virus production were infectious and generated infectious virus.

Transfection assays and virus rescue were carried out as described previously[24]. Subsequently either virus from transfected cultures or the proviral DNA (described in Fig. 12) were assayed for transforming function on quail embryo fibroblasts. DNA or virus from cultures transfected by L5MH2, the three mht-deletions and d myc-SX each transformed quail fibroblasts (Fig. 12). About 10^2 focus-forming units per ml were obtained from media of cultures directly transfected with the transforming plasmids. No focus forming activity was detected in medium from cultures transfected with the myc-deletion d myc-SacI and the myc frameshifts myc-fm 1 and 2.

Several foci generated by each virus strain were picked and allowed to grow into microcolonies. These foci consisted of cells that appear smaller than most primary cells. Fig. 13 shows typical micro-colonies of cells transformed by wild type MH2 (Fig. 13A), by the mht deletion mutant, d mht-Stu I (Fig. 13B), and by the in-frame myc deletion d myc-SX (Fig. 13C). Variations in cell morphology and sociology were observed among cultures of completely transformed cells which had been derived from individual foci generated by the same wild type or mutant virus (not shown). Nevertheless typical cultures of cells transformed by the mht-deletion and the myc in-frame deletion mutants of MH2 were indistinguishable in morphology and growth properties from cultures transformed by wild type MH2 (Fig. 13A-C). However, preliminary data suggest that quail cells directly transformed by DNA of mht-deletions d mht-SacI and d mht-BH form denser foci, of apparently more adherent cells under liquid medium than wild type MH2 (compare Fig. 13D and E, F).

Based on the result that primary cell cultures infected by the Δgag-mht deletion-frameshift mutants of MH2 are just as transformed as cells infected by wild type MH2, we conclude that the δgag-myc gene of MH2 transforms cells in primary cultures without complementation by the Δgag-myc gene. The results that the myc frameshift deletion mutant d myc-Sac I and the myc frameshift mutations myc-fm 1 and 2 failed to transform fibroblasts is entirely consistent with the conclusion stated and shows directly that δgag-mht has no transforming function by itself. Thus, based on the in vitro transformation assay of primary cells, we have no evidence that the Δgag-mht gene has any oncogenic function.

One significant point should be noted, the internal in-frame myc-deletion of MH2, d myc-SX, appears to be an exception because it is able to transform fibroblasts like the wild-type MH2. However this result is consistent with previous results, namely that iso-structural spontaneous myc deletions of avian carcinoma virus MC29, mapping in the same myc region that was deleted here in MH2, also retain fibroblast transforming function. Thus an internal 165 nucleotide myc domain that maps between the Sal I and Xho I sites of the δgag-myc gene of MH2 is not essential for fibroblast transforming function of the δgag-myc gene.

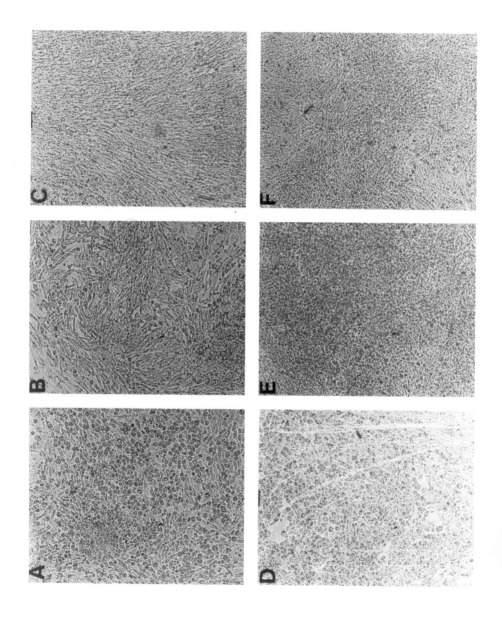

Figure 13. Morphology of primary quail embryo cells transformed by (A) wild-type MH2 pseudotyped with myeloblastosis associated virus (MAV-1), L5MH2 (MAV-1), (B) a mht-deletion of MH2, dmht-StuI (MAV-1), (C) an in-frame myc-deletion of MH2, myc-fm (MAV-1), (E) and (F) mht-deletions d mht-SacI and d mht-BH. The cells photographed are typical clonal colonies derived from foci of transformed quail cells. The cells shown in A-C were infected with virus produced by chick cells transfected with proviral DNAs (Figure 12). The cells photographed in D-F are quail primaries directly transformed with proviral DNAs.

D. **Proto-mht gene.** Now that we have been able to define the viral portion of the v-mht onc-gene, it became important for us to learn something about its cellular homolog, c-mht. Several clones had been derived from the normal chicken genomic DNA library that we found hybridizable to the v-mht probe. By subcloning and reconstruction experiments, we have been able to align these cellular sequences with the viral mht sequences and have subsequently determined that the viral homologous portion extends over a 16Kb stretch of the cellular genome[28]. Thus, by direct DNA sequence analysis we have confirmed that v-mht has the structural properties of a putative oncogene, that is, it possesses a cellular homolog. Further, we have analyzed high molecular weight DNA from a variety of different species digested with restriction enzymes that do not cut within v-mht. Southern blot analysis of these digests, using a v-mht-TaqI probe, (data not presented) detected distinct bands within the genomic DNA of chicken, mouse, hamster and man. All the restriction fragments within the species examined were different, with the exception of a PstI fragment which was common in chicken and hamster DNA. To determine whether the v-mht homologous cellular sequences are part of the c-myc locus of the chicken, remembering that v-mht in the MH2 virus is contiguous to v-myc, or derived from a different chromosomal site, endonuclease-digested genomic chicken DNA was hybridized using v-mht and c-myc DNA probes. Probes containing only the v-mht sequence hybridized to restricted fragments of chicken DNA which were different from the fragments of the c-myc locus. However digestion of the same DNA with Eco RI indicated that both myc and mht were contained with a 15 kb DNA fragment (data not shown) which could be due to a physical linkage of these genes or a sample comigration of the two onc-gene containing fragments. Upon hybridization of the v-mht probe to a cloned Eco RI fragment of chicken DNA containing the 5' end of the v-myc related portion as well as 10 kb upstream c-myc sequences, no hybridization was observed. Taken together these experiments would indicate that unlike the captured MH2 retroviral genome, the v-myc and v-mht related cellular genes are not physically linked.

By DNA sequence analysis and heteroduplexing to localize the v-mht homologous sequences in the chicken cellular genome, we have been able to demonstrate that the viral homologous mht onc-gene extends over a 16Kb stretch of cellular genomic nucleotides. Also, we have been able to show that this 16Kb region contains the v-mht related sequences within 11 exons that can be precisely defined (Fig. 14). Further, we have been able to detect in the genomic sequences, specific transcription termination signals in the last 3' exon as well as polyadenylation signals, indicating that the viral transduced portion of the genome is a truncated version of the 3' end of the normal cellular gene. Consequently, we have been able, from this study, to determine the points of recombination of the helper virus with the normal cellular mht sequences[29]. Additional evidence that the v-mht is a truncated segment of the normal cellular gene comes from northern-blot analysis of poly A selected chicken cellular RNA and probing this normal messenger with nick-translated DNA using portions of c-mht not contained within the viral homologous sequences. As can be seen in Figure 14 when probe segment b was used it did not hybriddize to the 4.0 Kb messenger RNA species indicating that this segment may be part of the intervening sequences region (IVS). However, when segment a, a region 5' to the v-mht homology, was used as a probe, it can be seen that there are now sequences hybridizable to the c-mht RNA, indicating that this segment (a) contains coding information (i.e., exons) which are not present in the v-mht onc-gene and the MH2 virus.

In other studies with MC29, AMV and E26 viruses we have also observed, consistently similar differences among the sizes of proto-onc genes, their corresponding proto-onc transcripts and the specific sequences transduced by these retroviruses. The most dramatic example of this is seen in the ets portion of the E26 viral genome, where the sequence captured by this virus is only 1.5 Kb and the cellular mRNA is five times larger 7.5 Kb[22].

Figure 14. Organization of c-mht and the analysis of the c-mht mRNA.
Aliquots of 5µg of poly A selected RNA was prepared and subject to Northern Blot Analysis. The origins of the probes for each lane are indicated by thick end lines, drawn and lettered, on the lower portion of the c-mht restriction map. Boxes indicate c-mht exons precisely defined by DNA sequence analysis. Blackened boxes indicate mht specific sequences which are not present in v-raf.

137

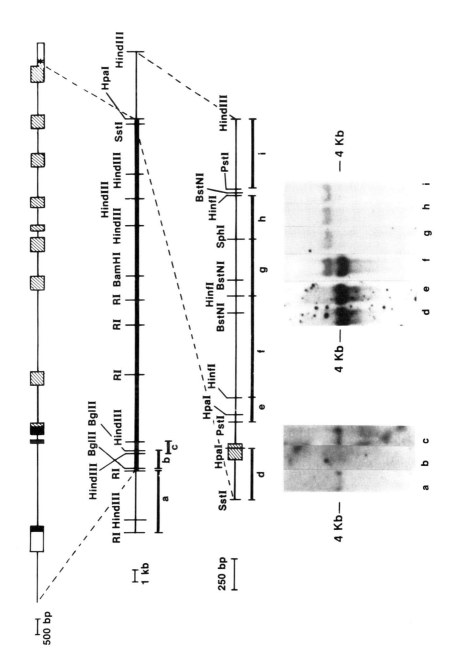

Genetic Organization of Chicken c-*mht* Gene

These findings again argue strongly that the transduction by the virus results in the "damaging" (i.e., truncation) of the normal cellular genes, in a functional sense. This alteration could perhaps lead to a truncated c-onc product fused to a portion of the viral protein, which in turn is able to compete with the normal undamaged c-onc protein, intracellularly. This competition could then result in the regulation of this highly conserved, normal protein's domain and possible target interactions with deplorable molecular consequences.

Finally, these collected experiments further confirm that v-mht possesses the features common to viable oncogenes, that is a viral transduced segment of a portion of a cellular homologous sequences which is highly conserved, in this case evolutionary throughout vertebrates being present in avians, rodents and man, and is actively expressed as a distinctive mRNA species at some stage in normal cells. Because of its conservation, it would suggest that c-mht may play an important role in cellular function. Interestingly, the human c-mht/raf homologous region has been assigned to chromosome number 3; deletions in the chromosomal band where this region maps are also associated with small cell lung carcinomas and other human malignancies[30]. The possibility exists, therefore, that chromosomal rearrangements or aberrant expression of c-mht may like other oncogenes be associated and involved in specific neoplasias thus justifying further intensive studies in this area.

VI. CONCLUSION

Numerous investigations into the cancer problem at the level of the cell have focused recently upon oncogenes; particularly those oncogenes recognized as captured by acute transforming retroviruses, which are able to convert normal cells into their malignant counterparts. By molecular cloning experiments, using the oncogenes of these acute transforming, we have initiated investigations into the structural organization of the acute avian leukemia viruses, and how this family of oncogenes may relate to their hosts and target organs, as well as their unique malignant specificities. Our interests in the MC29 family of acute transforming viruses as well as the AMV group, began with our successful isolation and cloning of the gene, responsible for transforming activity, the viral myc gene. We have noted, however, dramatic differences which exist between these groups of viruses; the MC29 group exhibiting a broad spectrum of oncogenicity causing leukemia to solid tumors in animals, and able to transform a variety of cells like fibroblasts and haematopoietic cells in tissue culture, the AMV group, on the other hand, displays a very narrow spectrrum of oncogenicity, causing only leukemia in animals and transforming haematopoietic cells in vitro. Even within the same MC29 family of viruses, differences exist; the MH2 viruses being notable, in that it contains two distinct onc-genes, one myc gene in common with this family group and another unique gene mht, which we have described in detail, and which shares a high degree of homology to another known, non-avian, viral transforming gene, v-raf. Thus, to comprehend the basis of the biological difference between these groups of specific acute trans-forming viruses, we focused our attempts to molecularly analyze the precise differences between the sequence structure and organization of these viruses at the integrated proviral level. In addition, we embarked upon comparative studies similarly characterizing the host animal, chicken, and human homologs of these genes, the cellular, proto-onc genes to help understand further how the vector helper viruses transduced these cellular genes from the host chromosome and what alteration had been sustained in the process, which may contribute to the malignant transforming potential of the retroviral varient. Not an incidental benefit has accrued from such studies, particularly in comparisons made with a wide variety of vertebrate cellular myc gene isolat-es comparing them to several defined myc containing avian retroviruses transforming genes. In particular, a unique codon emerges which may be of biological significance. This is a codon, where as a consequence of muta-tions, none of the three transforming viral sequences encode the amino acid residue found invarient at this locus, in all the cellular myc sequences determined to date, be it from fish, chicken, mouse or man. This evolution-ary conservation at position numbered 61 (defined from the first ATG in the avian exon II), belies some functional essentiality, which when mutated, may confer upon the viral agent capturing it some increased oncogenic poten-tial which would confer upon the infected cell some selective growth advant-age.

Needless to say, this site-specific mutational target becomes attractive as a model for myc transformation since it can be tested and evaluated by recombinant DNA techniques in conjunction with gene transfectional analyses. We are currently evaluating this transforming paradigm by altering v-myc and c-myc genes by site-specific mutagenesis; determining if such substitu-tions at this position would indeed effect changes in its oncogenic potential.

Although we initially cloned the viral myc gene and used it to compare and contrast this gene to its normal cellular homologs, our interest in the oncogenic diversity of the MC29 family of viruses and its variable disease specificities led us to discover the new oncogene mht and to conclude that this MC29 family virus, MH2, contains two distinct genes with oncogenic potential. One gene, related to the onc-gene v-myc, and the other, the Δ-gag-mht gene, closely related to the Δ-gag-raf transforming gene of the murine retrovirus MSV 3611. This finding led us to deduce that the number of cellular proto-onc genes are limited; essentially concluded because MH2 and MSV 3611, as well as other retroviruses from taxonomic groups, have transduced the same onc gene sequences from different animal species. Similarly, defining on a molecular basis the homology between a wide evolutionarily divergent number of proto-myc gene enabled us to make certain generalizations on the conservation of essential genomic regions in this oncogene rangings from fish to man. Having a trout myc probe also affords us a means of investigating a reversibly malignant teleost system, the lymphosarcoma of northern pike who characteristically succumb to malignant lymphomas during the winter months which reverse and disappear during warm weather months.

Further generalizations derived from our studies on proto-mht and myc genes and their expression have also led us to believe that viral onc genes are truncated sub-sets of proto-onc genes linked to sequences derived from one or more retroviral essential genes.

In complementary investigations, we have now focused our attentions towards difining the biological functions of the important onc-gene products. Such knowledge as we have accumulated has afforded us the capability to construct a number of oligopeptides specific to unique domains of our sequenced onc-genes. Such synthetic molecules enabled us to obtain peptide specific antibodies which can now be used to identify and localize intracellularly oncogene specific proteins. Additionally, we can have use of these oligopeptide antisera to confirm the production of our bacterially expressed oncogene proteins. It is thus anticipated that by a combined utilization of molecular probes derived from retroviral oncogenes to detect cellular homologous sequences in normal and malignant cells and subsequently identifying cellular onc-gene products, we will obtain important reagents with diagnostic potential and eventually also facilitate the functional characterization of these interesting genes.

VII. REFERENCES

1. Gilden, R. V., Rice, N. R. and McAllister, R. M. (1984) Gene Anal. Tech. 1, 23-33.
2. Vande Woude, G. F. and Gilden, R. V. (1985) In DeVita, V. T., Hellman, S. and Rosenberg, S. A. (Eds.) Cancer Principles and Practice of Oncology, J. B. Lippencott Co., Philadelphia, PA. Second Edition, Vol. 1, pp. 23-47.

3. Ascione, R., Sacchi, N., Watson, D. K., Fisher, R. J., Fujiwara, S., Seth, A. and Papas, T. S. (1986) Gene Anal. Tech. In Press.
4. Duesberg, P. H. (1985) Science 228, 669-677.
5. Bishop, J. M. and Varmus, H. (1984) In Weiss, R., Teich, N., Varmys, H. and Coffin, J. (Eds.) "RNA Tumor Virus" 2nd Edition, pp. 999-1108.
6. Bister, K. and Duesberg, P. H. (1982) In Klein, G. (Ed.) Advances in Viral Oncology, Raven Press, N.Y., 1, pp. 3-42.
7. Eva, A., Robbins, K. C., Andersen, P. R., Srinivasan, A., Tronick, S. R., Reddy, E. P., Ellmore, N. M., Galen, A. T., Lautenberger, J. A., Papas, T. S., Westin, E. W., Wong-Staal, F., Gallo, R. C. and Aaronson, S. A. (1981) In Yohn, D. S. and Blakeslee, J. R. (Eds.) Advances in Comparative Leukemia Research, Amsterdam, Elsevier/North Holland, pp. 381-384.
8. Watson, D. K., Psallidopoulos, M. C., Samuel, K. P., Dalla Favera, R. and Papas, T. S. (1983) Proc. Natl. Acad. Sci. USA 80, 3642-3645.
9. Lautenberger, J. A., Schulz, R. A., Garon, C. F., Tsichlis, P. N., Spyropoulos, D., Pry, T. W., Rushlow, K. E. and Papas, T. S. (1982) In Marchesi, V. T., Gallo, R. and Majerus, P. (Eds.) Differentiation and Function of Hematopoietic Cell Surfaces. New York, A. R. Liss, pp. 1-15.
10. Kan, N. C., Flordellis, C. S., Duesberg, P. H. and Papas, T. S. (1984) Proc. Natl. Acad. Sci. USA 81, 3000-3004.
11. Hayflick, J., Seeburg, P. H., Ohlsson, R., Pfeifer-Ohlsson, S., Watson, D., Papas, T. and Duesberg, P. H. (1985) Proc. Natl. Acad. Sci. USA 82, 2718-2722.
12. Van Beneden, R. J., Watson, D. K., Chen, T. T. and Papas, T. S. (1986) In Puett, D., Ahmad, F., Black, S., Lopez, D. M., Melner, M. H., Scott, W. A. and Whelan, W. J. (Eds.) Advances in Gene Technology: Molecular Biology of the Endocrine System. Cambridge, Cambridge University Press, pp. 156-157.
13. Murata, M., Richardson, J. S. and Susman, J. L. (1985) Proc. Natl. Acad. Sci. USA 82, 3073-3077.
14. Nominclature Committee of International Union of Biochemistry (1985) Eur. J. Biochem. 150, pp. 1-5.
15. MacLachlan, A. D. (1971) J. Mol. Biol. 61, 409-424.
16. Ramsay, G., Evan, G. I. and Bishop, J. M. (1984) Proc. Natl. Acad. Sci. USA 81, 7742-7746.
17. Papas, T. S. and Lautenberger, J. A. (1985) Nature 318, 237.
18. Varmus, H. E. (1984) Ann. Rev. Genet. 18, 553-612.

142

19. Kan, N. C., Flordellis, C. S., Garon, C. F., Duesberg, P. M. and Papas, T. S. (1983) Proc. Natl. Acad. Sci. USA 80, 6566-6570.

20. Hu, S. S. F., Moscovici, C. and Vogt, P. K. (1978) Virology 89, 162-178.

21. Pachl, C., Biegallse, B. and Linial, M. (1983) J. Virol. 45, 133-137.

22. Papas, T. S., Kan, N. C., Watson, D. K., Lautenberger, J. A., Flordellis, C., Samuel, K. P., Rovigatti, U. G., Psallidopoulos, M., Ascione, R. and Duesberg, P. H. (1985) In Neth, R., Gallo, R. C., Greaves, M. F. and Janka, G. (Eds.) Haematology and Blood Transfusion, Modern Trends in Human Leukemia VI. Berlin/Heidelberg, Springer-Verlag, Vol. 29, pp. 269-272.

23. Kan, N. C., Flordellis, C. S., Mark, G. E., Duesberg, P. H. and Papas, T. S. (1984) Science 223, 813-816.

24. Zhou, R-P., Kan, N. C., Papas, T. S. and Duesberg, P. H. (1985) Proc. Natl. Acad. Sci. USA 82, 6389-6393.

25. Graham, F. L. and Vander Eb, A. J. (1973) Virology 52, 456-467.

26. Perbal, B., Lipsick, J., Svoboda, J., Silva, R. and Baluda, M. (1985) J. Virol. 56, 240-244.

27. Robins, T., Bister, K., Garon, C., Papas, T. S. and Duesberg, P. H. (1982) J. Virol. 41, 635-642.

28. Flordellis, C. S., Kan, N. C., Psallidopoulos, M. C., Samuel, K. P., Watson, D. K. and Papas, T. S. (1983) In Whelan, W. J. and Schultz, J. (Eds.) 16th Annual Miami Winter Symposium, pp. 166-168.

29. Flordellis, C. S., Kan, N. C., Lautenberger, J. A., Samuel, K. P., Garon, C. F. and Papas, T. S. (1985) Virology 141, 267-274.

30. Bonner, T. O., O'Brien, S. J., Nash, W. G., Rapp, U. R., Morton, C. C. and Leder, P. (1984) Science 223, 71-74.

8

Molecular Mechanisms Involved in Human B and T Cell Neoplasia

Carlo M. Croce, Yoshihide Tsujimoto and Peter C. Nowell*

The Wistar Institute 3601 Spruce Street, Philadelphia, PA 19104

*The Department of Pathology and Laboratory Medicine
University of Pennsylvania, School of Medicine

I. INTRODUCTION

Since the discovery of the Philadelphia (Ph) chromosome in neoplastic cells of patients with chronic myelogenous leukemia[1], several other specific chromosomal alterations have been detected in human malignancies mainly in leukemias and lymphomas[2-4]. As a result of the introduction of a newly developed high resolution chromosome banding technique, it is now clear that nonrandom chromosomal alterations, predominantly chromosome translocations and inversions, occur in more than 90% of human hematopoietic malignancies[5].

While the association between specific chromosome translocations and certain human neoplasms is very consistent, for many years some investigators have considered such chromosomal changes epiphenomena of the malignant process, unrelated to the mechanisms involved in the pathogenesis of human neoplasms.

During the past four years, because of the demonstration of the translocation of cellular proto-oncogenes in Burkitt lymphoma[6] and chronic myelogenous leukemia[7-8], this view has been abandoned by most investigators and chromosomal changes are being considered to be directly involved in the pathogenesis of human neoplasms. In addition, the analysis of the chromosomal breakpoints in human tumors has provided increased understanding of the mechanisms responsible for oncogene activation[9,10] and of the molecular mechanisms involved in chromosome translocation[11,12].

II. BURKITT LYMPHOMA

Burkitt lymphoma is a very aggressive B cell malignancy, affecting predominantly children. Only recently Burkitt-like lymphomas have been detected in adults who are victims of the acquired immunodeficiency syndrome (AIDS)[13]. Burkitt lymphoma is endemic in a region of equatorial Africa, while it is sproadic in most of the other areas of the world. Interestingly, most of the African Burkitt lymphomas are positive for the Epstein-Barr virus (EBV) and express cytoplasmic or membrane bound immunoglobulins, while the sproadic cases are EBV negative and are immunoglobulin secretors[14]. These observations suggest that the cellular progenitors of African and sproadic Burkitt lymphomas may be B cells at different stages of B cell differentiation[14].

Approximately 75% of cases of Burkitt lymphomas carry a t(8;14) (q24;q32) chromosome translocation. The remaining 25% of cases carry either a t(8;22) (q24;q11)(16%) or a t(2;8) (p11;q24)(9%) chromosome translocation (Fig. 1). Thus the association between specific chromosome changes and Burkitt lymphomas is 100%. In 1979 we showed that the immunoglobulin heavy chain locus

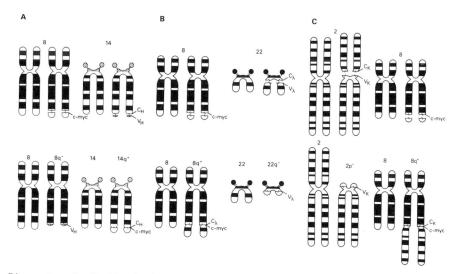

Figure 1. In Burkitt's lymphomas with the t(8;14) translocation, the c-myc oncogene translocates the the heavy chain locus (A), and a portion of the immunoglobulin locus (V_H) is translocated to chromosome 8. In Burkitt's lymphomas with the less frequent t(8;22) (B) and t(2;8) (C) translocations, the c-myc oncogene remains on the involved chromosome 8, but the genes for the immunoblobulin light chain constant regions (C_K or C_ω) translocate to a region 3' (distal) to the c-myc oncogene on the involved chromosome 8 ($8q^+$). Again with these translocations, the immunoglobulin loci are split so that sequences that encode for the variable portion of the immunoglobulin molecule (V_K or V_ω) remain on chromosome 2 or 22, respectively.

is on chromosome 14[15], and and in 1981 we showed that the locus for the lambda light chain is on chromosome 22[16]. On the basis of these findings we speculated that the genes for human immunoglobulin chains could be directly involved in the rearrangements observed in Burkitt lymphomas and in the pathogenesis of this disease[16]. The subsequent finding that the locus for immunoglobulin kappa chains maps at chromosome band 2q11[17,18] strengthened this speculation. Therefore, we have used somatic cell genetic techniques to determine whether the chromosome breakpoints in Burkitt lymphoma with the t(8;14) chromosome translocation involve directly the heavy chain locus (Fig. 1)[10]. The results of this analysis are summarized in Figure 1A.

As shown in this figure we found that hybrids carring the 8q⁻ chromosome contained the genes for the immunoglobulin heavy chain variable regions (V_H),
while the hybrids carrying the 14q⁺ chromosome contained the genes for the
constant regions of heavy chains (Fig. 1A). Thus the chromosome breakpoint
on band 14q32 observed in Burkitt lymphomas involve directly the locus for
immunoglobulin heavy chains[19].

Subsequently we found that the human homologue, c-myc of the v-myc oncogene
present in avian myelocytomatosis virus, is located at band 8q24, and is
translocated to the heavy chain locus on the 14q⁺ chromosome in Burkitt lymphomas with the t(8;14) chromosome translocation[6]. In these cases the translocated c-myc oncogene may remain in its germ line configuration or may
rearrange in its 5' region (Fig. 2)[6-20].

The c-myc oncogene is formed by three separated exons of which only the
second and the third are coding while the first exon codes for an untranslated
leader sequence (Fig. 2)[21]. The first ATG signal for protein synthesis is
at the beginning of the second exon and is followed by an open reading frame
that specifies a protein of 439 amino acids[21,22]. In Burkitt lymphomas with
the t(8;14) chromosome translocation the breakpoint may occur within the
first c-myc intron or 5' to the c-myc oncogene (Fig. 2B).

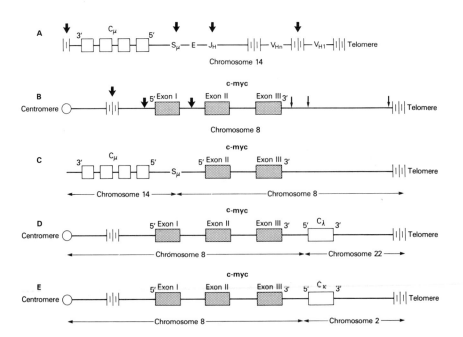

Figure 2. (A) A general diagram of an immunoglobulin heavy chain gene. The constant region (C) contains DNA segments that encode the common portion of immunoglobulin molecules, while the variable region (V_H) contains DNA segments that encode these portions of immunoglobulin molecules that differ from one another. During B cell differentiation, immunoglobulin gene rearrangement occurs so that one V_H gene segment comes to lie immediately adjacent to a D segment (not shown) and the D segment lies adjacent to a short coding segment (J_H). The elements labeled E is a DNA sequence that enhances promoter function, thereby increasing transcription of productively rearranged immunoglobulin gene. The S region contains a DNA sequence that is involved in another type of DNA rearrangement that is the basis for the class switch from secretion of one type of heavy chain to another. The symbol (|ı|ı|ı|) indicates that distances between adjacent parts of the chromosome are not defined. In Burkitt's lymphoma with the t(8;14) translocation the chromosome breakpoints within the heavy chain locus may occur in the region carrying V_H genes, in the region between J_H and V_H, in the heavy chain joining segment (J_H), in the switch region ($S\mu$), or may involve a different constant region coding segment. The arrows indicate possible sites for chromosomal breakpoints. (B) A general diagram of the c-myc gene. In Burkitt's lymphomas with the t(8;14) translocation, the chromosomal breakpoints on chromosome 8 are always 5' of the two coding exons (II and III) of the c-myc oncogene (thick arrows). In some cases the c-myc oncogene is decapitated by the chromosomal break, and the first exon of the gene remains on the 8q⁻ chromosome, while the coding exons translocate to chromosome 14 (line C). In Burkitt's lymphomas with the less frequent t(8;22) and t(2;8) translocations, the breakpoints are distal to the c-myc oncogene (thin arrows). (C) Example of a Burkitt's lymphoma with the t(8;14) translocation and a rearranged c-myc gene. The Cμ gene and the c-myc oncogene are inverted with respect to one another in that the transcriptional orientation of the c-myc and of the the Cμ genes are in opposite directions (5'->3'). (D) In Burkitt's lymphoma with the t(8;22) translocation, the c-myc oncogene remains on chromosome 8, while the portion of the lambda locus that encodes the constant region of a light chain translocates to the chromosomal region 3' (distal) to the c-myc oncogene (line B). (E) In Burkitt's lymphomas with the t(2;8) translocation, the c-myc oncogene also remains on chromosome 8, while the constant region of the kappa locus translocates to a chromosomal region 3' (distal) to the c-myc oncogene (line B).

There is also considerable heterogeneity of breakpoints within the heavy chain locus (Fig. 2A). The breakpoints may involve the chromosome region carrying V_H genes, or may involve J_H region or one of the switch (S) regions, predominantly the $S\mu$ region, but occasionally also an $S\gamma$ or an $S\alpha$ region (Figs. 2A and 2C).

In Burkitt lymphomas with the so-called variant t(8;22) and t(2;8) translocations, the breakpoints occur distally (3') to the involved c-myc locus, and the locus for either the lambda or the kappa light chains translocates to a region 3' (distal) to the involved c-myc oncogene (Figs. 1b and 1c)[10,23].

The consequences of these different types of translocations are essentially the same; the deregulation of the involved c-myc oncogene, that is transcribed constitutively at elevated levels because of its proximity to genetic elements within the three immunoglobulin loci capable of enhancing gene transcription in cis over considerable chromosomal distances[9,10,23,24,25].

We have also examined Burkitt lymphoma cells for the expression of the translocated and of the normal c-myc oncogene[26]. The results of this analysis indicated that in most Burkitt lymphomas only the c-myc oncogene involved in the translocation is transcribed, while the uninvolved c-myc gene on normal chromosome 8 is transcriptionally silent[26]. In a small minority of Burkitt lymphomas, however, the uninvolved c-myc oncogene is also expressed, but at very low levels[27]. We have used somatic cells genetic techniques to address the question of the consequences of chromosomal translocation in Burkitt lymphoma[9,10,23]. Somatic cell hybrids between mouse myeloma cells and Burkitt lymphoma cells were studied for the expression of the involved versus the uninvolved c-myc oncogene. The results of this analysis indicate that while the involved c-myc oncegene was expressed in the hybrids, the uninvolved c-myc oncogene on chromosome 8 was transcriptionally silent[9,10,23].

Human lymphoblastoid cells that expressed the normal c-myc oncogene were hybridized with the same mouse myeloma cells we hybridized with the Burkitt lymphoma cells[9]. The analysis of the hybrids carrying the human chromosome 8, where the c-myc oncogene resides, indicated that they were negative for human c-myc expression. Thus, there is a fundamental difference between the c-myc oncogene on normal chromosome 8 and the c-myc oncogene involved in one of the three different reciptocal chromosome translocations: the normal c-myc oncogene can be down-regulated in terminally differentiated B cells (e.g., mouse myeloma cells), while the c-myc oncogene involved in each of the three different translocations in the Burkitt tumor fails to respond to normal transcriptional control and is transcribed constitutively at elevated levels leading to agressive B cell neoplasms[9,10,23]. The interpretation was supported by the observation that the amplified c-myc oncogene of HL60 human promyelcytic cells was shut off in hybrids with mouse myeloma cells[9] and that the normal mouse c-myc oncogene was shut off in a Burkitt lymphoma back ground[28]. Additional somatic cell hybrid experiments also showed that the deregulation of the c-myc gene is B cell specific. Thus the results of the analysis of somatic cell hybrids indicated that the c-myc oncogene involved in the chromosome translocations behaved like an immunoglobulin gene, leading to its high constitutive expression in B cells.

III. CLONING GENES INVOLVED IN B-CELL NEOPLASIA

Translocations involving chromosome band 14q32 are often observed in non-Burkitt B cell malignancies. For example in a fraction B cells chronic lymphocytic leukemias (B-CLL), of diffuse B cell lymphomas[30-31] and of multiple myelomas, a translocation between chromosome 11 and 14 (t(11;14) (q13;q32) is observed[31]. In more than 80% of human follicular lymphomas, the most common human hematopoietic malignancy, a translocation between chromosomes 14 and 18 t(14;18)(q32;q21) is observed[32]. Since the breakpoints in these discorders involve band 14q32, we speculated that the human heavy chain locus could be involved[33]. By using somatic cell hybrids between mouse myeloma cells and human CLL cells with a t(11;14) chromosome translocation we found that the human heavy chain locus is split by the translocation in the leukemic cells[33]. We also found that similarly to the case of Burkitt lymphomas, the unproductively rearranged heavy chain gene is on the 14q+ chromosome. Then we cloned the DNA of this leukemia in a bacteriophage vector and screened the DNA library with a probe specific for the joining segment (J_H) of the heavy chain locus[34]. Positive clones were studied by restriction enzyme analysis to determine which clone contained the unproductively rearranged heavy chain gene. The sequences 5' to the involved J_H region of the 14q+ chromosome were then used as nucleic acid hybridization probes to DNAs derived from rodent-human hybrids[34]. Since the probes hybridized to DNA derived from chromosome 11, but not to DNA derived from the other human chromosomes, we concluded that we had cloned the joining between chromosome 11 and 14 on the 14q+ chromosome of this case of CLL[34].

As shown in Figure 3 a probe specific for the chromosome 11 breakpoint detected rearrangements in other B cell malignancies carrying this t(11;14) (q13;q32) chromosone translocation[11]. Thus this approach has provided us with a probe capable of detecting DNA rearrangement in B cell malignancies carrying this translocation, and we have proposed the name of bcl-1 (B cell leukemia and lymphoma-1) for this locus at band 11q13 that is involved in B cell tumors, carrying the t(11;14) chromosome translocation[11,34].

We have also taken advantage of a case of human pre B cell leukemia (380) carrying both a t(8;14) (q24;q32) and a t(14;18) (q32;q21) translocation[35] to clone the joining between chromosomes 14 and 18[36]. Screening of the DNA

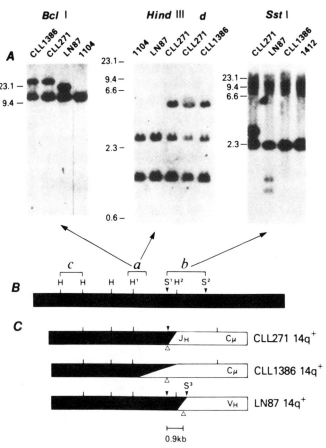

Figure 3. Southern blot hybridization of CLL 271, CLL 1386 and LN87 DNA with human chromosome 11-derived probes (A) and the maps of chromosome 14q+ in CLL 271, CLL 1386 and LN86 (C) of normal chromosome 11 (B).

library derived from 380 leukemic cells with a probe specific for the JH region resulted in the isolation of two classes of recombinant clones[36]. One class contained sequences derived from chormosome 8, while the other class contained sequences derived from chromosome 18[36]. We then used the chromosome 18 specific probe to clone the normal homologue on normal chromosome 18 and have used three different probes derived from this region of chromosome 18 to analyze human follicular lymphomas for DNA rearrangements[37]. One probe detected rearrangements in 2 out of 17 cases of follicular lymphoma. An additional probe, however, detected rearrangements in approximately 50% of human follicular lymphomas[37]. Thus, these two probes could detect rearrangements in approximately 60% of human follicular lymphomas[37]. Recently we have identified, with another probe a third region in the 18q21 band involved in rearrangement in approximately 20% of follicular lymphomas.

Thus by using three different probes we can detect rearrangements of this chromosomal segment in approximately 80% of human follicular lymphomas[37]. We proposed the name of bcl-2 (B cell leukemia/lymphoma 2) for the locus defined by these probes[35,36].

Analysis with a bcl-2 probe of mRNA expressed by various B cell neoplasms indicated the consistent presence of a 6 kb transcript (Fig. 4)[37]. Comparison of the levels of this bcl-2 transcript in pre B leukemic cells carrying the t(14;18) chromosome translocation versus pre B leukemic cells carrying the t(1;19) chromosome translocation indicated that in the leukemic cells with bcl-2 gene translocation the steady state levels of bcl-2 transcripts were 10-20 fold higher than in the other leukemic cells[37]. This result indicates that the juxtaposition of the bcl-2 gene to immunoglobulin enhancing elements results in deregulation of the involved bcl-2 gene, and its constitutive expression at elevated levels[32].

Thus by taking advantage of "chromosome walking" techniques and of the availability of leukemia and lymphoma cells carrying specific chromosomal translocations it is possible to isolate and characterize previously unrecognized genes that are involved directly in the neoplastic process in man (Fig. 4).

IV. CHROMOSOME TRANSLOCATION OCCUR AS MISTAKES DURING IMMUNOGLOBULIN GENE REARRANGEMENTS

Analysis of the chromosomal breakpoints involved in the t(11;14) and in the t(14;18) chromosome translocations have provided very important insights into the molecular mechanisms responsible for specific translocations in human B cells[11,12].

Analysis of the recombinant clones carrying the joinings between chromosomes 11 and 14 on the 14q+ chromosome of the leukemic cells in two cases of B-CLL indicated that in both cases the J_H segment of the heavy chain locus was involved in the rearrangement[11]. In Fig. 5 we compare the breakpoint sequences to the homologous sequences on normal chromosomes 11 and 14[11]. As shown in Fig. 5 the breakpoints on chromosome 11 in these two leukemias were separated by only 8 nucleotides, while the breakpoints on

152

chromosome 14 involved the 5' end of the heavy chain J_4 segment[11]. Interestingly, we observed stretches of extranucleotides at the joining sites that do not derive from either chromosome 11 and 14 (Fig. 5). The observation is of considerable importance, because Alt and Baltimore have previously described stretches of extranucleotides, for which they have proposed the name of N-regions, at joining sites in rearranged heavy chain genes[38]. These N-regions are presumably added by the enzyme terminal transferase (TdT)[38],

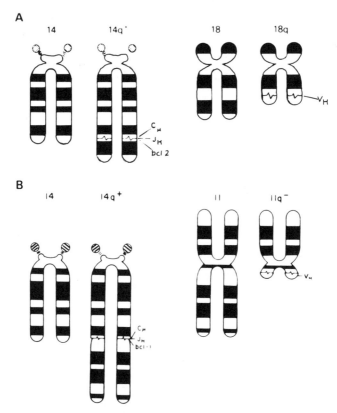

Figure 4.   Chromosome translocation in B cell lymphomas and leukemias of adults.   In follicular lymphomas with the t(14;18) translocation the bcl-2 gene, normally located on band q21 of chromosome 18 translocates to the heavy chain locus on chromosome 14 (A).   In lymphomas and leukemias with the t(11;14) translocation, the bcl-1 gene, normally located on band q13 of chromosome 11 translocates to the heavy chain locus chromosome 14 (B).

that is known to be expressed only in pre B and pre T cells. Thus this observation suggests that the t(11;14) chromosome translocations may be the result of mistakes in VDJ joining, where the VDJ joining enzyme joins separated segments of DNA on two different chromosomes instead of on the same chromosome[11,12].

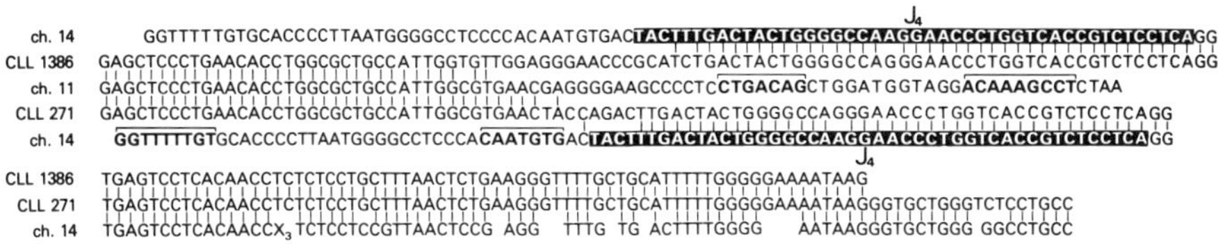

Figure 5. DNA sequences of the joining sites between chromosomes 11 and 14 in CLL 271, CDLL 1386 and of corresponding normal chromosome 11. Identical nucleotide sequences are shown by vertical lines. The boxed region indicates the J4 coding segment of the immunoglobulin heavy-chain gene. The DNA sequences shown by brackets on chromosome 14 indicate the conserved sequence 8mer-9mer.

It is known that the putative VDJ joining enzyme recognizes signal sequences that are heptamers and nonamers separated by a spacer of 12 nucleotides in the case of the 3' end of the diversity (D) segment and of 23 nucleotides in the case of the 5' end of the J_H segment of the heavy chain locus[39]. Thus, if the t(11;14) chromosome translocation is the result of a mistake in VDJ joining we should expect to observe a signal sequence (heptamer or nonamer) with a spacer of 12 nucleotides on normal chromosome 11 in close proximity to the breakpoints. As shown in Fig. 5, this is in fact the case[11]. Therefore, (i) since the breakpoints involve the 5' end of a J_H segment, (ii) since N-regions are present at joining sites and (iii) since signal sequences for VDJ joining are in close proximity to the breakpoints on chromosome 11, we conclude that the t(11;14) chromosome translocations are due to mistakes committed by the VDJ joining enzymes during immunoglobulin gene rearrangement at the pre B cell stage of differentiation[11].

Sequence analysis of t(14;18) chromosome breakpoints in follicular lymphomas and B cell leukemias carrying this translocation, indicated that this translocation is also the result of mistakes during the process of VDJ joining[12]. Furthermore, the fact that N regions are present at joining sites between chromosomes 14 and 18 sequences indicate that this translocation also accurs at the pre B cell stage of differentiation[12]. Then, why are follicular lymphoma cells mature B cells? Several possibilities may be considered to explain this paradox. Perhaps the substrate for the bcl-2 gene product is expressed at higher levels in mature B cells than in pre B cells. Another possibility is that enhancer strength is greater in mature than in pre B cells. Alternatively, an additional genetic change may occur in the involved B cells. This last possibility, however, does not explain why the malignant cells are mature B cells and not less-differentiated B cells.

V. INVOLVEMENT OF THE LOCUS FOR THE ALPHA CHAIN OF THE T CELL RECEPTOR IN
    HUMAN T CELL NEOPLASMS

By taking advantage of a mouse cDNA clone specific for the alpha chain of the T cell receptor, we have cloned the human homologous cDNA sequence and have mapped the human gene to chromosome 14 by using a panel of mouse x human somatic cell hybridids[40]. Using in situ hybridization, we then found that the locus maps at band 14q11[40]. This result is of considerable interest, because rearrangements, predominantly translocations and inversions, involving band 14q11 are very common in human T cell neoplasms[41]. Thus we speculated that in T cell leukemias and lymphomas with the inverted chromosome 14, inv(14) (q11;q32) or a t(14;14)(q11;q32) chromosome translocation the alpha chain gene may juxtapose to a putative oncogene normally located at band 14q32, for which we proposed the name of tcl-1[40].

Approximately 30% of human acute T cell leukemias (T-ALL) carry a t(11;14) (p13;q11) chromosome translocation[41]. To prove conclusively that the locus for the alpha chain of the T cell receptor is directly involved in the chromosome rearrangements observed in T cell neoplasms, we have hybridized mouse leukemic T cells with the leukemic cells of two patients with T cell ALL carrying this t(11;14) chromosome translocation[42]. The results of the analysis of the hybrids for the presence of human markers on chromosomes 11 and 14 and for the presence of specific human chromosomes are summarized in Table 1 and in Fig. 5. As shown in Fig. 6, the data indicated that the breakpoints directly involved the locus for the alpha chain of the T cell receptor[41]. Our results demonstrated that the genes for the variable regions ($V\alpha$) of the alpha chain of the T cell recpetor are proximal to the breakpoints, while the gene for the constant region ($C\alpha$) is distal[42]. Thus these results indicate that this locus is indeed involved in chromosome

Table 1.   Presence of the Vα and Cα Genes in Hybrids Between Mouse BW5147 Cells and Human T ALL Cells

Hybrids	Locus		Human Markers*					Human Chromosomes†			
	Vα	Cα	NP	LDH-A	c-H-ras	β-globin	bcl-1	14	14q-	11	11p+
517 A-A3	+	+	+	+	+	+	-	++	+++	-	-
517 B-D3	+	+	+	+	+	+	+	-	+	-	+
517 B-B1	-	-	-	+	+	+	+	-	-	-	+
517 B-A3	+	-	+	+	+	+	-	-	+	-	-
517 B-D3-G8	+	-	+	+	+	+	-	-	++	-	-
517 B-D3-G9	+	+	+	+	+	+	+	-	++	-	+++
517 B-DE-D2A	-	+	-	-	-	-	+	+	-	-	++
517 A-A3-A10	+	+	+	+	+	+	-	+	++	-	-
517 A-A3-G7	+	-	+	+	+	+	-	-	+++	-	-
515 BD2-CF3	+	-	+	+	+	+	-	-	+	-	-
515 BD2-CF6	+	-	+	+	+	+	-	-	+++	-	-

*NP, nucleoside phosphorylase; LDH-A, lactic dehydrogenase A. †Frequency of metaphases with relevant chromosomes; - = none; + = 10-30%; ++ = 30-50%; +++ = >50%. At least 25 metaphases were examined for each hybrid after trypsin-Giemsa staining. Selected metaphases were studied by the G11 technique to confirm the human origin or relevant chromosomes.

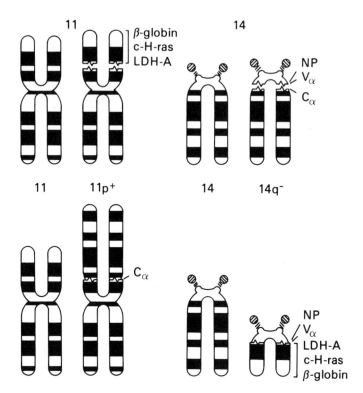

Figure 6.   The t(11;14)(q13;q11) translocation in ALL. The translocation breakpoint on chromosome 14 splits the locus for the alpha-chain of the T-cell receptor.   The Vα genes remain on the 14q⁻ chromosome, while the Cα genes translocate to the involved chromosome 11 (11p⁺). The gene for human nucleoside phosphorylase remains on the involved chromosome 14 (14q⁻). The genes LDH-A, β-globin, and c-H-<u>ras</u> translocate to the involved chromosome 14 (14q⁻).

rearrangements observed in T cell leukemia and lymphoma. We have also speculated that at band 11p13 there must be a putative proto-oncogene, for which we suggested the name of tcl-2, that is activated by its juxtaposition to the Cα locus[42].

This proposed mechanism of oncogene activation in T cell neoplasms through juxtaposition to the alpha locus of the T cell receptor is further supported by our recent investigation T cell leukemias carrying a t(8;14) (q24;q11) chromosome translocation[43]. By analyzing two independent cases we have shown that the breakpoints on human chromosome 8 are distal (3') to the c-myc oncogene[43] and that on chromosome 14 they involve directly the locus for the alpha chain of the T cell receptor[43]. Furthermore, analysis of the RNA produced by mouse-human hybrids derived from these tumors demonstrated that the c-myc oncogene juxtaposed to the translocated C alpha locus is deregulated and is transcribed constitutively at elevated levels[43]. Thus the mechanisms involved in the pathogenesis of human T cell neoplasms can closely parallel those observed in B cell neoplasia[43].

It is of considerable interest that leukemic T cells from patients positive for the human T cell leukemia virus (HTLV-1) often show the same chromosomal translocations involving the T locus that are present in HTLV-1 negative individuals[44]. This observation strongly suggests that the virus may play a role in the pathogenesis of these tumors by expanding the pool of T cells at risk for developing specific chromosomal translocations involving the locus for the alpha chain of the T cell receptor and cellular proto-oncogenes.

VI. CONCLUSIONS

Specific chromosomal translocation are involved in more than 80% of human B cell neoplasms. In all these cases the neoplastic phenotype is apparently the consequence of reciprocal chromosomal translocation involving the loci for human immunoglobulin chains and either well described cellular proto-oncogenes or putative proto-oncogenes. The juxtaposition of the proto-onco-genes to the immunoglobulin loci results in their transcriptional deregula-tion, because of their proximity to genetic elements within the human immuno-globulin loci capable of activating gene transcription in cis over consider-able chromosomal distances. Sequence analysis of the translocation break-points has provided important insights concerning the molecular mechanisms involved in chromosome translocation in B cells[32,39]. It appears that the reciprocal translocation contributing to B cell neoplasia are catalyzed by the same enzymes that are involved in physiological immunoglobulin gene rearrangements[32,39].

The analysis of human B cell leukemias and lymphomas has also provided considerable information concerning the possible scenarios for B cell neo-plastic transformation. It is clear that the Epstein Barr virus does not play a direct role in neoplastic transformation, but it may contribute by increasing the number of B cells at risk of developing chromosome translo-cations during immunoglobulin gene rearrangements[35].

Cytogenetic and molecular genetic analysis of T cell malignancies is beginning to provide a very similar scenario for neoplastic transformation.

158

The locus for the alpha chain of the T cell receptor is directly involved, and it apparently juxtaposes to proto-oncogenes or to putative proto-onco- genes leading to their transcriptional deregulation[43]. It seems quite likely that the enzyme system involved in rearrangements of the genes for the T cell receptor plays a cruicial role in the causation of these chromosomal translocations. Thus, the genetic basis of many human B and T may be quite similar. For the future, the challenge resides in trying to characterize specifically the role of both old and new proto-oncogenes in B and T cell proliferation, normal and neoplastic.

VII. REFERENCES

1. Nowell, P.C. and Hungerford, D.A. (1960) Science 132, 1497.
2. Rowley, J.D. (1973) Nature 243, 290.
3. Manolov, G. and Manolova, Y. (1972) Nature 237, 33.
4. Zech, L., Haglund, V., Nilsson, N. and Klein, G. (1976) Int. J. Cancer 17, 47.
5. Yunis, J. (1983) Science 221, 227.
6. Dalla Favera, R., Bregni, M., Erikson, J., Patterson, D., Gallo, R.C. and Croce, C.M. (1982) Proc. Natl. Acad. Sci. USA 79, 7824-7827.
7. DeKlein, A., van Kessel, A., Grosvel, G., Bartzam, C., Hagemeijer, A., Bootsma, D., Spurr, N., Heisterkamp, N., Groffen, J. and Stephenson, J. (1982) Nature 300, 765.
8. Groffen, J., Heisterkamp, N., Stephenson, J.R., van Kessel, A.G., DeKlein, A., Grosveld, G. and Bootsma, D (1983) J. Exp. Med. 158, 9.
9. Nishikura, K., ar-Ruishdi, A., Erikson, J., Watt, R., Rovera, G. and Croce, C.M. (1983) Proc. Natl. Acad. Sci. USA 80, 4822.
10. Croce, C.M., Theirfelder, W., Erikson, J., Nishikura, K., Finan, J., Lenoir, G. and Nowell, P.C. (1983) Proc. Natl. Acad. Sci. USA 80, 6922.
11. Tsujimoto, Y., Jaffe, E., Cossman, J., Gorham, J., Nowell, P.C. and Croce, C.M. (1985) Nature 315, 340.
12. Tsujimoto, Y., Gorham, J., Cossman, J., Jaffe, E. and Croce, C.M. (1985) Science 229, 1390.
13. Magrath, I., Erikson, J., Whang-Peng, J., Sieverts, H., Armstrong, G., Benjamin, D., Triche, T., Alabaster, I. and Croce, C.M. (1983) Science 222, 1094.
14. Douglass, E.C., Magrath, I.T., Lee, E.C., Whang-Peng, J. (1980) Blood 55, 148.
15. Croce, C.M., Shander, M., Martinis, J., Cicurel, L., D'Ancona, G.G., Dolby, T.W. and Koprowski, H. (1979) Proc. Natl. Acad. Sci. USA 76, 3416.

16. Erikson, J., Martinis, J. and Croce, C.M. (1981) Nature 296, 173.
17. McBride, D.W., Heiter, P.A., Hollis, G.F., Swan, D., Otey, M.C. and Leder, P. (1982) J. Exp. Med. 155, 1680.
18. Malcolm, S., Barton, P., Murphy, C., Fergusson-Smith, M.A., Bentley, D. L. and Rabbitts, T.H. (1982) Proc. Natl. Acad. Sci. USA 79, 4957.
19. Erikson, J., Finan, J., Nowell, P.C. and Croce, C.M. (1982) Proc. Natl. Acad. Sci. USA 79, 5611.
20. Dalla Favera, R., Martinotti, S., Gallo, R.C., Erikson, J. and Croce, C.M. (1983) Science 219, 963.
21. Watt, R., Staton, L.W., Marcu, K.B., Gallo, R.C., Croce, C.M. and Rovera, G. (1983) Nature 303, 725.
22. Watt, R., Nishikura, K., Sorrentino, J., ar-Rushdi, A., Croce, C.M. and Rovera, G. (1983) Proc. Natl. Acad. Sci. USA 80, 6302.
23. Erikson, J., Nishikura, K., ar-Rushdi, A., Finan, J., Emanuel, B.S., Lenoir, G., Nowell, P.C. and Croce, C.M. (1983) Proc. Natl. Acad. Sci USA 80, 7581.
24. Croce, C.M., Erikson, J., ar-Rushdi, A., Aden, D., Nishikura, K. (1984) Proc. Natl. Acad. Sci. USA 81, 3170.
25. Nishikura, K., Erikson, J., ar-Rushdi, A., Heubner, K. and Croce, C.M. (1985) Proc. Natl. Acad. Sci. USA 82, 2900.
26. ar-Rushdi, A., Nishikura, K., Erikson, J., Watt, R., Rovera, G and Croce, C.M. (1983) Science 222, 390.
27. Showe, L.C., Ballantine, M., Nishikura, K., Erikson, J., Kaji, H. and Croce, C.M. (1985) Mol. Cell. Biol. 5, 501.
28. Feo, S., ar-Rushdi, A., Huebner, K., Finan, J., Nowell, P.C., Clarkson, B. and Croce, C.M. (1985) Nature 313, 493.
29. Croce, C.M. and Nowell, P.C. (1985) Blood 65, 1.
30. Nowell, P.C., Shankey, T.V., Finan, J., Guerry, D. and Besa, E. (1981) Blood 57, 444.
31. Van den Berghe, H., Vermaelen, K., Louwagie, A., Criel, A., Mecucci, C. and Vaerman, J.P. (1984) Cancer Genet. Cytogenet. 11, 381.
32. Yunia J.J., Oken, M.M., Theologides, A., Howe, R.B. and Kaplan, M.E. (1984) Cancer Genet. Cytogenet. 604, 1.
33. Erikson, J., Finan, J., Rsujimoto, Y., Nowell, P.C. and Croce, C.M. (1984) Proc. Natl. Acad. Sci. USA 81, 4144.
34. Tsujimoto, Y., Yunis, J., Onorato-Showe, L., Erikson, J., Nowell, P.C. and Croce C.M. (1984) Science 224, 1403.

160

35. Pegoraro, L., Palumbo, A., Erikson, J., Falda, M., Giovanazzo, B., Emanuel, B.S., Rovera, G., Nowell, P.C. and Croce, C.M. (1984) Proc. Natl. Acad. Sci. USA 81, 7166.
36. Tsujimoto, Y., Yunis, J., Onorato-Showe, L., Nowell, P.C. and Croce, C.M. (1984) Science 224, 1403.
37. Tsukjimoto, Y., Cossman, J., Jaffe, E. and Croce, C.M. (1985) Science 228, 1440.
38. Desiderio, S.V., Yancopoulos, G.D., Paskind, M., Thomas, E., Boss, M.A., Landau, N., Alt, F.W., Baltimore, D. (1984) Nature 311, 752.
39. Tonegawa, S. (1983) Nature 302, 575.
40. Croce, C.M., Isobe, M., Palumbo, A., Puck, J., Erikson, J., Davis, M. and Rovera, G. (1985) Science 227, 1044.
41. Williams, D., Look, A.T., Melvin, S.L., Roberson, P.K., Dahl, G., Flake, T. and Strass, S. (1984) Cell 36, 101.
42. Erikson, J., Williams, D.L., Finan, J., Nowell, P.C. and Croce, C.M. (1985) Science 299, 784.
43. Erikson, J., Finger, K., Sun, L., ar-Rushdi, A., Nishikura, K., Minowada, J., Finan, J., Emanuel, B.S., Nowell, P.C. and Croce, C.M. (1986) Science, in press.
44. Sadamori, N., Kusana, M., Nishino, K., Tagawa, M., Yao, E., Yamada, Y.,Amagasaki, T., Kinoshita, K., Ichimuru, M. (1985) Cancer Genet. Cytogenet. 17, 279.

9

Involvement of Oncogene-Coded Growth Factors in the Neoplastic Process

Keith C. Robbins, C. Richter King, Neill A. Giese, Fernando Leal,
Hisanaga Igarashi and Stuart A. Aaronson

Laboratory of Cellular and Molecular Biology
National Cancer Institute
Bethesda, Maryland 20892

I. INTRODUCTION

Investigations of the genetic alterations that cause normal cells to become malignant have focused on a small set of cellular genes. Acute transforming retroviruses have substituted viral genes necessary for replication with discrete segments of host genetic information [1,2]. When incorporated within the retroviral genome, these transduced cellular sequences, termed onc genes, acquire the ability to induce neoplastic transformation. The discovery that independent virus isolates have recombined with the same or closely related cellular proto-oncogenes implies that only a limited number of cellular genes are capable of acquiring transforming properties.

The profound cellular alterations induced by activated cellular transforming genes have some similarities to those exhibited by cells in response to the growth promoting actions of hormones and growth factors. Each exerts pleiotropic effects on cellular metabolism, including the induction of sustained cell replication. Interest in understanding the actions of onc genes has led to concerted efforts to isolate, amplify, and sequence such genes. The present report summarizes investigations that have linked one oncogene to a cellular gene encoding a normal growth factor.

II. **Simian Sarcoma Virus.** Simian sarcoma virus (SSV) was isolated from a fibrosarcoma of a woolly monkey, and represents the only known sarcomagenic virus of primate origin[3]. The virus has been characterized in tissue culture[4], and its integrated DNA provirus has been cloned in infectious form[5] and sequenced[6]. Physical and biological characterization of its genome has localized its transforming gene to the cell-derived onc sequence, v-sis[7]. Moreover, antibodies prepared against small peptides derived from the v-sis sequence have been used to identify the 28,000 dalton v-sis gene product, p28^{sis}, in SSV transformed cells[6,7]. The molecular structure of SSV as well as the location and sequence of peptides used to prepare anti-p28^{sis} sera are shown in Figure 1.

III. **Predicted Amino Acid Sequence Homology Between p28^{sis} and Human Platelet-Derived Growth Factor.** Recent technological advances have led to a rapid proliferation of nucleotide sequence data, and thus predicted amino acid sequences for numerous proteins. Sequence data banks and computer programs have been developed in order to search for similarities among genes and the proteins they encode. By this approach, a segment of the predicted v-sis coded protein was shown to exhibit a high degree of match with the amino acid sequence of one peptide chain of human platelet-derived growth factor (PDGF)[8,9].

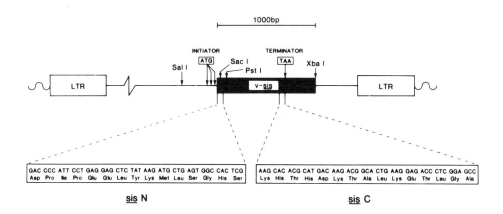

Figure 1. Major structural features of simian sarcoma virus (SSV) DNA. The cell-derived v-sis sequence of SSV is indicated as a darkened rectangle. Signals for translation of p28^{sis} are also indicated. The composition of sis-N and sis-C peptides was determined from the v-sis nucleotide sequence. LTR, long terminal repeat. bp, base pairs.

PDGF is a heat stable (100°C), cationic (pI, 9.8) protein[10]. It circulates in blood stored in the α granules of platelets and is released into serum during blood clotting[11]. It represents the major protein growth factor of human serum and is a potent mitogen for connective tissue and glial cells in culture[13,14]. Unreduced active PDGF exhibits multiple forms ranging in size from 28,000 to 35,000 daltons[10,15,16]. Reduction of PDGF produces inactive, smaller peptides ranging in size from 12,000 to 18,000 daltons[14,15].

Sequence analysis of the amino-terminal portions of both active human PDGF and its inactive, reduced peptides has revealed the presence of two homologous chains (PDGF-1 and PDGF-2) in PDGF preparations[17]. These peptides are identical at 8 of 19 positions near their amino termini, with no sequence gaps required for the homology alignment. Whether the active PDGF preparation is composed of a single protein formed by disulfide linkage of these two peptides or is composed of two proteins, each of which consists of a disulfidelinked homodimer is not yet known.

164

The predicted p28^{sis} sequence, starting at residue 67, demonstrated an
84% match to PDGF-2 over this same stretch. Furthermore, in the total of
70 PDGF-2 residues identified, 87.1% corresponded to the p28^{sis} sequence.
Taking into account the New World primate origin of v-sis[18], it was concluded that the v sis transforming gene arose by recombination between the
SSAV genome and a host cell gene for PDGF or a very highly related protein.
The observed amino acid differences between human PDGF-2 and v-sis could be
accounted for by the known degree of divergence between the genomes of
humans and cebids[19]. Moreover, a proteolytic cleavage signal (Lys-Arg)
is present at residues 65-66 in the p28^{sis} sequence, and the next residue
commences the homology between p28^{sis} and PDGF-2. Proteolytic processing
of p28^{sis} at or near residue 66 has been demonstrated to occur *in vivo*.
Presumably this cleavage removes an amino terminal peptide from the PDGF-2
related region of p28^{sis}[20].

IV. Mutagenesis of v-sis. Whereas the entire PDGF-2 sequence is encompassed within the v-sis gene product, there are three regions of p28^{sis}
which are unrelated to PDGF. These include the amino terminus of the transforming protein which is encoded by sequences derived from the helper virus
env gene as well as two v-sis cell-derived regions immediately flanking the
PDGF-2 homologous sequence. These distinct regions of predicted polypeptide
sequence suggest a multidomain structure for the v-sis transforming gene product.

Processing of the v-sis gene product in cells transformed by simian sarcoma
virus also reflects a multidomain structure. The primary v-sis translational
product, p28^{sis}, forms a dimeric structure soon after its synthesis and is
internally cleaved at both amino- and carboxy-terminal domains to yield a
protein analogous to a PDGF-2 dimer[20]. To determine the contributions of
these p28^{sis} domains to the transforming function(s) of the protein, we
subjected v-sis to *in vitro* mutagenesis.

The strategy for mutagenesis was based upon operational definition of
four regions of the sis transforming protein. As shown in Figure 2, these
included its helper virus env gene encoded amino terminus (A), its PDGF-2-
related region (C), and regions coded by the cell derived v-sis gene sequence
either upstream (B) or downstream (D) of the PDGF-2 coding sequence. Mutants
affecting each of these regions were constructed and analyzed by transfection
for their ability to transform NIH/3T3 cells[21].

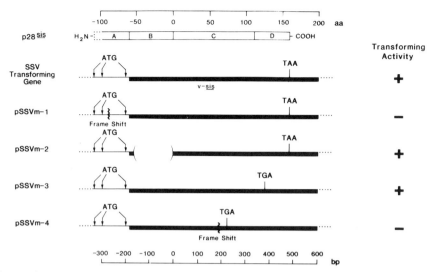

<u>Figure 2.</u> Structure of unaltered and mutant v-<u>sis</u> genes. The cell-derived v-<u>sis</u> sequences are shown schematically as heavy lines, and viral <u>env</u> gene-derived regions are indicated by thin lines. Potential translation initiation as well as translation termination codons for each mutant are shown. Codon locations are denoted based on the upstream boundary of the PDGF homologous region as position 0. Transforming activity refers to the ability of DNA clones to induce foci of transformation upon transfection of NIH/3T3 cells.

When regions of v-<u>sis</u> flanking the PDGF-2 coding sequence were removed, transforming activity was retained. Immunoprecipitation analysis of transformed cells containing pSSVm-2 or pSSVm-3 revealed a mutant v-<u>sis</u> gene product consistent in size with the each mutant's open reading frame. Moreover, both proteins formed dimer structures and were subsequently processed to a final product of 24,000 daltons. On this basis both final products were indistinguishable from the most mature form of the v-<u>sis</u> gene product, p24sis[21].

Nucleotide sequence comparison of the New World Primate-derived v-<u>sis</u> and human c-<u>sis</u> genes has revealed that their predicted amino acid sequences are more than 90% conserved in each of these two dispensible regions. This degree of evolutionary relatedness is greater than that observed for myoglobin[22] or fibrinopeptides A and B[23]. Thus, while these flanking sequences are dispensable for v-<u>sis</u> transforming activity, they may provide important function(s) in the maturation or storage of PDGF at its site of normal biosynthesis.

The fact that v-sis coded amino and carboxy terminal domains of p28sis are not necessary for transforming activity, implies that such activity must be localized within the PDGF-2-related domain. To test this possibility directly, we introduced a translation frame shifting mutation at codon position 66 localized within the PDGF-2-related coding sequence of v-sis (Fig. 2). This mutant, designated SSVm-4, did not induce focus formation upon DNA transfection.

By marker selection, we obtained cell populations containing SSVm-4 DNA. Immunoprecipitation analysis revealed a v-sis-coded gene product of 18,000 daltons which was specifically detected with anti-sis N serum. The electrophoretic mobility of this protein was identical whether analyzed under reducing or nonreducing conditions. These findings demonstrated that the PDGF-2-related domain of p28sis is required for SSV transforming activity and that v-sis coded amino acids between positions 62 and 128, not present in SSVm-4, must be necessary for dimer formation as well[21].

Other studies have shown that p28sis is synthesized on membrane bound polyribosomes and is immediately translocated across the endoplasmic reticulum membrane[24]. These studies have suggested the requirement of signal peptide coding sequences upstream of v-sis. As shown in Figure 2, mutation of the env gene sequence encoding the amino terminus of p28sis resulted in the loss of biologic activity. These findings are consistent with a recent report which described the requirement of this signal sequence for v-sis transformation[25]. The open reading frame of a cDNA clone derived from transcripts of the human sis proto-oncogene also predicts a signal-like peptide at an analogous position[26]. Thus, it is likely that processing of the normal human sis/PDGF-2 product, like that of its v-sis encoded counterpart, involves the use of a signal sequence for insertion into the endoplasmic reticulum.

V. Biosynthetic Pathway of the v-sis Gene Product. We have investigated the biosynthesis of the sis/PDGF-2 gene product in efforts to learn where this protein may interact with its cellular target(s). Our findings, summarized in Figure 3, document the biosynthetic pathway of the primary p28sis product. This protein is synthesized as a glycosylated precursor which dimerizes rapidly within the lumen of the endoplasmic reticulum to yield gp56sis. The unprocessed precursor then passes through the Golgi apparatus where its N-linked oligosaccharides are modified. After reaching a distal membrane location, processing of its amino and then its carboxy termini occurs, leading finally to a 24,000-dalton disulfide-linked dimer, p24sis.

Further localization studies have revealed that approximately 10% of total cellular v-sis-coded protein was detectable on the cell surface but that less than 1% could be found in cell culture fluids. Thus, the v-sis gene product is not quantitatively secreted from SSV-transformed cells[24].

Normal PDGF biosynthesis culminates with its storage in the alpha granules of platelets. Current understanding indicates that the Golgi apparatus is the site at which molecules are sorted for packaging or release. Our findings suggest that biosynthesis of the SSV transforming protein closely parallels that predicted for PDGF at least up to the point at which PDGF is packaged into granules. The peripheral membrane accumulation of the v-sis gene products in SSV-transformed fibroblasts may reflect the fact that fibroblasts lack differentiated functions required for normal storage of the molecule in granules.

As much as 10% of the steady-state levels of the v-sis gene product was detectable in physical association with the outer surface of the SSV-transformed cell membrane, indicating that some of the unprocessed dimer reaches an extracellular location. We have not yet determined which processing steps occur in association with the outer cell surface, nor have we identified the cell surface components to which the sis protein is bound. It is possible that some sis protein is nonspecifically extruded or released from the transformed cell and immediately sequestered at the cell surface. Another hypothesis derives from the novel synthesis of both the growth factor (sis/PDGF-2) and its receptor by the same cell. Known receptors for growth factors typically are synthesized in the endoplasmic reticulum and pass through the Golgi apparatus as they travel to the cell surface. Since the v-sis gene product exhibits this same biosynthetic pathway, this growth factor-like transforming protein may bind its receptor at a common intracellular location, with some of the complex reaching the cell surface.

Reports by several laboratories have documented the variable release of PDGF-like activity from certain SSV transformed cells (27-31). Whether the small amount of v-sis-coded protein released from SSV transformants can account for all of this PDGF-like activity remains to be determined. The fact that v-sis-coded proteins are not actively secreted does not exclude the possibility that those forms of the v-sis-coded protein released possess a very high specific activity for fibroblast mitogenesis. Alternatively, a novel PDGF-like growth factor distinct from the v-sis gene

168

product may be actively secreted from tissue culture cells in response to transformation by SSV. Such a hypothesis is consistent with reports that cells transformed by agents other than SSV also release a PDGF-like mito-gen[27,32]. In fact, SV40- and Ab-MuLV-transformed cells, which are among the highest secretors of such activity, lack detectable sis transcripts (unpublished observations). Approaches which involve purification and amino acid sequence analysis of the PDGF-like factors released from SSV transform-ed cells should aid in resolving this question.

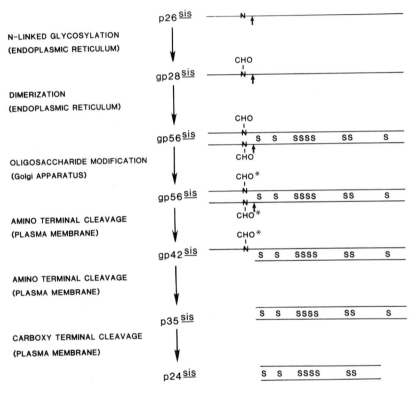

Figure 3. Summary of processing events affecting the v-sis translational product. Solid lines represent single polypeptide chains. N or S represent asparagine or cysteine residues, respectively. CHO and CHO* represent N-linked carbohydrate and modified N-linked carbohydrate, respectively.

Table 1. SSV Transforming Gene Product Possesses Fibroblast-Specific Mitogenic Activity

Mitogen	Protein added (µg)	Inhibiting peptide antibody[¶]	[³H]-thymidine incorporation[†]	
			BALB/MK	NIH/3T3
None	-	-	2,840	26,641
	-	sis-N	N.T.	29,125
	-	sis-N*	N.T.	27,555
SSV transformed cell membrane	20	-	2,976	497,111
protein	20	sis-N	2,676	244,023
	20	sis N*	2,702	484,275
	20	sis-C	2,462	110,260
	20	sis C*	2,814	486,970
Uninfected cell membrane protein	20	-	2,898	28,868
PDGF	0.003	-	2,485	255,621
EGF	0.001	-	195,320	362,514

*Indicates that antibodies were incubated with homologous peptide prior to inhibition study.

¶The amount of antibody required to precipitate all of the sis gene product recognized in membrane preparations was determined in parallel immunoprecipitation experiments using [³⁵S]-labeled HF/SSV cells as the source of membrane protein. The antibody concentration utilized was in two-fold excess.

†BALB/MK or NIH/3T3 cells were plated in 96 well culture dishes and grown to confluence without media changing. Sixteen hours after test samples were added, medium was supplemented with 2 µCi[³H]-Thymidine (New England Nuclear; specific activity 20 Ci/mmol) per well and incubated an additional 5 hr. Trichloroacetic acid insoluble material was measured by scintillation counting. EGF and PDGF receptor grades were purchased from Collaborative Research. Raw counts without substraction of background are shown.

N.T., not tested.

VI. The v-sis Gene Product Functions like PDGF. Utilizing SSV transformed cell membranes as the source of v-sis-coded protein, we have devised a
means of functionally characterizing cell-associated molecules that could
be unequivocally identified as products of the v-sis gene[33]. As shown
in Table 1, it was possible to demonstrate that v-sis translational products
synthesized by and associated with SSV transformed cells specifically induce
DNA synthesis in quiescent fibroblasts. Moreover, v-sis coded proteins
possessed the capacity to bind PDGF receptors and induce tyrosine phosphorylation of PDGF receptors. In each case, the v-sis coded nature of these
activities was established by specific inhibition with antibodies directed
against different regions of the v-sis gene product. These findings demonstrated that the SSV transforming protein is functionally equivalent to
PDGF.

In addition to the precursors, $p28^{sis}$, $p56^{sis}$, and $p42^{sis}$ which are recognized by anti-sis N serum, anti-sis C serum also detects $p35^{sis}$, a homodimer
species representing from 5-10% of the total v-sis gene product. By comparison of the residual PDGF-like activity following treatment by sis N and
sis C antiserum, we estimate that $p35^{sis}$ may be several-fold more active in
receptor competition or mitogenesis assays than less processed forms. All
of these studies established that processing at amino and carboxy termini
of this the $p56^{sis}$ dimer is not required for its PDGF-like functions,
although it appears that more mature forms may possess higher specific
activities[33].

VII. Evidence That SSV Transforming Activity Is Mediated By the PDGF
Receptor. As summarized above, v-sis translational products possess the
known functional activities of PDGF, including the ability to bind PDGF
receptors, stimulate PDGF receptor authophosphorylation, and induce DNA
synthesis of quiescent fibroblasts. If transformation by SSV were directly
mediated by the interaction of v-sis products with cellular PDGF receptors,
one should expect to observe a strict correlation between target cells
susceptible to SSV transformation and cell types possessing PDGF receptors.
To address this question, we investigated the ability of SSV to transform a
variety of cells in culture. We analyzed those cell types shown to possess
PDGF receptors, including fibroblasts and smooth muscle cells, as well as
cultures derived from epithelial or endothelial tissues, which lacked PDGF
receptors. As a control, we compared the transforming activity of SSV with
that of another acute transforming retrovirus, Kirsten-MSV, rescued by the
same helper virus.

Table 2. Susceptibility of Cell Types Which Possess or Lack PDGF
          Receptor to SSV Transformation

Tissue cell line	Presence of Surface PDGF Receptors	Transforming Activity	
		SSV	Ki-MSV
Fibroblast			
Mouse (NIH/3T3)	+	+	+
Human skin	+	+	+
Smooth muscle			
Bovine	+	+	+
Endothelial			
Bovine aorta	-	-	+
Epithelial			
Mink (MvlLu)	-	-	+

Biologic activity of rescued transforming virus was determined by direct focus or soft agar colony-forming assays. Foci or colonies were scored at 14-
21 days following infection.

As shown in Table 2, Kirsten-MSV efficiently transformed each of the target
cells analyzed. In contrast, SSV showed a more restricted pattern. We
observed high titered SSV transforming activity for fibroblasts and smooth
muscle cells. However, there was no discernible morphologic or detectable
growth alteration of either epithelial or endothelial cells in response to
SSV infection. The complete correlation between those assay cells susceptible to SSV transformation and those possessing PDGF receptors strongly
implies that SSV transforming activity is mediated by the obligatory interaction of its sis gene product with the PDGF receptor[33].

VIII. The Human sis Proto-Oncogene Is the Structural Gene For PDGF Polypeptide Chain 2. In view of the striking structural and functional similarities between human PDGF and the viral sis oncogene product, we have explored,
at the molecular level, the role of the human sis proto-oncogene in human
malignancies. In order to characterize the human sis/PDGF-2 locus, we isolated v-sis-related sequences from a bacteriophage library of normal human
DNA[34]. These clones represented a continuous stretch of approximately 30
kbp. By Southern blotting analysis and hybridization with a v-sis probe,
five v-sis homologous restriction fragments were identified within a 15-kbp
region. Nucleotide sequence analysis of the v-sis-related regions demonstrated that an open reading frame was contained within the first five c-sis
(human) exons. However, the 5'-most exon lacked a translation initiation

codon[34,35]. Thus, c-sis coding sequences are incompletely represented in SSV. This conclusion is further supported by the observation that a 4.2-kbp sis-related transcript is present in certain human tumor cells[36]. When the predicted c-sis (human) coding sequence was compared with that of the polypeptides representing PDGF-2, there was essentially complete homology[34,37,38]. These findings demonstrated that the c-sis (human) locus is the structural gene for PDGF-2.

IX. Expression Of the Normal Coding Sequence For Human sis/PDGF-2 Induces Cellular Transformation. The transcription of c-sis (human) was studied by using probes derived from introns and exons of the PDGF-2 gene. A 4.2-kb mRNA expressed in the A2781 human tumor cell line was detected by a v-sis probe and by c-sis probes representing each of the c-sis exons. The only other probe that hybridized to the same sized message was derived from a region 10 kbp upstream of the 5' most v-sis-related exon of human c-sis. This probe (pc-sis1) did not detect v-sis RNA, and thus might represent a non-sis-related exon of the c-sis transcriptional unit. Nucleotide sequence analysis of pc-sis1 was performed and revealed the presence of three open reading frames each of which was initiated by a methionine codon. Donor splice sites were found at positions within pc-sis1 that would allow for in-phase translation when spliced to the acceptor splice site in the first v-sis-related exon[39].

The DNA of a c-sis (human) phage clone, λ-c-sis clone 8, that contained all of the PDGF-2 coding sequences[34] was introduced into NIH/3T3 cells via transfection in order to study the structural requirements for c-sis gene expression. The sequences contained within λ c-sis clone 8 were incapable of transforming cells nor did they synthesize transcripts as determined by cotransfection experiments using a selectable marker gene (pSV2-gpt). Moreover, positioning a retroviral LTR upstream of the λ-c-sis clone 8 coding regions failed to confer transforming activity[39].

Since the putative upstream exon of c-sis (human) contained a potential amino terminal sequence for a PDGF/sis precursor, but not identifiable promoter signals, this segment was ligated in the proper orientation between the retroviral LTR and first exon of c-sis (human) clone 8. As shown in Figure 4, by transfection of NIH/3T3 cells with this molecular construct, transforming activity comparable to that of SSV DNA was observed (10^5 ffu/pmol)[39].

Transformants induced by the activated human sis/PDGF-2 coding sequence contained two major sis/PDGF-2 related protein species of 52,000 and 35,000 daltons, which were detected using anti-sis peptide serum and nonreducing

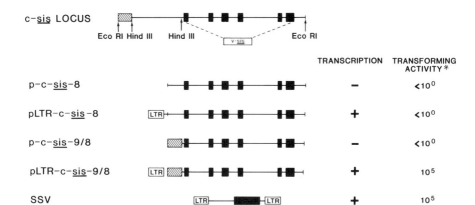

		TRANSCRIPTION	TRANSFORMING ACTIVITY*
p-c-<u>sis</u>-8		−	<10⁰
pLTR-c-<u>sis</u>-8	LTR	+	<10⁰
p-c-<u>sis</u>-9/8		−	<10⁰
pLTR-c-<u>sis</u>-9/8	LTR	+	10⁵
SSV	LTR LTR	+	10⁵

*Focus-forming units per pmol of PDGF-2 coding sequences

Figure 4. Expression of the normal PDGF-2 coding sequence in mouse fibroblasts induces morphologic transformation. Genomic DNA molecules cloned in
plasmid vectors were transfected onto NIH/3T3 cells and tested for transcriptional activation and transforming activity. A filled box indicates a c-sis/
PDGF-2 exon related to v-sis; a hatched box indicates the upstream c-sis/
PDGF-2 exon not related to v-sis; LTR, retrovirus long terminal repeat.

assay conditions. In contrast, a 26,000 dalton species, presumed to be the
primary translational product, was observed under reducing conditions. These
findings imply that the putative upstream exon sequences served to initiate
translation of a PDGF-2 precursor molecule, which underwent dimer formation
and subsequent processing. In light of the knowledge that the human sis gene
codes for PDGF-2 and our findings of highly efficient transforming activity by
the construct, we conclude that normal human PDGF-2 expressed in NIH/3T3 cells
is sufficient to induce transformation.

These studies have potentially important implications concerning the role
of normal genes coding for growth regulatory molecules in the neoplastic process. A number of growth promoting molecules have been shown to be released

by a variety of tumor cells[40-43]. In some cases, such molecules have been postulated to play a role in the neoplastic state of these cells. However, the alternative possibility exists that the expression of such factors is a secondary result of the genetic instability and dedifferentiated state known to exist in tumor cells.

Our findings establish that derepression of the coding sequence for a normal human growth factor can cause it to acquire transforming properties in an appropriate target cell. Moreover, when incorporated by a retrovirus, the v-sis/PDGF-2 transforming gene has been shown to induce fibrosarcomas and glioblastomas[44]. Many human glioblastomas and fibrosarcomas express sis/ PDGF-2 transcripts[36], whereas normal fibroblasts and glial cells so far analyzed do not. Thus, transcriptional activation of this gene could be involved in the induction of naturally occurring tumors of connective tissue origin. If so, it will be important to gain more detailed knowledge of the regulation of the human sis proto-oncogene in order to determine what mechanisms may lead to its transcriptional activation.

IX. REFERENCES

1. Bishop, J.M. (1982) in Ann. Rev. Biochemistry, Vol. 52, Snell, E.E., Boyer, P.D., Meister, A. and Richardson, C.C. eds., Academic Press, Palo Alto., 301-354.

2. Weiss, R.A., Teich, N., Varmus, H. and Coffin, R.J. (1983) in Molecular Biology of Tumor Viruses, RNA Tumor Viruses. 2nd edit., Cold Spring Harbor, New York.

3. Theilen, G.H., Gould, D., Fowler, M. and Dungworth, D.L. (1971) J. Natl. Cancer Inst. 47, 881-899.

4. Aaronson, S.A. (1973) Virol. 52, 562-567.

5. Robbins, K.C., Devare, S.G. and Aaronson, S.A. (1981) Proc. Natl. Acad. Sci. USA 78, 2918-2922.

6. Devare, S.G., Reddy, E.P., Law, J.D., Robbins, K.C. and Aaronson, S.A. (1983) Proc. Natl. Acad. Sci. USA 80, 731-735.

7. Robbins, K.C., Devare, S.G., Reddy, E.P. and Aaronson, S.A. (1982a) Science 218, 1131-1133.

8. Doolittle, R.F., Hunkapiller, M.W., Hood, L.E., Devare, S.G., Robbins, K.C., Aaronson, S.A. and Antoniades, H.N. (1983) Science 221, 275-277.

9. Waterfield, M.D., Scrace, G.T., Whittle, N., Stroobant, P., Johnsson, A, Wasteson, A., Westermark, B., Heldin, C.H., Huang, J.S. and Deuel, T.F. (1983) Nature 304, 35-39.

10. Antoniades, H.N., Scher, C.D. and Stiles, C.D. (1979) Proc. Natl. Acad. Sci. USA 76, 1809-1813.

11. Kaplan, D.R., Chao, F.C., Stiles, C.D., Antoniades, H.N. and Sher, C.D. (1979) Blood 53, 1043-1052.

12. Ross, R. Glomset, J., Karuya, B. and Harker, L. (1974) Proc. Natl. Acad. Sci. USA 71, 1207-1210.

13. Scher, C.D., Shepard, R.C., Antoniades, H.N. and Stiles, C.D. (1979) Biochim. Biophys. Acta 560, 217-241.

14. Heldin, C.H., Westermark, B. and Wasteson, A. (1979) Proc. Natl. Acad. Sci. USA 76, 3722-3726.

15. Heldin, C.H., Westermark, B. and Wasteson, A. (1981) Exp. Cell. Res. 136, 255-261.

16. Deuel, T.F., Huang, J.S., Proffit, R.T., Baenziger, J.U., Chang, D., and Kennedy, B.B. (1981) J. Biol. Chem. 256, 8896-8899.

17. Antoniades, H.N. and Hunkapiller, M.W. (1983) Science 220, 963-965.

18. Robbins, K.C., Hill, R.L. and Aaronson, S.A. (1982) J. Virol. 41, 721-725.

19. Wilson, A.C., Carlson, S.S. and White, T.J. (1977) Ann. Rev. Biochem. 46, 573-639.

20. Robbins, K.C., Antoniades, H.N., Devare, S.G., Hunkapiller, M.W. and Aaronson, S.A. (1983) Nature 305, 605-608.

21. King, C.R., Giese, N.A., Robbins, K.C. and Aaronson, S.A. (1985) Proc. Natl. Acad. Sci. USA 82, 5295-5299.

22. Dene, H., Sazy, J., Romero-Herrera, A.E. (1980) Biochim. Biophys. Acta 625, 133-145.

23. Wooding, G.L. and Doolittle, R.F. (1972) J. Hum. Evol. 1, 553-563.

24. Robbins, K.C., Leal, F., Pierce, J.H. and Aaronson, S.A. (1985) EMBO J. 4, 1783-1792.

25. Hannick, M. and Donoghue, D.J. (1984) Science 226, 1197-1199.

26. Josephs, S.F., Ratner, L., Clarke, M.F., Westin, E.H., Reitz, M.S. and Wong-Staal, F. (1984) Science 225, 636-639.

27. Bowen-Pope, D.F., Vogel, A. and Ross, R. (1984) Proc. Natl. Acad. Sci. USA 81, 2396-2400.

28. Owen, A.J, Pantazis, P. and Antoniades, H.R. (1984) Science (Wash.) 225, 54-56.

29. Huang, J.S., Huang, S.S., Deuel, T.F. (1984) Cell 39, 79-87.

30. Garrett, J.S., Coughlin, S.R., Niman, H.L, Tremble, P.M., Giels, G.M. and Williams, L.T. (1984) Proc. Natl. Acad. Sci. USA 81, 7466-7470.

31. Johnsson, A., Betsholtz, C., von der Helm, K., Heldin, C.-H. and Westermark, B. (1985) Proc. Natl. Acad. Sci. USA 82, 1721-1725.

32. Bleiberg, I., Harvey, A., Smale, G. and Grotendorst, G.R. (1985) J. Cell Physiol. 123, 161-166.

33. Leal, F., Williams, L.T., Robbins, K.C. and Aaronson, S.A. (1985) Science, in press.

34. Chiu, I.-M., Reddy, E.P., Givol, D., Robbins, K.C., Tronick, S.R. and Aaronson, S.A. (1984) Cell 37, 123-129.

35. Josephs, S.F., Dalla Favera, R., Gelmann, E.P., Gallo, R.C., and Wong-Staal, F. (1984) Science 219, 503-505.

36. Eva, A., Robbins, K.C., Andersen, P.R., Srinivasan, A., Tronick, S.R., Reddy, E.P., Ellmore, N.W., Galen, A.T., Lautenberger, J.A., Papas, T.S., Westin, E.H., Wong-Staal, F., Gallo, R.C. and Aaronson, S.A. (1982) Nature 295, 116-119.

37. Johnsson, A., Heldin, C.-H., Wasteson, A., Westermark, B., Devel, T.F., Huang, J.S., Seeburg, P.H., Gray, A., Ullrich, A., Scrace, G., Stroobant, P. and Waterfield, M.D. (1984) EMBO J. 3, 921-928.

38. Josephs, S.F., Guo, C., Ratner, L. and Wong-Staal, F. (1984) Science 223, 487-490.

39. Gazit, A., Igarashi, H., Chiu, I.-M., Srinivasan, A., Yaniv, A., Tronick, S.R., Robbins, K.C. and Aaronson, S.A. (1984) Cell 39, 89-97.

40. DeLarco, J.E. and Todaro, G.J. (1978) Proc. Natl. Acad. Sci. USA 75, 4001-4005.

41. Heldin, C.H., Westermark, B., and Wateson, A. (1980) J. Cell. Physiol. 105, 235-246.

42. Nister, M., Heldin, C.H., Wateson, A. and Westermark, B. (1982) Ann. N. Y. Acad. Sci. 397, 25-33.

43. Graves, D.T., Owen, A.J. and Antoniades, H.N. (1983) Cancer Res. 43, 83-87.

44. Wolfe, L.G., Deinhardt, F., Theilen, G.J., Rabin, H., Kawakami, T. and Bustad, L.K. (1971) J. Natl. Cancer Inst. 47, 1115-1120.

10

Serum-Free Selection of Onc Genes

Alan H. Beggs and George A. Scangos

Department of Biology
and Program in Human Genetics
The Johns Hopkins University
Baltimore, Maryland 21218

I. INTRODUCTION

In the past few years significant progress has been made in the understanding of the genetics of neoplasia as a result of two distinct but complementary methodologies: the study of retroviruses, and the transfer of
tumor DNA into NIH/3T3 cells. Despite the major advances made by these
techniques, they are subject to some limitations which are becoming increas-
ingly apparent. For example, although DNA from some human tumors is capable
of generating transformed foci of NIH/3T3 cells[1-9], approximately 80% of
human tumors and tumor cell lines tested are inactive in this assay[1-3,8].
Additionally, where the genes responsible for the transformation have been
identified, they have been predominantly of the _ras_ gene family[1-7], with
B-lym, T-lym, MNNG-HOS and neu more recently detected[10-13]. Consequently
little is known of the genetic or epigenetic changes which have occurred in
most human tumors. The standard focus forming assay is limited additionally
in that what is measured is a soft phenotype; i.e. loss of contact inhibition
does not provide insight into biochemical changes induced by onc genes.

There are many constraints on the types of genes which may be detected in
the NIH-3T3 focus forming assay: The genes must act dominantly; they must
not be so large that they are fragmented in the DNA isolation and transfection protocols; they must not be subject to species- or tissue-specific constraints which render them inactive in the recipient cells; the gene product
must be active and possess suitable targets in the recipient cells; a single copy of the gene must be capable of effecting transformation since the
transfer of multiple copies via genomic DNA is unlikely; the genes must not
repeat changes which are pre-existent in the recipient cells; and finally
the genes must induce focus formation. Thus, it is not surprising that many
tumor DNAs are negative in this assay.

Several groups have developed an alternative assay whereby 3T3 cells transfected with tumor DNA are injected into nude mice[14,15]. This protocol has
been successful in identifying several genes which would not have been detected by the standard focus forming assay. Thus, these genes were selected on
the basis of their ability to confer tumorigenicity to recipient cells.

In this chapter, we describe a novel selective system which we have developed to characterize a number of known onc genes representative of different
classes, and which may be useful for isolation of novel genes from tumors.
The selective system distinguishes transformed from non-transformed cells on
the basis of their respective freedom from and requirement for exogenous
peptide growth factors. We are using a serum-free medium developed by

McClure and coworkers[16,17]. This defined medium can be used to characterize the loss of specific requirements for growth factors and to directly identify genes in tumors which confer growth factor-independence. Several lines of evidence indicate that the genes detected by this system form a distinct and partially overlapping set with those detected by the focus forming assay, so that some of the genes which contribute to the transformed phenotype of human tumors and tumor cell lines but which do not induce focus formation may be detected. An addditional benefit to the use of defined media is that a more precise biochemical understanding of the role of the onc gene proteins can be gained in it than in complete medium containing serum.

The relationship of growth factors to oncogenesis was recognized many years ago by Temin, Todaro, and their coworkers[18,21]. The relationship of growth factors to onc genes has become clearer over the past year or two. Growth factors regulate the passage of normal cells through the cell cycle[22,23]. A common and fundamental property of many transformed cells is the lack of growth factor requirements, which at least partially explains their loss of growth control[19,23-27]. The peptide growth factors active on fibroblasts have been classified as competence factors [platelet-derived growth factor (PDGF), fibroblast growth factor (FGF)] or progression factors (insulin and the insulin-like growth factors IGF-I and IGF-II) on the basis of a growth stimulation assay using quiescent, contact inhibited cells[23]. The action of these factors was synergistic under these conditions, with Balb/C 3T3 cells requiring stimulation by factors from both groups in order to initiate DNA synthesis. In contrast, epidermal growth factor (EGF) has been classified in a separate group along with the transforming growth factor type-alpha[22]. Loss of growth control could occur as a result of inappropriate expression of these factors, because of altered receptors, or because of changes in the intracellular system which transduces the signal into DNA replication.

The finding that residues 67-175 of the virally-derived onc gene sis were virtually identical to the N-terminal 109 amino acids of the B chain of PDGF[22,28,29] clearly demonstrated the relationship between onc genes and growth factors. Sis is capable of inducing focus formation of NIH/3T3 cells[30] and the addition of PDGF to contact-inhibited cells results in a transient transformed phenotype[31,32], suggesting that the two proteins have similar activities. Furthermore, some tumor cell lines, including osteosarcoma and glioma derived lines secrete a mitogenic peptide very similar to PDGF[33-35].

A similarly dramatic finding was the demonstration that the onc gene erbB was similar to the intracellular and transmembrane domains of the EGF receptor[36]. Since the erbB protein appears similar to a truncated EGF receptor, it has been speculated that the lack of a regulatory EGF-binding domain may turn the protein constitutively on, thus contributing to the transformed phenotype[22]. More recently, the c-fms proto-onc gene has been shown to be closely related to the receptor for macrophage growth factor CSF-1[37]. The PDGF, EGF and insulin receptors have protein kinase activity[38-44], a property shared by a class of onc genes[22]. Growth factor receptors as well as some onc gene products such as abl[45], src[46] and fps[47] are membrane-associated proteins. These data, supported by nucleotide and protein sequence analyses[22] suggest structural and functional relationships between growth factor receptors and the tyrosine kinase family of onc genes.

One interesting class of growth factors are the transforming growth factors (TGFs). TGF-alpha, orginally detected in Moloney murine Sarcoma Virus transformed cells[18] is synthesized by a large number of human and rodent transformed cells[48-50]. TGF-alpha binds to the EGF receptor[51] and is placed in the same growth factor family as EGF[52]. TGF-alpha can stimulate the growth of fibroblasts in medium devoid of EGF and PDGF[28], and is required in conjunction with TGF-beta and PDGF for the growth of cells in soft agar[53,54].

Finally, the nuclear onc genes such as myc[55,56] and fos[57,59] may represent steps in the transduction of signals from the growth factor-receptor to the nucleus so that their inappropriate expression may mimic a constitutive "on" state and thus contribute to oncogenesis. Armelin et al.[60] have demonstrated that myc was an intracellular mediator of the PDGF-induced growth response. Futhermore, both myc and fos have been shown to be transcribed soon after stimulation of fibroblasts by PDGF[61-63].

These data taken together clearly demonstrate that inappropriate expression or structural alterations of growth factors, growth factor receptors, or intracellular machinery involved in transducing the growth factor signals, could and probably does contribute to the transformed phenotype. One of the characteristics of cells which possess altered genes in these pathways may be that they no longer require one of more growth factors for cell division. Selection for genes which confer growth factor-independence on NIH-3T3 cells may detect altered genes in the DNA of human tumors and tumor cell lines. Furthermore, a determination of the ability of known onc genes to relieve growth factor requirements will add to the understanding of onc gene function.

II. MATERIALS AND METHODS

A. Serum-free media preparation.

McClure's Serum-Free (MSF) medium was prepared essentially as described[17] with a few minor modifications. Three 1 liter packets of DME (GIBCO #430-2100) and one 1 liter packet of Ham's F-12 (GIBCO #430-1700) were combined with 4.8g sodium bicarbonate, 1.6g L-histidine, 80ml of 0.75M HEPES (pH 7.9), 0.2ml 1M 2-aminoethanol, and 40μl 5×10^{-4}M sodium selenite in 4 liters of laboratory grade deionized water. This basal medium was filter sterilized through a 0.22μm millipore filter using a 5% CO_2 positive pressure filtration apparatus and stored up to one month at 4°C. At use, the medium was supplemented with 2mM L-glutamine, 50U/ml penicillin, 50μg/ml streptomycin, 100μg/ml kanamycin sulfate (all GIBCO) and appropriate protein additives. Aliquots of insulin and FGF (both from Collaborative Research) were stored at -70°C as 100X stocks (200 g/ml and 2500 g/ml respectively). Human transferrin (Sigma Chem. Co.) was stored at -20°C as a 100X stock of 500μg/ml. Oleic acid/BSA was not used. Instead, linoleic acid/BSA (Collaborative Research) was used occasionally at a final concentration of 2.5μg/ml of linoleic acid.

B. Cell culture.

NIH/3T3 cells, orginially derived in the laboratory of G. Todaro, were maintained at 37°C under 5% CO_2/95% air in alpha-MEM supplemented with 10% calf serum (CS), L-glutamine, and antibiotics (all GIBCO). Fresh cultures were initiated from frozen stocks every few months. The human and mouse tumor cell lines SK-HEP-1 (ATCC HTB 52), Wiltu-1 (ATCC HTB 50) and C127 (ATCC CRL 1616), were obtained from the American Type Culture Collection, and the SV40-transformed human fibroblasts (GM4429A) were obtained from L. Grossman. All of these cell lines were carried under conditions recommended by the supplier.

C. Growth curves.

Growth curves were carried out by plating $1-2 \times 10^4$ cells in growth medium with serum into triplicate 60mm Petri dishes which had a 5mmx5mm grid (in 1mm increments) scratched in the bottom. After attachment, the cells were washed extensively with phosphate buffered saline (PBS) and fed experimental medium. Cells were fed fresh medium every two days and time points were obtained by counting the number of cells within the grid using a phase concrast microscope. To obtain the last time point, the plates were trypsinized and cells were counted in a hemacytometer. Growth was expressed as the ratio of cell number at time x to time zero (Nx/No).

D. ^{3}H-thymidine incorporation.

Incorporation of tritiated thymidine was measured in an assay adapted from Shipley and Ham[64]. 10^5 cells per well were plated in Falcon 24-multiwell plates in Dulbeccos Modified Egale Medium with 10% CS and allowed to remain confluent for two days. On day three, the wells were washed with PBS and the cells were incubated with MSF plus transferrin for six hours. Medium was removed and fresh MSF with transferrin and experimental supplements plus 1μCi/ml tritiated methyl thymidine (40-60Ci/mmole, Amersham) was added. At the end of a 24 hour labeling period, the medium was removed and the wells were washed twice with 1ml PBS. Following the wash, 75μl of PBS were added to each well and the cells were harvested by swabing the wells with cotton tipped applicators. Incorporated counts were then precipitated onto the cotton fibers by immersing the applicators in 10% trichloroacetic acid (TCA) for 20 minutes and 5% TCA for 10 minutes, both at 4°C. Following a 15 minute rinse in 95% ethanol, the cotton tips were air dried and counted in Aquasol (New England Nuclear) in a Beckman model LS100C liquid scientillation counter. All points were done in quadruplicate.

E. Plasmids.

Plasmids DNA was isolated by the method of Guerry et al.[65]. Plasmids p9.1[66] and H-1[67] (provided by T. Papas) contain the genomes of avian myelocytomatosis virus (MC29) and Harvey murine sarcoma virus respectively. Plasmid pSSV-11[30] (from K. Robbins) contains a proviral clone of simian sarcoma virus. Finally pdBPV-1 (142-6), which contains the genome of bovine pappiloma virus (BPV) type 1, was kindly provided by P. Howley[68].

F. Gene transfer assay.

NIH/3T3 cells were plated at 3×10^5 cells per 100mm Petri dish one day prior to transfer. 0.01-1.0μg plasmid DNA and 30μg salmon sperm carrier DNA were coprecipitated onto the cells by the calcium phosphate technique[69]. One day later, the cells were washed with PBS and fed selective medium. The medium was changed every 2-3 days for 2-3 weeks after which the cells were fixed with 70% ethanol and stained with 0.5% crystal violet.

III. CHARACTERIZATION OF MCCLURE'S SERUM-FREE MEDIUM

A. Rationale.

To characterize the growth factor requirements of transformed cells and to develop an alternative to the standard NIH/3T3 cell focus forming assay, we characterized a serum-free, defined medium developed by McClure and coworkers[16,17]. McClure reported that Balb/C 3T3 cells grew well in this medium when it was supplemented with fibroblast growth factor (FGF), insulin, and transferrin, but failed to grow when the FGF was removed. SV40-transformed 3T3 cells, in contrast, had lost their FGF-dependence[17]. This medium, which we have termed MSF (McClure's Serum Free) medium seemed to provide the basis for a selective system based on growth factor independence. The rationale was that if a given onc gene was capable of conferring growth factor independence, then cells transfected with that gene might grow in MSF medium lacking FGF, insulin, or both. In order to determine if the medium was suitable, we tested the ability of NIH/3T3 cells and several contact-inhibited and density-indendent cell lines to grow in the medium.

B. Growth of tumor cell lines in MSF medium.

To determine the spectrum of cell types capable of growth in MSF medium, and to assay for the lack of an FGF requirement, we performed growth curves on an SV40 transformed human fibroblast line from a patient with xeroderma pigmentosum (GM4429A)[70] and several tumor cell lines (Fig. 1). Growth in alpha-MEM with 5 or 10% fetal bovine serum (FBS) was compared to growth in MSF supplemented with 2μg/ml insulin and 5μg/ml transferrin (MSF-IT). The SV40 transformed line (GM4429A) grew quite well in the absence of FGF, indicating that MSF supports the growth of human as well as murine SV40 transformed cell lines. These cells exhibited a slightly lower saturation density in MSF but were capable of continuous proliferation in this medium for at least several weeks. SK-HEP-1, a human hepatoma line[71], is another example of a cell line capable of extended growth in the absence of FGF. After a short lag time, these cells grew in MSF-IT at virtually the same rate as in the presence of 10% FBS. In contrast, Wiltu-1, derived from a Wilms tumor[72], ceased growth after one day in MSF-IT. These cells rapidly became quiescent and after five or six days in this medium, they began to die and slough off. This line is contact inhibited and it does not form tumors in nude mice, however, it is clearly an established line with mutliple chromosome abnormalities. The karyotype has been reported to be hypodiploid to hyperdiploid including large subtelocentric and large telocentric marker chromosomes[72].

Both SK-HEP-1 and GM4429A were density independent for growth and capable of forming foci. In contrast, C127, a mouse adenocarcinoma line, is strongly contact inhibited, and in fact, these cells are often used as recipients in a focus forming assay for bovine papilloma virus[73]. Initially, these cells grew slowly in MSF-IT, but after several passages in this medium, they grew with a doubling time of 25 hours in MSF-IT and 22 hours in alpha-MEM with

184

5% FBS (Fig. 1). Throughout these experiments, they remained contact inhibited. This was important because it illustrated the point that loss
of contact inhibition and the ability to grow without FGF are not equivalent phenotypes. Thus, selection for transformed cells in media lacking
FGF may yield contact inhibited, but growth factor independent, cells which
would not be detected in the standard focus forming assay.

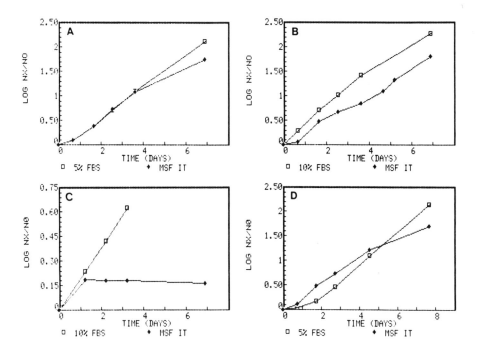

Figure 1. Growth curves of SV40 transformed human fibroblasts and murine
and human tumor cell lines in MSF-IT and alpha-MEM plus FBS. A, GM4429A.
B, SK-HEP-1. C, Wiltu-1. D, C127.

C. NIH/3T3 cells provide a defined system in which to study the loss of growth factor requirements.

Since we wished to examine the action of specific onc genes in relieving growth factor requirements, we needed a cell system with a defined set of requirements. Stiles et al.[23] have shown that for optimal growth, Balb/C 3T3 fibroblasts require two classes of growth factors, termed competence and progression factors. To determine if our NIH/3T3 cells maintained similar requirements, we tested their growth in MSF medium in the presence of absence of insulin (a progression factor) and varying amounts of FGF (a competence factor). A dose response curve for FGF with or without 2μg/ml insulin revealed that these cells have an absolute requirement for FGF and a less stringent requirement for insulin (Fig. 2). In the absence of FGF, the cells became quiescent within two days and eventually sloughed off and died. The rate of cell death was density dependent, with sparse cells dying off faster than dense ones.

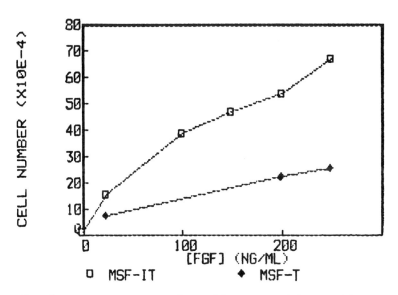

Figure 2. Dose response curve for cell growth with or without insulin in the presence of varying amounts of FGF. 1x10^4 NIH/3T3 cells were plated in duplicate 35mm Petri dishes in medium with 10% CS. After attachment, cells were washed extensively and fed MSF-IT or MSF-T (MSF with 5μg/ml transferrin) and FGF as indicated. Cells were fed every two days for seven days after which they were trypsinized and counted in a hemacytometer. Data are plotted as average number of cells per dish.

The assay described above, was done using growing cells actively traversing the cell cycle while the original experiments of Stiles et al.[23] were performed on quiescent cells. To determine if there was any difference in the effects of insulin and FGF on growing versus quiescent 3T3 cells, we measured the amount of ^{3}H-thymidine incorporated in contact inhibited quiescent cells fed with FGF and/or insulin (Table 1). Again, the cells exhibited a stringent requirement for FGF while the removal of insulin resulted in roughly a two-fold reduction in ^{3}H-thymidine incorporation. Thus, our NIH/3T3 cells required both competence (FGF) and progression (insulin) factors for optimal growth in MSF medium. The removal of either one or the other resulted in a detectable reduction in the growth capacity of cells in that medium. Other experiments have shown that removal of transferrin had no apparent effect on cell growth in our assays, however, this component was included in most experiments in order to ensure optimal conditions for growth.

Table 1. Effects of removing FGF and insulin on DNA synthesis in quiescent NIH/3T3* cells.

Factors Present[#]	Factors Missing	Incorp. CPM + SE[†]
10% Calf serum	None	67,295 + 2230
FGF & Insulin	None	87,870 + 5804
FGF	Insulin	45,125 + 2315
Insulin	FGF	3,895 + 258
None	FGF & Insulin	2,935 + 134

*The cells used in this experiment were previously transfected with pBR322 and pSV2neo[80]. Their growth factor requirements were indistinguishable from those of the parental NIH/3T3 cell line.
#FGF = 25µg/ml, insulin = 2 µg/ml.
†SE = Standard error.

IV. A GENE TRANSFER ASSAY TO DETECT ONC GENES WHICH RELIEVE GROWTH FACTOR REQUIREMENTS.

To determine if MSF medium was a suitable selective system, and to gain insight into the function of known onc genes, serum-free selection was used to characterize the growth factor requirments of NIH/3T3 cells transfected with plasmids containing various viral genomes. In these experiments, plasmids containing avian myelocytomatosis virus MC29 (myc), Harvey murine sarcoma

virus (H-ras), and simian sarcoma virus (sis) proviral genomes, as well
as bovine papilloma virus were applied to NIH/3T3 cells. Plasmid pBR322
provided a baseline for the frequency of spontaneous transformants. Growth
in alpha-MEM + 5% FBS was used to select for loss of contact inhibition and
focus formation while MSF-IT and basal MSF selected, respectively, for independence from FGF or from insulin and FGF.

Figure 3 illustrates differences between the morphology of foci generated
in media with serum and colonies selected in MSF medium. Note that while

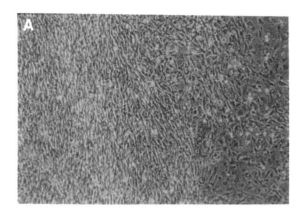

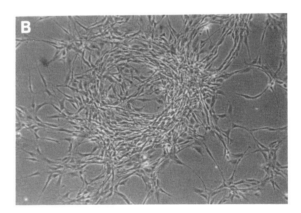

Figure 3. Phase contrast micrographs of a representitive focus grown in
alpha-MEM + 5% FBS (A) and a representitive colony selected in MSF-IT (B)
NIH/3T3 cells were transfected with plasmid H-1 containing a vH-ras gene.

focus formation occurs on a background of quiescent contact inhibited cells, selection in MSF kills off nontransformed cells leaving isolated colonies of transformed ones. The morphology of these colonies varies from fully contact inhibited and flat to density independent and highly refractile.

In one gene transfer experiment, pSSV-11, containing a v-sis gene, induced an average of 20 and 34 colonies per plate when transformants were selected in MSF-IT and MSF-T respectively. However, addition of 2.5 μg/ml linoleic acid/BSA to MSF-IT resulted in a complete absence of colony formation. We attribute this to the fact that BSA inhibits attachment of cells to the dish[17] resulting in the loss of dividing cells when the plates are fed. Therefore, we conducted all other experiments without using the linoleic acid/BSA supplement.

The four viral constructs tested each had a distinct response in the different selective systems employed (Fig. 4). Plasmid p9.1, which contains a myc gene, was negative for focus formation and the ability to induce FGF independence. Plasmid pdBPV-1(142-6), on the other hand, was positive in the focus forming assay but did not confer FGF-independence. H-1, containing an H-ras gene, was equally proficient at inducing focus formation and FGF independence. Removal of insulin and transferrin as well as FGF consistently reduced the number of macroscopic colonies 4-5 fold. By contrast, pSSV-11 was equally active in all three conditions, and showed no apparent insulin/transferrin requirement. Equal numbers of colonies were generated by sis regardless of the presence of absence of insulin and transferrin (Fig. 4).

Plasmid H-1 contains the Harvey murine sarocma virus (Ha-MuSV) genome. Our data show that the vH-ras gene was efficient at transforming 3T3 cells to FGF independence. The greater number of colonies in MSF-IT when compared to alpha-MEM + 5% FBS is probably due to satellite colony formation since the vH-ras transformed cells are less adherent in MSF than in complete medium. In contrast to plates transfected with v-sis, the vH-ras transfected plates have strikingly fewer colonies when selected in basal MSF (Fig. 4). If scored under a dissecting microscope, many small colonies of less than 50 cells were seen, although, upon extended incubation of these plates the colonies did not continue to grow. We interpret this to mean that while insulin and transferrin have no effect on the efficiency of initial transformation by vH-ras, their absence caused cells to grow much more slowly or abort after a limited number of divisions. Growth curve and ^{3}H-thymidine incorporation studies on H-ras transfected cells selected in serum indicate that the limiting factor for these cells in insulin (Beggs and Scangos, submitted). The ability of H-ras transfected cells to form colonies in medium

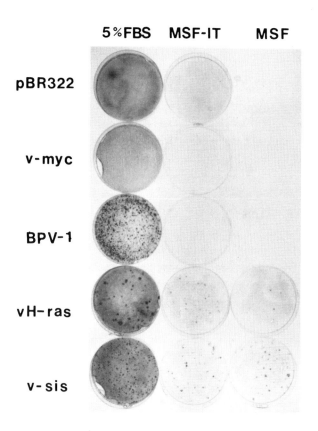

5%FBS MSF-IT MSF

pBR322

v-myc

BPV-1

vH-ras

v-sis

Figure 4. Focus and colony forming ability of various viral constructs in complete medium or MSF medium lacking FGF or FGF and insulin. NIH/3T3 cells were transfected with plasmids containing the indicated onc genes as described in Materials and Methods. Plates were stained and photographed after three weeks of growth in the indicated medium.

lacking insulin may be dependent on the dosage of the ras gene product, p21. To examine this question, were currently assaying transformants selected under the various conditions for levels of p21 expression.

Recently, several groups have shown that there is extensive homology between the sis gene of simian sarcoma virus and the PDGF β-chain[28,29]. Since then, sis transformed cells have been shown to secrete a mitogen with properties very similar to those of PDGF[74,75]. As illustrated in Figure 4, cells transfected with pSSV-11[30] formed foci and colonies with approximately equal facility in all conditions tested. These data suggest that, in addition to FGF independence, sis transformation also induced insulin independence. This interpretation is supported by growth curves on isolated transformants which demonstrate that the insulin requirement of NIH/3T3 cells is abolished by sis transformation (Beggs and Scangos, submitted). Furthermore, growth curve studies by ourselves (unpublished data) and others[76] suggest that PDGF partially relieves the insulin requirement of growing fibroblasts. Clemmons et al.[77] have shown that PDGF induces human fibroblasts to secrete endogenous somatomedin C (EGF I). A similar mechanism could explain the apparent loss of the insulin requirement in sis transformed NIH/3T3 cells.

Bovine papilloma virus [pdBPV-1 (142-61)] was very efficient at inducing foci in the presence of serum (Fig. 4). Dvoretzky et al.[78] have shown that BPV-1 infected 3T3 and C127 cells will form foci, grow in soft agar, and form tumors in nude mice. In addition, BPV-1 transformed C127 cells exhibited significantly better growth in 3% serum than their nontransformed counterparts. Thus, by several stringent criteria, BPV-1 infected fibroblasts are fully transformed. Our serum free colony forming assay, however, clearly demonstrates that transformation by BPV-1 did not alter the stringent requirement for FGF. The growth factor requirement of BPV-1 transformed cells may be related to the fact that BPV induces primarily benign fibro-papillomas in cattle[79].

C127 cells and BPV-1 transformed 3T3 cells represent complementary subsets of the transformed phenotype. C127 cells were contact inhibited but capable of FGF independent growth. Conversely, BPV-1 transformation relieved contact inhibition without affecting the FGF requirement. This dissociation of FGF independence from loss of contact inhibition supports the notion that these two traits may be under separate control in some transformed cell lines.

Plasmid p9.1 contains the integrated proviral genome of avian myelocy-tomatosis virus (MC29)[66]. Using this construct, we were unable to detect biological activity in our assay (Fig. 4). This may reflect a true lack of activity by myc or alternatively, it may be a property of the particular construct used. A recent report has successfully demonstrated myc activity in PDGF free medium[60], but only after construction of myc genes under the control of strong promoters. These data suggest that the inactivity of our construct may have been due to insufficient levels of myc protein and that other myc constructs might be active in the medium.

Recently, we have conducted similar experiments using plasmids containing transformation defective and helper viruses without active onc genes. No

detectable activity was observed for any of these constructs under any conditions indicating that the action of the viral clones represented activity
of the onc genes they carry and not a nonspecific effect of the viral LTRs
(Beggs and Scangos, submitted).

V. SUMMARY

We have described the development of a selective system useful for the
identification and characterization of onc genes capable of conferring
growth factor independence. The use of defined, serum-free media allows us
to select for transformed cells which have lost specific growth factor requirements. We have used this system to show that several cloned onc genes
generate different transformed phenotypes with respect to growth factor requirements. BPV-1 is active in relieving contact inhibition, yet these
transformed NIH/3T3 cells retain their stringent requirement for FGF. In
contrast, sis and H-ras were equally proficient at relieving contact inhibition and the requirement for FGF. Sis induced equal numbers of colonies
regardless of the presence or absence of insulin, however, H-ras-mediated
colony formation decreased four-fold when insulin was removed. This suggests that H-ras is less efficient in relieving the insulin requirement
than is sis. To determine if colony formation by H-ras is a function of
dosage, we are conducting experiments to measure the level of expression of
p21 in transformants selected with and without insulin in the media.

We have also presented data to show that loss of contact inhibition and
loss of growth factor requirements are dissociable phenotypes under se-
prate control in some cells. Thus, it should be possible to use this selective system to identify transforming genes in tumor DNA. Since some of
these genes may be undetectable by the standard focus forming assay, selection in MSF medium may prove to be a useful tool for identifying and elucidating the action of activated cellular onc genes.

VI. ACKNOWLEDGEMENTS

This work was supported by award 1N-11V from the American Cancer Society
and CA 40572 from the National Institutes of Health. AB was supported by
NIH training grant GM 07813. GS is a Leukemia Society of America Scholar.

VII. REFERENCES

1. Perucho, M., Goldfarb, M., Shimizu, K., Lama, C., Fohg, J., and Wigler,
    M. (1981) Cell 27, 467-476.
2. Pulciani, S., Santos, E., Lauver, A. V., Long, L. K. Robbins, K. C.,
    and Barbacid, M. (1982) Proc. Natl. Acad. Sci. USA 79, 2845-2849.
3. Krontiris, T., and Cooper, G. (1981) Proc. Natl. Acad. Sci. USA 78,
    1181-1184.

4. Shih, C., Padhy, L. C., Marray, M., and Weinberg, R. (1981) Nature 290, 261-263.

5. Pulciani, S., Santos, E., Lauver, A. V., Long, L. K., and Barbacid, M. (1982) Nature 300, 539-542.

6. Der, C. J., Krontiris, T. G., and Cooper, G. M. (1982) Proc. Natl. Acad. Sci. USA 79, 3637-3640.

7. Murray, M. J., Shilo, B., Shih, C., Cowing, D., Hsu, H. W., and Weinberg, R. A. (1981) Cell 28, 355-361.

8. Lane, M. A., Sainten, A., and Cooper, G. M. (1982) Cell 25, 873-880.

9. Lane, M. A., Sainten, A., and Cooper, G. M. (1981) Proc. Natl. Acad. Sci. USA 78, 5185-5189.

10. Diamond, A., Cooper, G., Ritz, J., and Lane, M (1983) Nature 305, 112-116.

11. Lane, M., Sainten, A., Doherty, K., and Cooper, G. (1984) Proc. Natl. Acad. Sci. USA 81, 2227-2231.

12. Cooper, C. S., Park, M., Blair, D. G., Tainsky, M. A., Heubner, K., Croce, C. M., and Vande Woude, G. F. (1984) Nature 311, 29-33.

13. Schechter, A. L., Stern, D. F., Vaidyanathan, L., Decker, S. J., Drebin, J. A., Greene, M. I., and Weinberg, R. A. (1984) Nature 312, 513-516.

14. Blair, D. G., Cooper, C. S., Oskarsson, M. K., Eader, L. A., and Vande Woude, G. F. (1982) Science 281, 1122-1125.

15. Fasano, O., Birnbaum, D., Edlund, L., Fogh, J., and Wigler, M. (1984) Molec. Cell Biol. 4, 1695-1705.

16. Wolfe, R. A., Sato, G. H., and McClure, D. B. (1980) J. Cell Biol. 87, 434-441.

17. McClure, D. B. (1983) Cell 32, 999-1006.

18. DeLarco, J., and Todaro, G. (1978) Nature 272, 356-358.

19. DeLarco, J., and Todaro, G. (1978) Proc. Natl. Acad. Sci. USA 75, 4001-4005.

20. Temin, H. (1967) The Wistar Symposium Monograph; No. 7 p. 103-116.

21. Temin, H. J. (1970) Cell. Physiol. 75, 107-120.

22. Heldin, C-H. and Westermark, B. (1984) Cell 37, 9-20.

23. Stiles, C., Capone, G., Scher, C., Antoniades, H., Van Wyk, J., and Pledger, W. (1979) Proc. Natl. Acad. Sci. USA 76, 1279-1283.

24. Scher, C., Pledger, W., Martin, P., Antoniades, H., and Stiles, C. (1978) J. Cell. Physiol. 97, 371-380.

25. Stiles, C. (1983) Cell 33, 653-655.

26. Ozanne, B., Fulton, R., and Kaplan, P. (1980) J. Cell. Physiol. 105, 163-180.

27. Kaplan, P., Anderson, M., and Ozanne, B. (1982) Proc. Natl. Acad. Sci. USA 79, 485-489.

28. Doolittle, R. F., Hunkapiller, M. W., Hood, L. E., Devare, S. G., Robbins, K. C., Aaronson, S. A., and Antoniades, H. N. (1983) Science 221, 275-277.

29. Waterfield, M. D., Scrace, T., Whittle, N., Stroobant, P., Johnsson, A., Wasteson, A., Westermark, B., Heldin, C.-H., Huang, J. S., and Deuel, T. F. (1983) Nature 304, 35-39.

30. Robbins, K. C., Devare, S. G., Reddy, E. P., and Aaronson, S. A. (1982) Science 218, 1131-1133.

31. Mellstrom, K., Hoglund, A.-A., Nister, M., Heldin, C.-H., Westermark, B., and Lindberg, U. (1983) J. Muscle Res. Cell Motil. 4, 589-609.

32. Westermark, B., Heldin, C.-H., Ek, B., Johnsson, A., Mellstrom, K., Nister, M., and Wasteson, A. (1983) in "Growth and Maturation Factors, 1. G. Guroff, ed. New York, John Wiley and Sons, p. 73-115.

33. Heldin, C.-H., Westermark, B., and Wasteson, A. (1980) J. Cell. Physiol. 105, 235-246.

34. Betsholtz, C., Heldin, C.-H., Nister, M., Ek., B., Wasteon, A., and Westermark, B. (1983) Biochem. Biophys. Res. Commun. 117, 176-182.

35. Nister, M., Heldin, C.-H., Wastaeson, A., and Estsermark, B., (1984) Proc. Natl. Acad. Sci. USA 81, 926-930.

36. Downward, J., Yarden, Y., Mayes, E., Scrace, G., Totty, N., Stockwell, P., Ullrich, A., Schlessinger, J., and Waterfield, M. D. (1984) Nature 307, 521-527.

37. Sherr, C. J., Rettenmier, C. W., Sacca, R., Roussel, M. F., Look, A. T., and Stanley, E. R. (1985) Cell 41, 665-676.

38. Glenn, K., Bowen-Pope, D. F., and Ross, R. (1982) J. Biol. Chem. 257, 5172-5276.

39. Ek, B., Westermark, B., Wasteson, A., and Heldin, C.-H. (1982) Nature 295, 419-420.

40. Das, M., Miyakawa, T., Fox, C. F., Pruss, R. M., Aharonov, A., and Herschman, H. R. (1977) Proc. Natl. Acad. Sci. USA 74, 2790-2794.

41. Buhrow, S. A., Cohen, S., and Staros, J. V. (1982) J. Biol. Chem. 257, 4019-4022.

42. Cohen, S., Ushiro, H., Stoscheck, C., and Chinkers, M. (1982) J. Biol. Chem. 257, 1523-1531.

43. Kasuga, M., Zick, Y., Blithe, D. L., Karlsson, F. A., Haring, H. U., and Kahn, C. R. (1982) J. Biol. Chem. 257, 9891-9894.

44. Roth, R. A., and Cassell, D. J. (1983) Science 219, 299-301.

45. Witte, O. N., Rosenberg, N., Shields, A., and Baltimore, D. (1979) J. Virol. 31, 776-784.

46. Courtneidge, S. A., Levinson, A. D., and Bishop, J. M. (1980) Proc. Natl. Acad. Sci. USA 77, 3783-3787.

47. Feldman, R. A., Wang, E., and Hanafusa, H. (1983) J. Virol. 45, 782-784.

48. Kaplan, P. L., and Ozanne, B. (1982) Virology 123, 372-380.

49. Twardzik, D. R., Rodaro, G. J., Marquardt, H., Reynolds, F. H., and Stephenson, J. R. (1982) Science 216, 894-897.

50. Wsardzik, D. R., Todaro, G. J., Reynolds, F. H., and Stephenson, J. R. (1983) Virology 124, 201-207.

51. Carpenter, G., Stoscheck, C. M., Preston, Y. A., and DeLarco, J. E. (1983) Proc. Natl. Acad. Sci. USA 80, 5627-5630.

52. Marquardt, H., Hunkapillar, M. W., Hood, L. E., Twardzik, D. R., DeLarco, J. E., Stephenson, J. R., and Todaro, G. J. (1983) Proc. Natl. Acad. Sci. USA 80, 4684-4688.

53. Anzano, M. A., Roberts, A. G., Smith, J. M., Sporn, M. B., and DeLarco, J. E. (1983) Proc. Natl. Acad. Sci. USA 80, 6264-6268.

54. Assoian, R. K., Grotendorst, G. R., Miller, D. M., and Sporn, M. B. (1984) Nature 309, 804-809.

55. Alitalo, K., Ramsay, G., Bishop, J. M., Ohlsson Pfeifer, S., Colby, W. W., and Levinson, A. (1983) Nature 306, 274-277.

56. Donner, P., Greiser-Wilke, I., and Moelling, K. (1982) Nature 296, 262-266.

57. Finkel, M. P., Biskis, B. O., and Jinkins, P. B. (1966) Science 151, 698-701.

58. Curran, T., Macconell, W. P., van Straaten, F., and Verma, I. M. (1983) Molec. Cell. Biol. 3, 914-921.

59. Van Beveren, C., van Straaten, F., Curran, T., Muller, R., and Verma, I. M. (1983) Cell 32, 1241-1255.

60. Armelin, H. A., Armelin, C. S., Kelly, K., Steward, T., Leder, P., Cochran, B. H., and Stiles, C. D. (1984) Nature 310, 655-660.

61. Greenberg, M. E., and Ziff, E. G. (1984) Nature 311, 433-438.

62. Kruijer, W., Cooper, J. A., Hunter, T., and Verma, I. M. (1984) Nature 312, 711-716.

63. Muller, T., Bravo, R., Burckhardt, J., and Currant, T. (1984) Nature 312, 716-720.

64. Shipley, G. D., and Ham, R. G. (1981) In Vitro 17, 656-670.

65. Guerry, P., Leblanc, D. J., and Falkow, S. (1973) J. Bacteriol. 116, 1064-1066.

66. Reddy, E. P., Reynolds, R. K., Watson, D. K., Shultz, R. A., Lautenberger, J. and Papas, T. S. (1983) Proc. Natl. Acad. Sci. USA 80, 2500-2504.

67. Ellis, R. W., DeFeo, D., Maryak, J. M., Young, H. A., Shih, Y., Chang, E. H., Lowy, D. R., and Scolnick, E. M. (1980) J. Virology 36, 408-420.

68. Sarver, N., Byrne, J. C., and Howley, P. M. (1982) Proc. Natl. Acad. Sci. USA 79, 7147-7151.

69. Loyter, A., Scangos, G. A., and Ruddle, F. H. (1982) Proc. Natl. Acad. Sci. USA 79, 422-426.

70. Kuhnlein, U., Tsang, S. S., Lokken, O., Tong, S., and Twa, D., (1983) Bioscience Reports 3, 667-674.

71. Fogh, J., and Trempe, G. E. (1975) in Human Tumor cells in vitro, J. Fogh ed., Plenum Press, New York, pp. 115-159.

72. Fogh, J. (1978) Natl. Cancer Inst. Mongr. 49, 5-19.

73. Sarver, N., Byrne, J. C., and Howley, P. M. (1982) Proc. Natl. Acad. Scie. USA 79, 7147-7151.

74. Deuel, T. F., Huang, J. S., Huang, S. S., Stroobant, P., and Waterfield, M. (1983) Science 221, 1348-1350.

75. Owen, A. J., Pantazis, P., and Antoniades, H. N. (1984) Science 225, 54-56.

76. Powers, S., Fisher, P. B., and Pollack, R. (1984) Mol. Cell. Biol. 4, 1572-2576.

77. Clemmons, D. R., Underwood, L. E., and Van Wyk, J. J. (1981) J. Clin. Invest. 67, 10-19.

78. Dvoretzky, I., Shober, R., Chattopadhyay, S. K., and Lowy, D. R. (1981) Virology 103, 369-375.

79. Lancaster, W. D., and Olson, C. (1978) Virology 89, 372-379.

80. Southern, P. F. and Berg. P. (1982) J. Molec. Appl. Gen. 1, 327-341.

11

The Role of Ionic Signals in Early Gene Induction
During T Cell Activation

Kathleen Kelly and Brenda Underwood

Immunology Branch, National Cancer Institute, Building 10,
Room 4B017, Bethesda, Maryland 02115

198

I. INTRODUCTION

The mechanism whereby a quiescent lymphocyte is activated to proliferate and express differentiated functions is a fundamental question for understanding immune regulation and growth control. The binding of ligands such as antigen, mitogenic lectins, and some cell surface-specific antibodies to their membrane receptors on lymphocytes generates a transmembrane signal resulting in a variety of metabolic changes culminating after 24 hours in DNA synthesis[1,2]. One initial consequence of transmembrane signalling is the expression of mRNA species novel to activated cells. For example, the cellular proto-oncogene c-myc[3], the T cell growth factor, IL-2[4], and the IL-2 receptor[5,6] increase expression within approximately 1, 12, and 6 hours, respectively, following mitogenic stimulation of T cells. In addition, here we describe the rapid and transient expression of an additional mRNA species, c-fos, between 30 and 90 minutes after mitogen addition to human T cells. Such increases occur in the presence of protein synthesis inhibitors[3,6], indicating that mRNA induction is a direct result of the signals that follow receptor binding and as such probably represent primary transcriptional events.

The involvement of ion channels in T cell activation is suggested indirectly by reports of membrane depolarization[7,8], hyperpolarization [8,9], increased ion fluxes across the membrane[10], and increases in intracellular free calcium[9,11] following mitogenic stimulation. Using the gigaohm seal recording technique, the existence has been demonstrated in human T lymphocytes of a voltage-gated potassium (K^+) channel that resembles delayed rectifier K^+ channels of nerve and muscle[12]. The role of such channels in T lymphocyte activation is suggested by two lines of evidence. First, in voltage-clamped T lymphocytes, the T cell mitogen, PHA, causes K^+ channels to open upon depolarization more rapidly and at more negative potentials[12]. Thus, an immediate consequence of PHA binding to T cells may be an effect upon K^+ channel gating. Second, DNA synthesis is inhibited in PHA-stimulated T cells by the K^+ channel blockers tetraethylammonium (TEA), 4-aminopyridine (4AP) and quinine at doses that block K^+ currents in voltage-clamped lymphocytes[12,13]. However, because these blockers inhibit protein synthesis[13], their effect upon the earliest activation events cannot be directly assessed utilizing assays based upon the expression of specific protein species or DNA synthesis. Therefore, in order to establish a causal relationship between ionic signals mediated by K^+ channels and T cell activation, we have examined the effect of K^+ channel blockers upon PHA-induced gene transcription. We show here that concentrations of K^+ channel blockers that inhibit K^+ current flow in patch-clamped human T cells and mitogenesis in PHA-stimulated peripheral blood lymphocytes (PBL) do not inhibit PHA-induced increases in steady state levels of c-fos, c-myc, and IL-2 receptor mRNA.

II. MATERIALS AND METHODS

Reagents: Purified PHA (Difco Laboratories, St. Louis, MO) was prepared as a stock solution in PBS and stored at -20 prior to use. Verapamil (Searle Pharmaceuticals, Chicago, IL) was supplied as a sterile, purified aqueous solution. 4AP (Sigma Chemical Co., St. Louis, MO) was recrystallized in methanol three times prior to use.

Cell Culture: Heparinized peripheral venous blood was obtained from healthy volunteers. Mononuclear cells were isolated by Ficoll-Hypaque density gradients, washed thoroughly and cultured in RPMI 1640 supplemented with 10% fetal calf serum (Gibco Laboratories, Grand Island, NY) and 30 μ g/ml gentamycin. Cell cultures were maintained at 37° in a humidified atmosphere of 10% carbon dioxide.

Lymphocyte Proliferation: Two hundred thousand lymphocytes in 0.2 ml of medium were incubated for four days in microtiter plates in the presence or absence of PHA and titrated amounts of K^+ channel blockers. Six hours before harvesting the cultures with an multiple automated cell harvester, 1.0μ curie of ^{3}H-thymidine was added per well. Incorporated thymidine was determined by scintillation counting.

Isolation of Cellular RNA and Northern Blot Analysis: RNA was isolated by guanidine isothiocyanate extraction and cesium chloride gradient centrifugation according to the method of Chirgwin et. al.[14]. RNA was size fractionated on 1% agarose-formaldehyde gels[15] and transferred to nitrocellulose. Purified DNA fragments were nick-translated to an average specific activity of 5.0×10^8 cpm/μg and hybridized to immobilized RNA as previously described[16]. Probes used are as follows: c-myc- Cla I-Eco R1 fragment encompassing the third exon of human c-myc[16], v-fos - 1.3 kb Pvu II-Bgl II fragment from the v-fos coding region of the FBJ virus[17], human IL-2 receptor- 700 b.p. Eco R1-linkered cDNA insert[5], and human β -2 microglobulin- 600 b.p. cDNA insert[18]. Hybridized filters were washed in 0.1 x SSC at 55° for c-myc, IL-2 receptor, and β -2 microglobulin probes and at 45° for the v-fos probe.

III. RESULTS

c-fos mRNA Levels are Regulated by PHA in T Cells. c-myc and c-fos are two members of a small class of proto-oncogenes that encode nuclear proteins[19,20]. c-myc is an inducible gene that is regulated in a cell-specific manner by agents that initiate a proliferative response; for example, PDGF in fibroblasts[3], Concanavalin A in T cells[3], and partial hepatectomy in liver[21]. Similarly to c-myc, c-fos gene transcription is induced in fibroblasts by PDGF, but with more rapid and transient kinetics[22,23]. In order to investigate the generality of c-fos induction by growth promoting agents, we have assayed the steady-state levels of c-fos mRNA in human PBL before and at various times after treatment with PHA. As shown by the Northern blots presented in Figure 1, c-fos mRNA is not detectable in quiescent PBL, is transiently induced within 30 minutes following PHA addition, and again is undetectable by three hours after stimulation. Also, immunoprecipitation studies using anti-fos specific antisera have shown that c-fos protein synthesis closely parallels c-fos mRNA levels (K. Kelly and T. Curran, manuascript in preparation). In Figure 1 a kinetic profile of the identical RNA samples hybridized with a c-myc probe is shown for comparison. c-myc mRNA begins to increase within 1 hour after PHA stimulation and, in contrast to c-fos, remains at an induced level at three hours (Figure 1) and several hours thereafter (data not shown). A control β 2-microglobulin probe demonstrates that equal amounts of mRNA are assayed from each sample. In a manner similar to c-myc, c-fos mRNA induction is enhanced in the presence of 10 µg/ml of cycloheximide.

K[+] Channel Blockers do not Inhibit PHA-Induced Gene Expression. The classic K[+] channel blockers 4AP, TEA, and quinine inhibit PHA-induced mitogenesis in a dose-dependent manner with roughly the same potency as for channel blockade[12,13]. 4AP appears to block voltage-gated K[+] channels in distinction to Ca^{2+}-activated K[+] channels[24], while TEA and quinine block both types of K[+] channels[24,25]. It also has been reported that organic or "slow" calcium channel antagonists such as verapamil and diltiazem block K[+] currents in human T cells[26]. In order to establish the concentration of channel blockers required to inhibit PHA-induced mitogenesis in fresh human PBL using our culture reagents, cells were cultured with 1 µg/ml PHA and titrated concentrations of various K[+] channel blockers. The incorporation of ^{3}H-thymidine 96 hours after PHA and blocker addition are shown in Table 1. The concentrations required to produce a 50% inhibition of [3]-H thymidine incorporation are similar to published values[13,26].

Figure 2 shows the effect upon early gene induction of two K[+] channel blockers, verapamil and 4AP, utilized at concentations that completely inhibit K[+] current flow and PHA-induced mitogenesis. c-myc and IL-2 receptor mRNA's are undetectable in nonstimulated human PBL and are quantitatively induced with the expected kinetics in PHA-stimulated cultures.

TABLE 1

Inhibition of PHA-Induced T Cell Proliferation

PBL + Additives	^{3}H-Thymidine Incorporation (cpm)	% Inhibition
Media	1108	--
PHA	39077	--
PHA + Verapamil		
12.5 μM	26446	32
25.0 μM	19489	50
50.0 μM	6796	83
100.0 μM	625	100
PHA + 4AP		
1.2 mM	39243	0
2.5 mM	24963	13
5.0 mM	2284	94
10.0 mM	809	100
PHA + Quinine		
12.5 μM	47363	0
25.0 μM	33849	13
50.0 μM	25934	34
100.0 μM	7277	82

PBL were cultured in microtiter plates with the addition of PHA and K$^+$ channel blocking drugs at the initiation of culture. Cells were labeled with ^{3}H-thymidine for 6 hours prior to the harvesting of cultures at 96 hours. All values represent the average of quadriplicate wells.

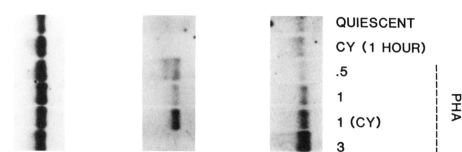

Figure 1. Analysis of c-myc, c-fos, and beta-2 microglobulin mRNA levels at various times after the addition of PHA to PBL cultures. PBL were cultured in the presence or absence of 1 µ g/ml PHA and 10 µg/ml cycloheximide (Cy) as described in Materials and Methods. At various times after the addition of PHA, cell aliquots were harvested and RNA was extracted and purified. 10 µg of total RNA were assayed from each sample by Northern blot analysis. The molecular weight of each RNA species was determined relative to 18s and 28s ribosomal RNA.

c-myc mRNA levels are marginally diminished in the presence of 4AP and verapamil at two hours after PHA addition and are unaffected at four hours. Similarly, IL-2 receptor mRNA is unaffected or slightly increased in the presence of channel blockers at four and 15 hours after adding PHA to the cultures. 150 µM quinine gives identical results to those obtained with 4AP and verapamil (not shown). Also, c-fos induction at 60 minutes is unaffected by all three K+ channel blockers (not shown). Thus, these channel blockers appear to inhibit mitogenesis as a result of effects upon activation steps unlinked to or subsequent to specific mRNA induction.

IV. DISCUSSION

The activation of a quiescent, G0 T cell by agents that initiate a proliferative response requires the translation of novel proteins that are similar to those termed competence genes in other systems[27]. The synthesis of mRNA's encoding such proteins occurs as a primary event, independent of protein synthesis, spanning between one and several hours following transmembrane signaling. Some of the competence genes induced in T cells such as IL-2 and the IL-2 receptor are unique to lymphocytes[4,5], while others

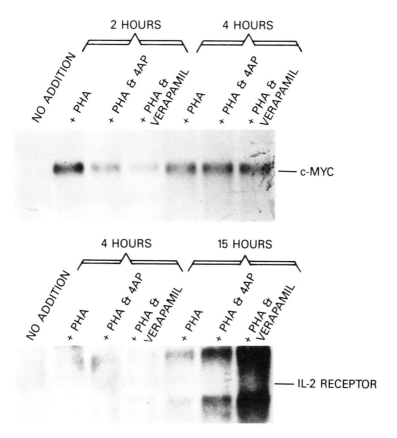

Figure 2. Analysis of c-myc and IL-2 receptor mRNA accumulation in PBL at various times after the addition of PHA and the effect of K⁺ channel blockers on this process. PBL were cultured in the presence or absence of 1 μg/ml PHA and the presence or absence of either 100 μM Verapamil or 10 mM 4AP. K⁺ channel blockers were preincubated with PBL cultures for 30 minutes at 37°. At various times after the addition of PHA (time 0), cells were harvested and RNA was extracted and purified. 10 μg of total RNA were assayed from each sample by Northern blot analysis. Equal amounts of RNA from each sample were assayed, as shown by a comparison of ribosomal RNA band intensity after staining with ethidium bromide and by hybridization analysis with a control beta-2 microglobulin probe (not shown).

such as the proto-oncogene c-myc are induced in lymphoid and other cell types[3,21,22]. We show here that the c-fos proto-oncogene is included in this latter category of genes and is as yet the earliest transcriptional event observed in activated T cells. The rapid and transient induction of c-fos observed in fibroblasts is mimicked in T cells suggesting that the physiological milieu necessary for c-fos gene regulation is present and most likely similar in both cell types. Although transcription and mRNA accumulation occurs with variable kinetics for each member of the competence gene family[6], the occurrence of transcriptional induction in the presence cycloheximide indicates that the transcription of a gene expressed later (e.g. c-myc) is not dependent upon translation of a mRNA expressed earlier (e.g. c-fos).

Because competence gene mRNA expression is one of the earliest functional indications of transmembrane signaling, assaying the relationship between putative, initial transmembrane signals susceptible to biochemical blockade and gene induction allows the examination of a sequence of obligatory steps. Voltage-gated K[+] channels appear to be the main ion channel in human T cells[12] and have been hypothesized to play either an active or a permissive role in T cell activation prior to mitogen-induced protein synthesis[13]. We have utilized various K[+] channel blockers to show that functioning K[+] channels are not required for the induction of several so called competence genes. Therefore, ionic signals mediated through K[+] channels appear to effect a step unlinked to or subsequent to mRNA accumulation for the particular competence genes that were assayed. The inhibition of protein synthesis resulting from K[+] channel blockade[13] may well be sufficient to explain their nonpermissive effect upon PHA-induced mitogenesis. Whether protein synthesis inhibition is a specific or nonspecific effect of K[+] channel blockade has yet to be established. Of course we cannot rule out that the induction of some other essential competence gene is affected by K[+] channel blockade.

A variety of accumulated data points to a role for increased intracellular free calcium in lymphocyte transmembrane signaling[28]. However, calcium channels have not been detected in human T cells[12,29], and therefore, it has been suggested that K[+] channels could serve as a route of calcium entry[13]. One K[+] channel antagonist, Verapamil, utilized in these studies blocks passive calcium channels in other tissues[30] and inhibits mitogen-induced $^{45}Ca^{2+}$ influx in human PBL[26]. Since verapamil blockade does not inhibit the induction of the competence genes analyzed here, the previous hypothesis that calcium influx through K[+] channels plays a critical role in early signaling seems unlikely.

In summary, we and others have described a number of genes that are transcriptionally regulated as a primary event following transmembrane signaling in T lymphocytes. As shown here, assaying transcriptional induction of these so called competence genes in the presence of specific biochemical blockers, allows a direct assessment of sequential signals required for T cell activation.

V. REFERENCES

1. Erard, F. Nabholz, M., Dupuy-D'Angeac, A. and MacDonald, H.R. (1985) J. Exp. Med. 162, 1738-1743.
2. Meuer, S.C., Hussey, R.E., Cantrell, D.A., Hogdon, J.D., Schlossman, S.F., Smith, K.A. and Reinherz, E.L. (1984) Proc. Natl. Acad. Sci. USA 81, 1509-1514.
3. Kelly, K., Cochran, B., Stiles, C.D. and Leder, P. (1983) Cell 35, 603-610.
4. Efrat, S., Pilo, S. and Kaempfer, R. (1982) Nature 297, 236-239.
5. Leonard, W.J., Depper, J.M., Crabtree, G.R., Rudikoff, S., Pumphrey, J., Robb, R.J., Kronke, M., Svetlik, P.B., Peffer, N.J., Waldman, T.A. and Greene, W.C. (1984) Nature 311, 626-631.
6. Kronke, M., Leonard, W.J., Depper, J.M. and Greene, W.C. (1985) J. Exp. Med. 161, 1593-1598.
7. Kieffer, H., Blume, A.J. and Kaback, H.R. (1980) Proc. Natl. Acad. Sci. USA 77, 2200-2204.
8. Felber, S.M. and Brand, M.D. (1983) Biochem. J. 210, 885-891.
9. Tsien, R.Y., Pozzan, T. and Rink, T. (1982) Nature 295, 68-71.
10. Segel, G.B., Simon W. and Lichtman, M.A. (1979) J. Clin. Invest. 64, 834-841.
11. Hesketh, T.K., Moore, J.P., Morris, J.D.H., Taylor, M.V. and Metcalfe, J.C. (1985) Nature 482-484.
12. DeCoursey, T.E., Chandy, K.G., Gupta, S. and Cahalan, M.D. (1984) Nature 307, 465-468.
13. Chandy, K.G., DeCoursey, T.E., Cahalan, M.D., McLaughlin, C. and Gupta, S. (1985) J. Exp. Med. 160, 369-385.
14. Chirgwin, J.M., Przybyla, A.E., MacDonald, R.J. and Rutter, W.J. (1979) Biochemistry 18, 5294-5299.
15. Lehrach, H., Diamond, D., Wozney, J.M. and Boedtker, H. (1977) Biochemistry 16, 4743-4751.
16. Battey, J., Moulding, C., Taub, R., Murphy, W., Stewart, T., Potter, H., Lenoir, G. and Leder, P. (1983) Cell 34, 779-787.
17. Curran, T., Peters, G., Van Beveren, C., Teich, N.M. and Verma, I. (1982) J. Virology 44, 674-682.
18. Suggs, S.V., Wallace, R.B., Hirose, T., Kawashima, E.H. and Itakura, K. (1981) Proc. Natl. Acad. Sci. USA 78, 6613-6617.
19. Persson, H. and Leder, P. (1984) Science 225, 718-721.
20. Curran, T., Miller, A.D., Zohas, L. and Verma, I.M. (1984) Cell 36, 259-268.

21. Makino, R. Hayashi, K. and Sugimura, T. (1984) Nature 310, 697-698.
22. Greenberg, M.E. and Ziff, E.B. (1984) Nature 311, 433-437.
23. Muller, R., Bravo, R., Burckhardt, J. and Curran, T. (1984) Nature 312, 711-716.
24. Schwartz, W. and Passow, H.A. (1983) A. Rev. Physiol. 45, 359-374.
25. Fishman, M.C. and Spector, I. (1981) Proc. Natl. Acad. Sci. USA 78, 5245-5249.
26. Birx, D.L., Berger, M. and Fleisher, T.A. (1984) J. Immunol. 133, 2904-2909.
27. Cochran, B.H., Reffel, A.C. and Stiles, C.D. (1983) Cell 33, 939-947.
28. Lichtman, A.H., Segel, G.B. and Lichtman, M.A. (1983) Blood 61, 413-422.
29. Matteson, D.R. and Deutsch, C. (1984) Nature 307, 468-471.
30. Lee, K.S. and Tsien, R.W. (1983) Nature 302, 790-793.

12

Molecular Evolution of <u>Ets</u> Genes From Avians to Mammals

and Their Cytogenetic Localization to Regions Involved in Leukemia

Takis S. Papas, Dennis K. Watson, Nicoletta Sacchi,

Stephen J. O'Brien and Richard Ascione

Laboratory of Molecular Oncology
Division of Cancer Etiology
National Cancer Institute
Frederick, MD 21701

208

I. SUMMARY

The mammalian homologues of the ets-region from the transforming gene of avian erythroblastosis virus, E26, consists of two distinct domains located on different chromosomes. Using somatic cell hybrid panels, the mammalian homolog of the 5' v-ets-domain (ets-1) was mapped to chromosome 11 in man, to chromosome 9 in mouse, and to chromosome D1 in cat. The mammalian homolog of the 3' v-ets domain (ets-2) was similarly mapped to human chromosome 21, to mouse chromosome 16, and to feline chromosome C2. To better define the human proto-ets domains, the genomic DNA was molecularly cloned and sequences analyzed. The ets-related sequences of human DNA on chromosomes 11 and 21 were found to be discontiguous, unlike that of the chicken and avian E26 virus genome, except for a small overlap region. We conclude that the ets sequence shared by the virus, the chicken and man is likely to contain at least two dissociable functional domains, identifiable as ets-1 and ets-2. The human ets-1 locus is transcriptionally active and encodes a single mRNA of 6.8 kb, while the second locus, human ets-2 encodes three mRNAs of 4.7, 3.2 and 2.7 kb. By contrast, the chicken homolog, having a contiguous ets-1 and ets-2 sequence, is primarily expressed in normal chicken cells as a single 7.5 kb mRNA.

Because chromosome translocations have been associated with different human disorders, we have used our human probes with two panels of rodent-human cell hybrids to study specific translocations occurring in acute myeloid leukemias (AML). The human ets-1 gene was found to translocate from chromosome 11 to 4 in t(4;11)(q21;q23) and the human ets-2 gene was found to translocate from chromosome 21 to 8 in t(8;21)(q22;q22). Both translocations were found associated with the altered expression of ets.

II. INTRODUCTION

Transforming genes, or proto-onc genes, represent a class of conserved cellular genes which may play an important role in tumorigenesis. These genes were initially defined as transduced RNA segments in transforming retrovirus genomes, and have also been described and delineated by focus induction after transfection of mouse 3T3 cells with genomic DNA extracted from human tumors[1-5]. The limited number of proto-oncogenes (circa 30), described to date, has attracted considerable research emphasis over the past few years as an experimental model and an opportunity in which to study neoplastic transformation from both a genetic and molecular perspective. As a result of these extensive analyses, there are now at least five documented modes of oncogene activation associated with tumorigenesis.

These include: 1) transduction of portions of proto-oncogene transcripts by retroviruses, thereby placing the oncogene under regulatory control of strong promoters in the viral long terminal repeats (LTRs) gene segment[1-5]; 2) chromosomal insertion of an infecting retrovirus genome adjacent to a proto-oncogene similarly altering their control of transcription[5,6]; 3) translocation of cellular oncogenes to chromosomal regions of differential regulation[7,8]; 4) amplification of oncogene containing segments, thereby increasing the gene dosage of the oncogene[9-11]; and 5) point mutation, with concomitant alteration of regulation and/or expression, in the cellular coding sequence[2].

The ets sequence was identified as a second cellular sequence transduced by the avian replication-defective retrovirus, E26. The 5.7-kilobase (kb) RNA genome of E26 contains: in addition to partial retroviral gag and env genes, a truncated part of the myb oncogene originally identified in avian myeloblastosis virus (AMV) and an E26-specific sequence, ets Fig. 1[12,13]. The nucleotide sequence of a 2.46-kb DNA region of E26 has revealed a contiguous gag-myb-ets open reading frame encoding for a 135-kilodalton (kd) protein, p135[14,16]. E26 induces both myeloblastosis and erythroblastosis in vivo and transforms erythroid and myeloid precursors in vitro. The myeloid oncogenic property that E26 and AMV has in common is thought

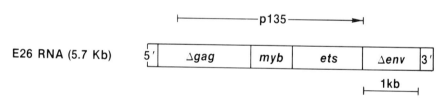

Figure 1. Genomic organization of the avian E26 acute transforming virus.

to be encoded by the common myb domain, while the unique erythroblastosis of E26 is thought to be encoded by the singular ets domain of the tripartite viral onc-gene[14,15] or may perhaps be due to a cooperative effect of myb and ets.

We would like to present, in this review, an overview of the ets gene and outline the major findings resulting from the research carried out in our laboratory. Data emanating from this laboratory that has been recently submitted for publication has resulted in the following conclusions regarding the ets oncogene: 1) There are two separable genes in mammals which we have termed respectively, ets-1 and ets-2. These genes are structurally distinct, transcriptionally active and each situated on unique chromosomal loci; 2) ets-1 and ets-2 map at syntenic homologs in mammals; with ets-1 located in man on chromosome 11 mapping on chromosome 9 in mouse, and the chromosome D1 in cat. The ets-2 similarly, mapped to human chromosome 21, is located on mouse chromosome 16, and the feline chromosome C2; 3) we have precisely defined by sequence analysis, the human domains of both ets-1 and ets-2. The ets-1 is homologous to the viral 5' (v-ets) domain while the ets-2 is homologous, to the 3' v-ets domain. The ets related human DNA sequences, on chromosome 11 and 21, are discontiguous except for a small overlap region; 4) (a) Both ets-1 and ets-2 map in humans to a chromosomal region having few known disease associations. Specifically, the human ets-1 was found to translocate from chromosome 11 to chromosome 4 in the t(4;11)(q21;q23) leukemia. This translocation is, in fact, characteristic of a specific subtype of leukemia that often is found in newborns and may be congenital; (b) similarly the human ets-2 gene was found to translocate from chromosome 21 to chromosome 8 in the translocation t(8;21) (q22;q22), found in AML-M2 patients; (c) both translocations were found to be associated with expression of ets genes different from the expression in normal lymphocytes raising the possibility that these genes may play a role in the pathogenesis of these leukemias.

III. RESULTS

Conservation of dual domains of ets in Mammalia.

A. Human (Hu) proto-oncogene: Hu-ets-1 maps to chromosome 11 and Hu-ets-2 maps to chromosome 21. In order to identify the human proto-oncogene homologs of v-ets, a nearly full length v-ets molecular clone, E1.28 (Fig. 2A), was used as a probe in a Southern blot[17] analysis of human and rodent DNA. Four fragments of 8.2, 6.2, 3.6 and 0.83 kb, were detected following Eco R1 digestion of human DNA (Fig. 2A). The segregation of three of these fragments (8.2, 6.2 and 3.6 kb) was examined using DNA from a panel of 50 independent somatic cell hybrids which had been genetically characterized by electrophoretic typing of previously assigned isozyme loci and by karyotype analysis using both G-11 and G-trypsin staining procedures [18,19]. These hybrids, which were prepared by PEG mediated fusion of normal human lymphocytes with HPRT resistant mouse (RAG) or Chinese hamster (E36) fibroblasts, retained the entire rodent genome but lost human chromosomes in varying combinations.

Two of the Hu-ets fragments produced by Eco R1 digestion (6.2 and 8.2 kb) were concordantly retained, or lost in the hybrid panel. The 3.6 kb fragment segregated independently from the others (Fig. 2A), suggesting that at

least two chromosomes contained sequences homologous to v-ets. This observation has been confirmed by the molecular cloning of two ets genes, the
characterization and DNA sequences of which are discussed in detail elsewhere[20].

Subclones of human DNA sequences homologous to different portions of the
v-ets gene were employed in our mapping experiments. The H33 clone, which
is homologous to the 3' portion of v-ets, hybridized to the 3.6 kb human
Eco R1 fragment, but not to the 0.83, 6.2 or 8.2 kb fragments (Fig. 2B).
Two additional cloned human sequences, pRD6K and pRD700, were shown to be
homologous to contiguous 5' portions of v-ets. These probes recognized the
Eco R1 fragments of 6.2 and 0.83 kb, respectively, but did not cross-hybri-
dize with H33. The human DNA segment homologous to the 5' regions of v-ets,
and characterized by the 0.83 and 6.2 kb Eco R1 fragments is referred to as
Hu-ets-1. The human locus homologous to the 3' region of v-ets, for which
the 3.6 kb Eco R1 fragment is diagnostic, is termed Hu-ets-2.

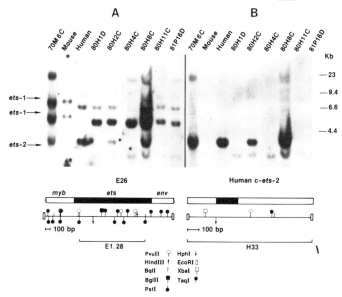

Figure 2. Analysis of human ets-1 and ets-2. Restriction maps of avian
provirus and of the H33, c-ets-2 clone are presented below the autoradio-
graphs, with ets specific sequences indicated as solid bars[14,20]. a)
DNA from mouse x human (70 series) and Chinese hamster x human (80 and 81
series) somatic cell hybrids were digested with Eco R1 and probed with a
molecular clone of the avian v-ets gene (E1.28). b) The same gels probed
with H33, a molecular clone of the Hu-ets-2 probe which recognizes the 3.6
kb fragment, but not the 0.8, 6.2 and 8.2 kb fragments which are diagnostic
for Hu ets 1.

212

The chromosomal positions of ets-1 and ets-2 in the human genome were determined by correlating the presence of the diagnostic Eco R1 fragments in the hybrid panels using both the E1.28 (v-ets) and H33 (Hu-ets-2) specific molecular clones as probes. The presence the Hu-ets-1 locus was 92-97% 97% concordant with human chromosome 11 and the chromosome 11 isozyme markers LDHA and ACP2, but was highly discordant (33-58%) with each of the other human chromosomes (Fig. 3A-Top). Similarly, the presence of Hu-ets-2 marker was 100% concordant with the presence of human chromosome 21 and its isozyme marker SOD1 (Fig. 3A-Bottom). These data support the localization of the Hu-ets-1 proto-oncogene on chromosome 11 and the Hu-ets-2 locus on chromosome 21. The assignment of Hu-ets-1 to chromosome 11 is also consistent with the recent study of de Taisne et al.[21], who reported the assignment of an ets proto-oncogene to 11q23-24.

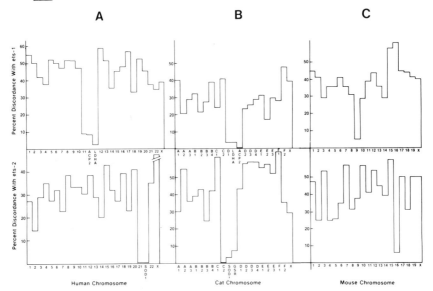

Figure 3. Analysis of the association of ets-1 and ets-2 diagnostic fragments with segregant chromosomes in three panels of somatic cell hybrids in the human panel, A, consists of 40 hybrids; B, the feline panel 38 hybrids; and C, the murine panel with 16 hybrids[22]. Chromosome scores represent the consensus result of karyotyping (G-banding) and isozyme scores. Thirty-six isozyme systems diagnostic for human chromosomes and 24 systems diagnostic for feline chromosomes were tested for each appropriate hybrid. (Assignment of feline LDHA and ACP2 to feline chromosome D1 is a corrected assignment, S.J. O'Brien et al., in preparation).

In situ hybridization of the H33 (Hu-ets-2) clone to the normal human chromosome preparations confirmed our assignment of the Hu-ets-2 to chromosome 21 and further localized the gene to the long arm (Fig. 4). In an analysis of 89 metaphase spreads from normal human peripheral blood cells, 37 grains were found situated on chromosome 21; 34 of these were located on the terminal portion of chromosome 21. These labeled sites, each consisting of one to three grains, represented 20% of all labeled sites distributed throughout the 89 metaphase spread. Compilation of grain positions from multiple (N=50) labeled No. 21 chromosomes revealed a clustering of grains on segments 21.1-22.3. On the basis of the significant labeling of this region on the long arm of chromosome 21, we can conclude that the Hu-ets-2 gene is located in the 21q22.1-22.3 region.

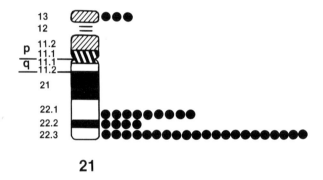

Figure 4. Diagrammatic representation of in situ hybridization of ets-2 demonstrates the distribution of 37 grains which fell on human chromosome 21 in 89 metaphase spreads after in situ hybridization using the Hu-ets-2 as a probe (H33).

B. Assignment of the feline ets-1 to chromosome D1 and ets-2 to C2. The domestic cat homologues of the viral ets sequence were resolved following digestion, with Xba I, of genomic DNA from cat x rodent cell hybrids; and hybridization with one of two probes: (1) H33, specific for Hu-ets-2, and (2) pRD700, specific for Hu-ets-1. The somatic cell hybrid panel used for the cat mapping experiment were expanded and analyzed for chromosomal complement by the same techniques that were employed in the human analysis[18,19]. Two Xba I fragments (6.8 and 11.0 kb) were detected in cat DNA, and these segregated independently in the hybrid panel[22]. Interestingly, both fragments were resolved with the H33 (Hu-ets-2 specific) probe. The RD700 probe, which is specific for Hu-ets-1, preferentially detected a 4.0 kb band. This fragment was 96-100% concordant with feline chromosome D1 and its included markers LDHA, ACP2 (Fig. 3B-Top), but highly discordant, 18-47%, with the 18 additional feline chromosomes. The appearance of the 11.0 kb Xba-I feline fragment in the panel was 93-100% concordant with the presence of chromosome C2 and its isozyme markers, SOD1 and GSR, but highly discordant, 25-70%, with other cat chromosomes (Fig. 3B-Bottom). These data permit the assignment of the ets-1 cat homologue to chromosome D1 and ets-2 to chromosome C2.

C. Assignment of mouse ets-1 to chromosome 9 and ets-2 to chromosome 16. The murine homologues of v-ets were visualized as three fragments with Eco R1 5.1, 6.8 and 15 kb, and with Pst I 2.9, 7.8 and 9.8 kb[22], using both the v-ets (E1.28) and the Hu-ets-2 (H33) clones as probes. The Hu-ets-1 specific pRD700 probe, described above, recognized only the 7.8 kb Pst I fragment[22]. A previously characterized panel of mouse x Chinese hamster (E36) hybrids were employed to study these chromosomal associations of the murine ets loci (19). These hybrids retain the entire Chinese hamster chromosomal complement, but lose mouse chromosomes in different combinations. DNA was extracted from each of 16 hybrids and were concomitantly studied by isozyme and karyologic analysis to determine the murine chromosomal complement.

The murine DNA fragments segregated as two distinct loci in the hybrid panel[22]. The Pst I fragment which is diagnostic for Hu-ets-1 (7.8 kb) was 94% concordant with mouse chromosome 9, but discordant, 30-70%, from the Hu-ets-2 (2.9 and 9.8 kb) segments and each of the 19 other mouse chromosomes, (Fig. 3C-Bottom). The 2.9 kb segment diagnostic for Hu-ets-2 was also 94% concordant with mouse chromosome 16 but highly discordant, 37%, (Fig. 3C-Top) with Hu-ets-1 and the 19 other mouse chromosomes (25-60%). Additionally, one of the hybrids positive for Hu-ets-2 contained no other mouse chromosome except for chromosome 16. Thus these data permit the assignment of ets-1 and ets-2 to murine chromosome 9 and 16, respectively.

D. Retention of homologous syntenic loci in Mammalia. With the recent rapid expansion of the human, murine and feline gene maps, a more complete picture of chromosomal homologies between these species is emerging[23]. Over 100 homologous genes have been mapped in both mouse and man, and a comparative analysis of the two gene maps has revealed that considerable rearrangements have occurred since these species shared a common ancestor[23,24,25]. The cat has fewer loci mapped than the mouse, but the extent of retention of homologous syntenic groups to man seems to be two to three times greater than between man and rodents[19,23]. The Hu-ets-1 locus is mapped at chromosome 11q in man; to the human chromosome 11 homolog in the cat (D1) and to the murine homologue of human 11q, which is chromosome 9. The diagram in Figure 5 shows the homologous loci mapped to their respective linkage groups in the three mammalian species. Similarly, the Hu-ets-2 locus mapped to human chromosome 21, is located on its murine counterpart at chromosome number 16, and its feline homologue, chromosome C2. This conservation of the linkage position of the two proto-oncogene domains, in the same chromosomal positions, in the three species indicates that their duality has persisted since the divergence of mammals began over 100 million years ago.

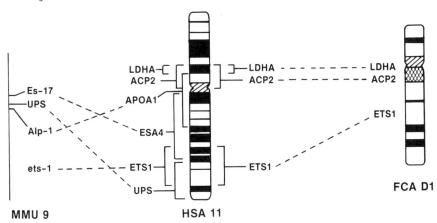

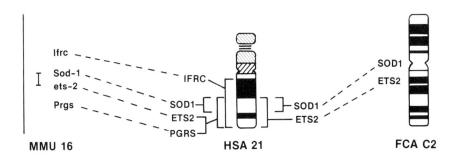

Figure 5. Diagram of regional positions of homologous loci on chromosomes to which ets-1 and ets-2 have been assigned in man, mouse, and cat. All the loci have been regionally assigned in the human map and several have been positioned in mouse. Modified from genetic maps of man, mouse and cat[22]. Basis for homology of included genes is discussed in references (23) and (24).

216

III. The ets sequence from the transforming gene of avian erythroblastosis virus, E26, has unique domains on human chromosomes 11 and 21; both loci
are transcriptionally active.

A. Human ets homologs are dispersed to chromosomally separate loci. In
order to characterize the chromosomal organization of human ets sequences,

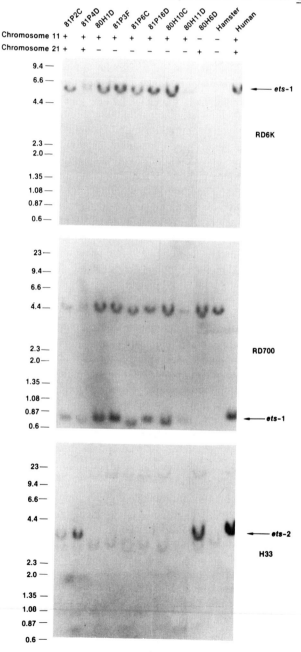

Figure 6. Hybridization of molecularly cloned Hu-ets probes to EcoRI digests of normal human lymphocytes x E36 Chinese hamster somatic cell hybrids.

Lambda phage containing ets equivalents of human DNA were selected from two different human libraries using the Bgl I v-ets clone as a screening probe. One recombinant phage, λRD3, was obtained from a human rabdomyosarcoma library; the other, λH33, from a human placenta library. Two fragments of ets DNA sequences from λRD3 were subcloned into pBR322, and were designated pRD6K and pRD700. Another subclone of ets DNA derived from λH33 library was termed pH33. The sizes and bordering restriction sites of these clones are diagrammed in Fig. 7. Samples of DNA prepared from somatic cell hybrids between hamster and human human cells were digested with EcoRI and fragments were resolved on 0.8% agarose gels. Immobilized DNA[17] was hybridized under stringent conditions (50% formamide, 5 X SSC, 42°C) with human ets probes (A) RD6K, (B) RD700, and (C) H33. The presence or absence of chromosome 11 and 21 is indicated by symbols (+,-) under the hybrid cell line name. ets-1 and ets-2 denote sequences derived from human chromosome 11 and chromosome 21 loci, respectively.

human DNA was digested with Eco R1 and subjected to size-fractionation by agarose gel electrophoresis; the fragments were blotted onto a nitrocellulose filter and hybridized with the three Hu-ets specific clones. As illustrated in Fig. 6, different Hu-ets subclones (cf. Fig. 7), specific for different regions of v-ets recognized different fragments in human genomic DNA. The RD6K probe recognized a 6.2 kb Eco R1 fragment in human DNA; RD700 recognized a 0.83 kb fragment; and H33 resolved a 3.6 kb fragment. Since each Hu-ets subclone recognized a distinct human fragment, it was possible that chromosomally separate DNA segments, each homologous to different portions of the v-ets oncogene, existed in the human genome. To explore this possibility, DNA from a panel of hamster x human somatic cell hybrids which segregrate human chromosomes in different combinations[22,26,27] were examined with the Hu-ets clones. These results (Fig. 6) indicated that the RD6K hybridized specific to 6.2 kb Eco R1 fragment and the RD700 to 0.83 kb Eco R1 fragment, both concordantly associated in these hybrids, suggesting they reside on the same human chromosome. The H33 specific 3.6 kb Eco R1 fragment was highly discordant with the other two fragments, suggesting a minimum of two chromosomally distinct and nonoverlapping ets loci present in the human genome. We have subsequently assigned these two loci termed Hu-ets-1 (defined by homology to RD6K and/or RD700) and Hu-ets-2 (defined by homology to H33) to human chromosomes 11 and 21 respectively[22]. In addition, this data demonstrates the chromosomal specificity of Hu-ets probes.

B. Determination of the point of dispersion of v-ets homologous sequence in Hu-ets-1 and Hu-ets-2. By hybridization analyses, we have shown above that Hu-ets-1 and Hu-ets-2 contain unique subsets of v-ets homologous sequence. We have determined the partial nucleotide sequence of ets-1 (RD700) and ets-2 (cDNA 14 and H33). By alignment of these sequences with those of v-ets from E26 (Fig. 8), one can see three regional domains of homology; two related uniquely to Hu-ets-1 and Hu-ets-2 and a third which defines the overlap between the v-ets related sequences of these loci. Each human ets clone contains a region that is closely related to and is colinear with viral ets (Fig. 7, 8). The human ets sequences are bordered by regions of non-homology, compared to viral ets, which appear to extend the reading frame in the 5' and 3' directions (Fig. 8). However, our data does not distinguish between the possibilities that these sequences of non-homology are either coding regions or are non-coding introns. No splice donor signal can be detected at the 3' border of Hu-ets-2 and v-ets, suggesting that the open reading frame extends beyond this border. Hu-ets-2 encodes thirteen unique amino acids beyond this border; in contrast, the viral gene encodes sixteen unique amino acids. Thus, the viral transforming protein (p135) and the Hu-ets-2 gene product are predicted to have different carboxyl-termini. Tentative splice acceptor and donor signals can be identified at the borders of overlap between the Hu-ets-1 (pRD700) sequence and viral ets. Further work analyzing human ets-1 cDNA clones would help to define the specific coding regions of this gene.

Comparison of the predicted amino acid sequences of Hu-ets-1 and Hu-ets-2 with their viral equivalents (Fig. 8) demonstrated 98% and 95% homology, respectively. This strong evolutionary conservation implies that these genes must perform some important cellular functions.

To determine whether chicken equivalents of the viral ets, c-ets, map in one locus or are scattered over several loci, proto-ets clones were selected from two chicken genomic libraries and characterized. One recombinant phage, termed λC51, was selected using a viral ets probe, and was found to contain a chicken DNA insert of approximately 15 kb (manuscript in preparation). To estimate the complexity of the c-ets sequence of λC51, the clone was hybridized with either a 5' (537 bp Hph I-Pvu II) or 3' (169 bp Hind III-Bgl I) viral probe (Fig. 7). Both probes hybridized to the λC51 DNA insert, indicating that sequences complementary to both Hu-ets-1 and Hu-ets-2 exist within this 15 kb of chicken DNA.

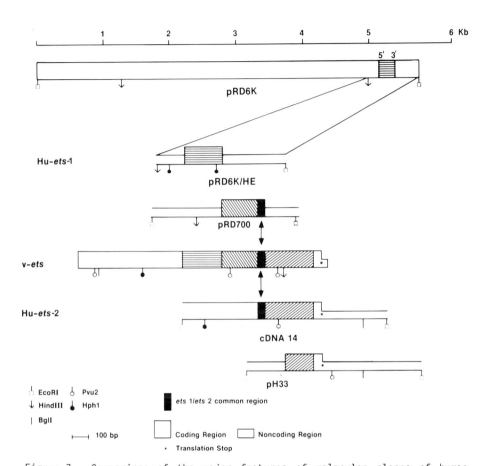

Figure 7. Comparison of the major features of molecular clones of human Hu-ets-1 and Hu-ets-2, and the ets-specific region of the E26 virus.

The previously sequenced v-ets portion of E26[14] is diagrammed and alligned with the subclone, pRD700, derived from a molecular clone, λRD3, from the human Hu-ets-1 locus, and two subclones cDNA 14 and pH33 derived from the human Hu-ets-2 locus.

Allignment was determined by sequence analysis (Fig. 8). The Hu-ets-1 subclone is diagrammed above the v-ets sequence and the Hu-ets-2 subclones are shown below the v-ets sequence.

Another subclone from λRD3, pRD6K (insert utilized for probe in data presented in Figures 1 and 4) has not been localized by sequence analyses but has homology to the 537 bp Hph I - Pvu II fragment of v-ets (that is, immediately 5' to the portion of v-ets alligned with pRD700).

220

```
           Phe Leu Pro Pro Pro Leu Pro Pro
Hu-ets-1   T C CTA CCT CCT  C T A CC  C ⌐        .  C  G    1420      T  .  A     .         T T     T      C C
v-ets      ATG TGC ATG GGA CGT GTC AGT CGA GGT AAA CTG GGT GGC CAG GAC TCC TTT GAG AGC ATA GAG AGC TAC GAC AGC TGT GAC CGC CTG ACA
           Met Cys Met Gly Arg Val Ser Arg Gly Lys Leu Gly Gly Gln Asp Ser Phe Glu Ser Ile Glu Ser Tyr Asp Ser Cys Asp Arg Leu Thr

                                                     Asn
Hu-ets-1        1480              .A  T        A C        . T  T         T C .  C           T  G  T        .
v-ets      CAG TCC TGG AGC AGC CAG TCC TCC TTC CAG AGC CTG CAG CGC GTC CCC TCC TAC GAT AGC TTT GAC TCA GAG GAC TAC CCC GCC GCC CTG
           Gln Ser Trp Ser Ser Gln Ser Ser Phe Gln Ser Leu Gln Arg Val Pro Ser Tyr Asp Ser Phe Asp Ser Glu Asp Tyr Pro Ala Ala Leu

                                                                                                  Leu
Hu-ets-1        1570          .                        G  G  C  T  .     C C  T          1630          T
v-ets      CCC AAC CAC AAG CCC AAG GGC ACC TTC AAG GAC TAT GTT CGA GAT CGG GCT GAC ATG AAC AAG GAC AAG CCT GTC ATT CCT GCC GCT GCC
Hu-ets-2   T       T A G CCA A    T  TCT TT  AAG G T T    ATC CAA GAG AGG A T  AC CCA G   G GC A G    A  A  T  A      A     TG
           Pro Asn His Lys Pro Lys Gly Thr Phe Lys Asp Tyr Val Arg Asp Arg Ala Asp Met Asn Lys Asp Lys Pro Val Ile Pro Ala Ala Ala
           Leu                   Lys                                                       Gly                                  Val

           |cDNA 14                                                   |pRD700
                                          Arg Arg    Pro Ala Ala ***
Hu-ets-1   A   T      .         ⌐LT   G C C   T CC  GCT GCT  AG                     .                    .
v-ets      CTC GCC GGC TAC ACA GGC AGT GGA CCC ATC CAA CTG TGG CAA TTC CTG CTG GAG CTG CTC ACT GAC AAG TCC TGT CAG TCC TTC ATC AGC
Hu-ets-2   G                 T         A        T  T  G            G T  C               A T A    A    C  A
           Leu Ala Gly Tyr Thr Gly Ser Gly Pro Ile Gln Leu Trp Gln Phe Leu Leu Glu Leu Leu Thr Asp Lys Ser Cys Gln Ser Phe Ile Ser
                             Phe                                                                            Ser

                             .                          .                 1800            .                      .
v-ets      TGG ACG GGT GAT GGC TGG GAG TTC AAG CTT TCC GAT CCA GAT GAG GTG GCC AGG CGG TGG GGC AAG AGG AAA AAC AAG CCC AAG ATG GAC
Hu-ets-2       T  A  C  A        T   .  CG   C   C                      A                    C  C          A          T          A
                             Ala                                                                                                Asn

                     .                  .                              .     |pH33
Hu-ets-1        1850                                                         ▸                    .         1900.
v-ets      TAT GAG AAG CTG AGC CGT GGT CTG CGT TAC TAT TAC GAC AAG AAC GTC ATC CAC AAG ACG GCC GGC TAC GTC TAC CGC TTC GTC
Hu-ets-2   C                   G  C TA  C                             A                T G  G           G                G
                                                                      Ile                Ser

                     .              .1950                            ▭                     .                   2000.
v-ets      TGC GAC CTG CAG AGC CTG CTG GGC TAC ACA CCA GAG GAG CAC TCA TCA GCA TCT GGC TTG ACG TCC AGC ATG GCG TGC AGC TCC TTT TGA
Hu-ets-2        C     A  T        G T  G  C          A TG CAC G C ATC CTG    G C CA  C   GA   C   A GA T A
           Cys Asp Leu Gln Ser Leu Leu Gly Tyr Thr Pro Glu Glu His Ser Ser Ala Ser Gly Leu Thr Ser Ser Met Ala Cys Ser Ser Phe ***
                                Asn                 Phe         Leu His Ala Ile Leu     Val Gln Pro Asp Thr Glu Asp ***
```

Figure 8. Comparison of nucleotide sequences of human Hu-ets 1, Hu-ets-2 and the viral transforming gene of E26 (v-ets).

Nucleotide sequence of the E26 ets-homologous domains of Hu-ets molecular clones are alligned with v-ets. The complete line of nucleotides, the numbering and predicted amino acids are from that previously presented for v-ets proceeding in the 5' and 3' direction[14]. The nucleotide and amino acid changes found in the human ets-1 gene (pRD700) are aligned above this partial viral sequence, while those found in the human ets-2 gene (cDNA 14, pH33) are presented below the viral sequence. Brackets indicate 5' and 3' junctions of viral and cellular flanking DNA. The large arrows define the region of overlap between Hu-ets-1 and Hu-ets-2. Presumptive splice donor (⌐) and acceptor (⌐) signals are indicated. The symbol (I) defines the junction between the last two Hu-ets-2 exons.

C. Hu-ets-1 and Hu-ets-2 are both transcriptionally active. To determine whether the human ets loci are transcriptionally active and to estimate the complexity of the human ets genes, we have analyzed ets-specific mRNAs. For this purpose poly(A) selected RNA from human cells was size fractionated by electrophoresis in an agarose gel, transferred to nitrocellulose paper and then hybridized with ^{32}P-labeled DNA specific probes for Hu-ets-1, or Hu-ets-2. The results show a 6.8 kb Hu-ets-1 mRNA and three distinct Hu-ets-2 mRNA species of 4.7, 3.2 and 2.7 kb (Fig. 9A). From these data we can draw the following conclusions: (i) Both human ets loci are transcriptionally active. (ii) The Hu-ets-1 appear to be a single gene of maximal coding complexity of 6.8 kb and Hu-ets-2 may be a single gene with alternate initiation or splice signals with a complexity of 4.2 kb. (iii) There is only a slight overlap between the ets-related sequences of Hu-ets-1 and Hu-ets-2 encoding 14 amino acids where 12 are conserved between these two loci.

Similar studies with RNA from chicken cells, using a v-ets probe which contains ets-1 and ets-2 contiguous sequences, identifies primarily a single major transcribed species of approximately 7.5 kb. A minor component, however, was observed which does not correspond to any human mRNA species identified (Fig. 9B); similar results have been reported by others[13].

IV. Hu-ets-1 and Hu-ets-2 genes are transposed in acute leukemias with (4;11) and (8;21) translocations.

A number of leukemias of the myelomonocytic lineage show chromosome abnormalities in the very regions where the human-ets genes reside (Fig. 10)[28]. Acute leukemia associated with the (4;11) chromosome translocation occurs more frequently in infants and young adults and has a rapid course and a poor prognosis (Table 1)[29-37]. Notably, the 4;11 leukemia is found in newborns strongly suggesting that it may be congenital in origin[28]. This leukemia has for some time been classified as a form of acute lymphocytic leukemia (ALL), FAB L1 or L2, based primarily on the morphological appearance of the leukemic cells. However, the nature of this leukemia is controversial since none of the features noted has been definitive for lineage assignment of the leukemic cells. The (4;11) blasts do not express surface or cytoplasmic immunoglobulin (SIg or CIg) nor do they form E rosettes with sheep erythrocytes. Most do not have the common acute lymphocytic leukemia antigen (CALLA). The enzyme terminal deoxynucleotidyl transferase (TdT) is often expressed. Blasts from different patients have been shown to react with monoclonal antibodies recognizing B lymphoid antigens, HLA-DR and, p24/BA-2 as well as myelomonocytic antigens (CDW13/MCS2, Leu-M1, 2D1, 1C2). Immunoglobulin heavy and light chain gene rearrangements have been detected in

222

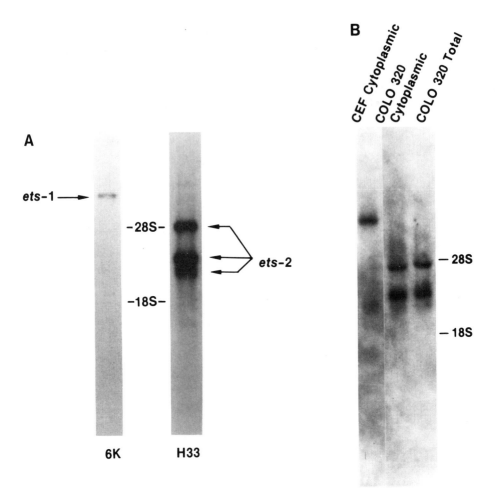

Figure 9. Human ets-1 and ets-2 loci are transcriptionally active.

A. Polyadenylated RNA prepared from HeLa cells was resolved on 1.5% formaldehyde-agarose gels and hybridized to RD6K (purified DNA from pRD6K, ets-1) or H33 (purified DNA from pH33, ets-2) probes under stringent conditions[20]. Mobility of the 28S and 18S ribosomal RNA's are as indicated.

B. Expression of c-ets in chicken embryo fibroblasts (CEF) and human COLO-320 cells. Total cell RNA was also prepared from COLO-320 cells. Samples (20 μg) were resolved on 1.2% formaldehyde-agarose gels. CEF RNA was hybridized to a v-ets probe (1.28 kb Bgl I fragment) and COLO 320 RNA samples were hybridized to H33 under stringent condition (as described in Figure 6).

Chromosome Aberrations Commonly Found in ANLL

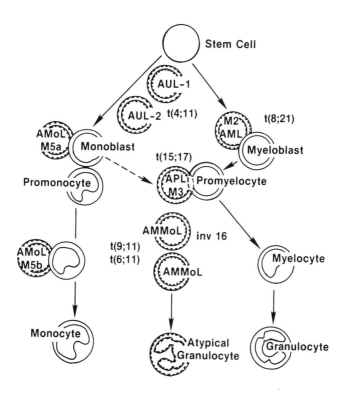

Figure 10. Non-random cytogenetic abnormalities associated with subtypes of human acute myeloid leukemias representing the malignant transformation of different myelomonocytic maturation stages.

Table 1

Clinical characteristics of (4;11) leukemia

NEWBORN/INFANTILE TYPE:	age 0-2 yr
Congenital	Longest survival: 14 mo
JUVENILE/ADULT TYPE:	age >11 yr
	Longest survival: 41 mo
DISEASE COURSE:	Rapid, with a median survival of 8 mo
COMPLETE REMISSION:	Rare and short: ca. 3 mo
THERAPEUTIC RESPONSE:	Poorly responding to ALL-type therapy

This Table has been based on data reported in literature (29-37).

(4;11) cells. This would suggest a commitment toward the B lineage. Nevertheless, (4;11) cells express certain myelomonocytic antigens and can be
induced to display monocyte features by phorbol ester treatment. It has
also been shown that the in vitro growth pattern of (4;11) cells is more
comparable to ANL than to ALL blasts. Taken together, the features of
(4;11) blasts (Table 2) suggest that the malignant transformation may have
involved a very undifferentiated percursor cell of the myelomonocytic lineage
or a common lymphoid/myeloid precursor. The 11q23 region, where Hu-ets-1
is located, participates in a number of translocations, (Table 3) involving
a second variable chromosome in acute myeloid leukemias, thus suggesting
that this region must contain critical myeloid transformation gene(s).
These leukemias result from the expansion of elements of the myelomonocytic
lineage with various degrees of maturation. We focused primarily on the
t(4;11)(q21;q23) translocation (Fig. 11A) that represented a consistent feature of a subtype of infant-associated leukemia thought to be congenital
(cf. Table 1) (28). The peculiar ultrastructural and immunologic characteristics of these leukemic blasts implicate a bone marrow precursor with the
ability to differentiate either towards the myeloid or lymphoid lineage
(cf. Table 2). The 21q22 region where Hu-ets-2 resides is involved in the
translocation (8;21)(q22;q22) (Fig. 11B), commonly found in acute myelogenous
leukemia with morphology M2 (Table 4)[38]. This region (21q22) is also implicated in Down's syndrome[39]. These patients with three (or more) chromosome
21 show a marked incidence of acute leukemia, particularly ANLL[40]; whereas
infants may present benign, reversible leukemoid reactions. This association suggests that trisomy 21 may be predisposing factor for leukemic transformation.

Table 2

Features of (4;11) leukemic blasts

MORPHOLOGY:	L1 and L1 according to FAB classification
IMMUNOLOGIC PHENOTYPE:	HLA-DR+ CALLA- T- cIg-
	variable expression of B-cell antigens
	variable expression of myelomonocytic antigens
	TdT: positive in most cases
IMMUNOGLOBULIN GENES:	Rearrangements of heavy and light chain genes
ULTRASTRUCTURE:	Basophil or mast cell morphology
IN VITRO GROWTH:	Similar to ANL blasts; myelomonocytic features can be induced by phorbol ester

This Table has been based on data reported in literature[29-37].

Table 3

Acute Leukemias with 11 q23 rearrangements

Diagnosis	Chromosome Rearrangement
AUL	t(4;11)(q21;q23)
ANLL	t(9;11)(p21-22;p23)
ANLL	t(10;11)(*;q23)
ANLL	t(6;11)(q27;q23)
ANLL	t(11;17)(q23;q27)
ANLL	t(11;19)(q23;q13)

*Variable breakpoints on chromosome 10.

Our data demonstrates that both Hu-ets-1 and Hu-ets-2 genes translocate from their normal position as a consequence of rearrangements involving the 11q23 and 21q22 breakpoints. This conclusion is based on analysis of two panels of somatic cell hybrids retaining, in a chinese hamster cell background, either the normal or the recombinant chromosomes deriving from the (4;11) and (8;21) translocation (Fig. 11 A and B).

Chinese hamster fibroblasts, A3, were fused with an established leukemia cell line, RS4;11[41], presenting the (4;11)(q21;q23) translocation. A number of cell hybrids[42] have been isolated in selective HAT medium and subsequently identified cytogenetically by the R-banding technique and assayed biochemically for the presence of markers of chromosome 4 and 11 e.g., lactate dehydrogenase A (LDHA) - chromosome 11; phosphoglucomutase-2 (PGM2)

Table 4

Features of t(8;21)(p22;q22) Leukemia

PERCENTAGE OF ALL de novo M2 LEUKEMIAS:	16%
GEOGRAPHIC DISTRIBUTION:	more frequent in Japan and South Africa
MALE/FEMALE RATIO:	3/1
REMISSION RATE:	75% (complete) 15.9% (partial)
AGE DISTRIBUTION (yr)	
<1	0
2-19	26.8
20-39	26.4
40-59	31.7
>60	17.1
MEDIAN SURVIVAL FROM DIAGNOSIS:	9.5 mo

Based on data of the Fourth International Workshop on chromosomes in Leukemia (1982).

- chromosome 4. The calcitonin growth factor-related peptide gene located in the 11 pter-11q12 region was detected by a specific DNA probe. The human ets-1 probe RD6K[22] was used to identify Hu-ets-1 sequences in DNA isolated from these cell hybrids.

The human 3.0 kb Pst I fragment, identified by the RD6K probe, is seen to be present in hybrids containing either the intact 11 or the recombinant 4q-chromosomes (Fig. 12, Lanes 3, 5, 6 and 7). The same is true for a 6.2 kb Eco RI fragment. This experiment left unresolved whether the chromosomal breakpoint is within or outside of the Hu-ets-1 gene. Nevertheless, Southern blot analysis of DNA from three t(4;11) leukemias, from the (RS4;11) cell line, two (9;11)(p22;q23) leukemias, (AMMoL-M4 and AMMoL-M5 respectively) and of the diploid myelomonocytic cell line HL-92[43] with a deletion [(11)(q23)] did not demonstrate any rearrangements of Hu-ets-1 using a variety of restriction enzymes (data not shown). This analysis suggests that the breakpoint must occur outside of the 12 kb region containing the above restriction fragments.

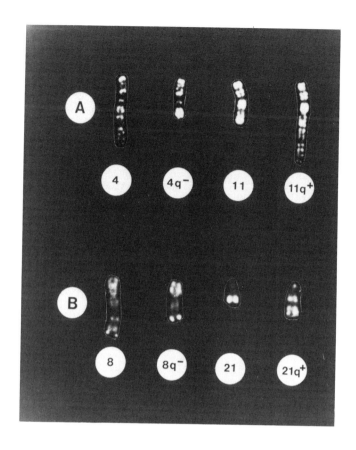

Figure 11. Partial karyotype analysis showing the normal and recombinant chromosomes resulting from: A) the reciprocal translocation t(4;11)(q21;q23), and B) the reciprocal translocation t(8;21)(q22;q22).

We have used a similar approach to investigate whether the Hu-ets-2 gene translocates in t(8;21) AML-M2 leukemia. The usual, 8 and 21 chromosomes, as well as the recombinant derivatives 8q and 21q+ of the t(8;21) leukemia have been isolated in a chinese hamster cell background. This panel of cell hybrids has been characterized by extensive segregation analysis; isozyme analysis using markers specific for chromosomes 8 and 21; (e.g., the glutathione reductase activity (GSR) for chromosome 8; the soluble superoxide dismutase (SOD-1 for chromosome 21), and probes for c-myc (8q24) and c-mos (8q22) genes[45-48]. DNA extracted from these cell hybrids was

228

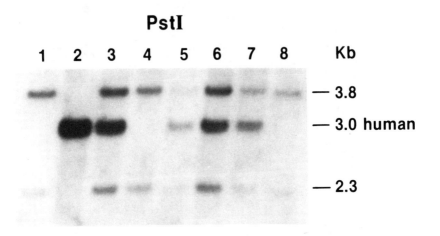

PstI

| 1 | 2 | 3 | 4 | 5 | 6 | 7 | 8 | Kb |

— 3.8

— 3.0 human

— 2.3

Figure 12. Southern blot analysis of human lymphocytes, A3 chinese hamster fibroblasts and A3 x t(4;11) leukemic cells. The DNAs were digested with Pst I and subjected to electrophoresis in a 0.8% agarose gel. Blot hybridization analysis with a human ets-1 specific (RD6K) probe (C10) was carried out under stringent conditions (50% formamide, 5 x SSC, 42°C; washings: 2 x SSC, 0.5% SDS at 65°C, 0.1 x SSC at 25°). The human 3.0 kb Pst I fragment is detected in hybrids containing either the chromosome 11 or 4q⁻. Lane 1, A3 fibroblasts; Lane 2, human lymphocytes; Lane 3, hybrid 30A (Chr. 11); Lane 4, hybrid 27B (Chr. 11q⁺); Lane 5, hybrid 5B (Chr. 4q⁻ and 11q⁺); Lane 6, hybrid 11B (Chr. 4q⁻); Lane 7, hybrid 17A (Chr. 4 and 4q⁻); Lane 8, hybrid 12B (Chr. 4 and 11q⁺).

subjected to Southern-blot analysis utilizing the Hu-ets-2 genomic probe (H33) and another ets-2 probe designated cDNA 14[22]. The 3.8 kb Eco RI fragment of the Hu-ets-2 gene is present in the cell hybrid containing the recombinant chromosome 8q⁻, but not in the hybrid containing the chromosome 21q⁺, indicating that the Hu-ets-2 gene was transposed from chromosome 21 to chromosome 8 (Fig. 13). Similarly, the Bam HI 6.8 kb fragment, the Pst I 12 kb fragment, and the Hind III 3.5 kb fragment were present in the

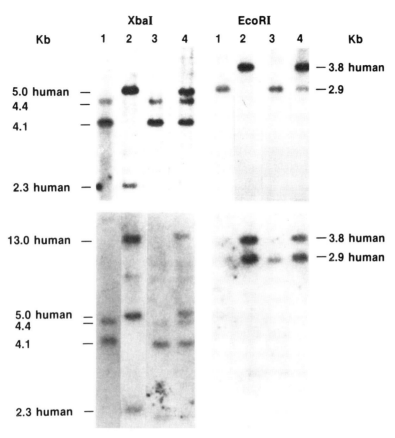

Figure 13. Southern blot analysis of human lymphocytes, A3 chinese hamster fibroblasts x t(8;21) leukemic cell hybrids. The DNAs were digested with Xba I and EcoRI and subjected to electrophoresis in a 0.8% agarose gel. Blot-hybridization analysis with human ets-2 specific probes, H33 (top) and cDNA 14 (bottom) was carried out as described in Fig. 12 legend. Lane 1, Chinese hamster cells; Lane 2, human lymphocytes; Lane 3, 21-8Ab5-23 (21q⁺) hybrid; Lane 4, 13b1S816 (8q⁻) hybrid. The EcoRI 3.8 kb and Xba I 5.0 kb human fragments are detectable only in the 8q⁻ hybrid.

hybrid with chromosome 8q⁻ but not in the one with chromosome 21q⁺ (data not shown). In the Xba I digest (Fig. 13, bottom) only the human 5.0 kb fragment, but not the 2.3 kb fragment, was detectable in the 8q⁻ containing hybrid. Thus, the Xba I site of the Hu-ets-2 gene may have been eliminated a consequence of translocation. Similar results utilizing the same as blots with the cDNA 14 probe were obtained. With this cDNA 14 probe, we were able to detect a 2.9 kb human Eco R1 fragment and an additional 13 kb Xba I fragment that was associated only with the cell hybrid containing the 8q⁻ chromosome. Thus, we concluded from these experiments that at least 20.3 kb of the Hu-ets-2 gene had been translocated to chromosome 8. DNA from eight t(8;21) AML-M2 patients were subjected to Southern blot analysis[17] using the same restriction enzymes as above; no Hu-ets-2 gene rearrangement were detected. Moreover, the ³H-labeled Hu-ets-2 probe, H33, hybridized specifically to the 8q⁻ chromosome of fresh leukemic cells from t(8;21) AML-M2 patients[49]. In situ hybridization analysis of fresh leukemic cells having another translocation (9;11)(p21;q23) which involves the 11q23 region, after probing with the v-ets 1.28 kb Bgl I fragment[14], shows the translocation of ets sequences from chromosome 11 to chromosome 9[49]. This translocation is usually associated with acute myelomonocytic leukemia (AMMoL-M4) and acute monocytic leukemia (AMoL-M5)[50].

We next determined if the translocation of human ets-1 and ets-2 affected the transcription patterns of these genes. This study could only be performed on a limited number of patients which were cytogenetically characterized. In particular, fresh bone marrow blasts specimens were needed to preserve the integrity of the RNA. We were, nonetheless, able to assay for the expression of mRNA in fresh leukemic samples. Total RNA was isolated from leukemic cells and compared to normal human lymphocyte RNA in Northern blot experiments. In one AUL t(4;11) leukemia we observed only low levels of Hu-ets-1 mRNA (Fig. 14A); similar results were also obtained using RNA from the RS4;11 cell line (data not shown). In two t(8;21) AML-M2 leukemias we did not observe all the human ets-2 mRNA species present in normal control lymphocytes (Fig. 14B), and known to be present in several other tissues and cell lines of human origin[22]. The 4.7 kb and 3.2 kb mRNA species were notably absent in one patient sample, and the 4.7 kb species was absent in the other. The expression of Hu-ets-2 gene in the t(8;21) cells is also much lower than observed in the control lymphocytes. It may be possible that the altered expression of ets-1 and ets-2 genes is a consequence of the translocations observed. Alternatively, this finding might represent the typical expression of ets genes in the normal cell counterparts of these leukemic blasts. Myeloid precursor cells, which are impossible to identify and isolate from normal bone marrow using present-day technology, would be the ideal controls for these studies rather than lymphocytes.

These studies indicate that the Hu-ets-2 gene translocates to the 8q⁻ chromosome which has been suggested[51] to be the critical recombinant

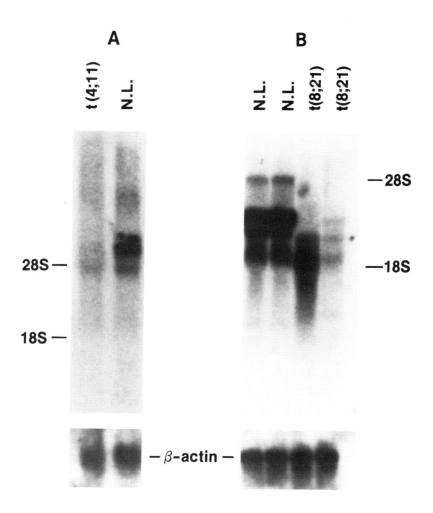

Figure 14. Northern blot analysis of total RNA extracted from: A) blast cells derived from a t(4;11) AUL patient and normal lymphocytes (N. L.), and B) blasts cells derived from two t(8;21) AML-M2 patients and normal lymphocytes. In all cases, RNA was extracted by the guanidinium/cesium chloride method and resolved on 1.2% formaldehyde-agarose gels (C33). Hybridization was performed under stringent conditions (as described in Fig. 12) using the (A) ets-1 (RD6K) and (B) ets-2 (H33) probes. The same blots (bottom) have been rehybridized with a β-actin cDNA probe to compare the amount of RNA in these samples.

chromosome in the t(8;21) translocation; particularly based upon the circumstantial cytogenetic evidence that this chromosome is the one constant in both the simple and complex translocations. Notably, at the 8q22 breakpoint site another proto-oncogene, c-mos resides which does not translocate to the other recombinant chromosome 21q+[46], supporting the previous supposition that the 8q⁻ is the critical chromosome.

Similarly the 11q23 region is also believed to be critical, since this region is a constant one, participating in translocations involving a second variable chromosome. It has been suggested by Rowley[31] that these translocations can bring together two types of genes, one related to growth control (proto-oncogene) in a certain hematopoietic cell and in a specific differentiative stage; and another gene, coding for a protein critical to that cell, at that particular stage. In this context, 11q23 can be hypothesized to contain the locus for a growth-regulatory factor (i.e., Hu-ets-1 product), whereas the regions of the other chromosome (i.e., 4q21 or 9p22) could contain the loci for myeloid stage specific genes. The molecular characterization of the breakpoints, as well as the identification of the human ets-1 and ets-2 gene products are necessary in order to establish whether these genes, with the discussed cytogenetic abnormalities, play a crucial role in the development of some acute leukemias.

V. DISCUSSION

At least three different prototype transforming retroviruses have been described which contain two distinct oncogenes encompassed by helper viral sequences. These include: MH2 which contains v-myc and v-mht; avian erythroblastosis virus which contains v-erb A and v-erb B; and E26 which contains v-myc and v-ets. We have shown that the v-ets segment of E26 is derived from two domains which are themselves encoded on different chromosomes in mammals. In addition to E26, two additional oncogenic viruses, GR-FeSV and FBR-MSV, contain hybrid onc genes that include genetic elements from two different cellular genes and from essential retrovirus genes[52-54]. Diagnostic genomic clone probes for the two domains (termed ets-1 and ets-2) have been used to demonstrate transcriptional activity of both loci[20] and to chromosomally map to chromosome homologs in different mammals[22]. The genes do not overlap, in man, and have been assigned to chromosomes 11 and 21, respectively.

This dispersal of mammalian proto-ets sequences is in contrast to the organization in chicken from which the E26 virus was orginally isolated. Avian c-ets has a genomic complexity of at least 40-50 kb (15) which encodes a 7.5 kb ets transcribed RNA[13,20]. This single RNA transcript is resolved in RNA blots with both ets-1 and ets-2 specific probes, suggesting that the two domains are contiguous in the chicken's genome. The biologically active viral ets mRNA is a truncated 1.5 kb version of the chicken message. Since v-ets is a rather small subset of the chicken proto-ets locus, as well as of the two mammalian proto-ets loci, the relative contribution of the myb, ets-1 and ets-2 domains to viral transformation is not yet obvious. Transduction of a 1.6 kb sequence from chicken proto-ets by the retrovirus that generated E26 is so far the only hint that proto-ets has oncogenic potential. The transforming gene of E26 appears to be one of the most complex examples of how proto-onc genes and retroviruses generate viral onc genes.

Our data suggest that the ets region shared by E26, the chicken and man, contains at least two dissociable domains. This is deduced from the observation that the human complement of viral ets related sequence is distributed between two different genes located on two different chromosomes. Further, the high degree of conservation of the ets-related genes in chicken and man suggest that these genes encode functions essential to the cell. It thus appears that the transforming gene of E26, which is derived from three different progenitor genes, may contain four functional domains, Δgag, myb and two ets domains corresponding to human ets-1 and ets-2. We are now constructing E26 deletion mutants to determine the functionality of ets-1 and ets-2 domains.

Our results delineating the expression of ets 1 and ets 2 in human cells present evidence for multiple RNA species. The Hu-ets-1 probe reveals one 6.8 kb transcript, while the Hu-ets-2 probe detected three distinct RNA species of 4.7, 3.2 and 2.7 kb. This findings suggests functionally distinct proteins are potentially translatable from these multiple mRNAs. This observation in human cells is marked contrast to that seen with chicken cell RNA; hybridization with the v-ets probe showed only one major RNA species of 7.5 kb. Taken together these data indicate that in the chicken only one gene product is functionally transcribed, whereas in man as a result of evolutionary divergence, the ets 2 domain became part of another gene which was transcriptionally active, expressing a series of mRNA's with perhaps differing function(s). This hypothesis is further substantiated by our observations that ets-1 and ets-2 genes behave separately, each having unique loci in the mouse and cat, as well as man.

In addition to establishing conservation of linkage groups and the occurrence of two distinct ets-related loci in three mammalian orders, our work suggests that ets encodes separate transcriptionally active and perhaps functionally distinct products. These genes and their encoded products, could have presumably been separate and functionally distinct prior to the evolutionary radiation of the Mammalia. We are presently preparing specific antibodies against synthetic oligopeptides derived from the predicted ets sequences and bacterially expressed ets gene products, in effort to characterize the various gene products. These reagents will also assist in the determination of this respective biological function which, by analogy with other oncogene products, are expected to be involved at some critical point in the control of normal cellular growth and/or function.

A restricted number of chromosome regions are implicated in human cancers; these regions presumably contain genes whose disarrangement is crucial to the establishment of neoplasia[55]. It has been known for sometime that there is a specifically of certain translocations associated with hematopoietic tumors[51]. This may result in a proliferative advantage conferred by the recombinant chromosome(s) to a hematopoietic cell, when in a particular differentiative stage and within a particular lineage[56]. We now know that several proto-oncogenes[57] and other genes such as those coding for immunoglobulins[58] and T-cell receptor[59] map at, or are in close proximity to, breakpoints characteristic of translocations and inversions that occur in certain leukemias. These features support the above concept that cytogenetic accidents occurring at a particular differentiative stage may initiate a cascade of molecular alterations that results in the leukemic transformation. Two well defined examples of chromosome translocation which have repercussions at the molecular level are: gene deregulation in Burkitt's lymphomas with (8;14), (8;22) and (2;8) translocations involving the c-myc locus with the heavy and light chain Ig loci[60]; production of a chimeric protein in chronic myelogenous leukemia (CML) with the (9;22) translocation (Philadelphia chromosome). In the latter case a fusion product of bcr-abl genes is found[61].

It is well known that the human chromosomes have numerous fragile sites perhaps conferring a propensity towards forming breakpoints; thus 20 of the 51 fragile sites so far identified map at or close to the breakpoints found associated with 16 of 31 characterized cytogenetic abnormalities identifiable in various leukemias, lymphomas and certain solid-tumors[57].

Constitutive fragile sites have been recognized on human chromosome 11 and 21 at or near the same bands (11q23.3 and 21q22) that map close to the Hu-ets region. In addition, a number of known human acute leukemias particular of the myelomonocytic lineage present specific chromosome aberrations involving the 11q23.3 and 21q22 bands. Taken together these data make our investigations into the involvement of the <u>ets</u> gene very promising and support the use ofthe Hu-<u>ets</u> probes to study the pathogenesis of the above mentioned leukemias.

Subregional assignment of Hu-<u>ets</u>-2 to the 21q22.3 band is of additional importance because it is this region of chromosome 21 which is thought to be pathogenetic for Down's syndrome. Down's syndrome is the most frequent identifiable genetic cause of mental retardation and is associated with a large number of developmental abnormalities. Individuals with this syndrome are markedly at risk for the development of acute leukemia. A congenital leukemia or leukemoid reaction may occur in Down's syndrome neonates which spontaneously resolve, raising the possibility that some alteration of auto-crine stimulation of haematopoeitic cells could be involved. Some of these neonates have been mosaic for trisomy 21 and in these cases the leukemic-like cells were all of the trisomic clone. This finding suggest that (a) gene(s) on chromosome 21 is involved in the growth and/or differentiation of haematopoeitic cells.

Finally not to mitigate the value of other approaches towards the resolu-tion and evaluation of oncogenes in human malignances, it would seem from these studies which also presents evidence for the taxonomic divergence of three distinct proto-oncogenes to three unique chromosomal loci, along with a concomitant dispersion of gene products; that the rationale for using re-troviral vectors and genes for such investigations related to human disease, remains strongly justifiable.

VI. REFERENCES

1. Duesberg, P.H. (1983) Nature 304, 219-226.
2. Varmus, H.E. (1984) Ann. Rev. Genet. 18, 553-612.
3. Bishop, J.M. (1983) Ann. Rev. Biochem. 52, 301-354.
4. Weinberg, R.A. (1980) Ann. Rev. Biochem. 49, 197-226.
5. Varmus, H.E. (1982) Cancer Surv. 2, 301-319.
6. Hayward, W.S., Neel, B.G. and Astrin, S.M. (1981) Nature 209, 475-479.
7. Klein, G. (1983) Cell 32, 311-315.
8. Groffen, J., Stephenson, J.R., Heisterkamp, N., de Klein, A., Bartram, C.R. <u>et al</u>. (1984) Cell 36, 93-99.
9. Kohl, N.E., Kanda, N., Schreck, R.R., Burns, G., Latt, S.A. <u>et al</u>. (1984) Cell 35, 359-367.
10. Schwab, M., Alitalo, K., Klempnauer, K.H., Varmus, H.E., Bishop, J.M. <u>et al</u>. (1983) Nature 305, 245-248.

11. Little, C. D., Nau, M. M., Carney, D. N., Gazdar, A. F. and Minna, J. D. (1983) Nature 306, 194-196.

12. Duesberg, P. H., Bister, K. and Moscovici, C. (1980) Proc. Natl. Acad. Sci. U.S.A. 77, 5120-5124.

13. Leprince, D., Gegonne, A., Coll, J., deTaisne, C., Schneeberger, A., Lagrou, C. and Stehelin, D. (1983) Nature 306, 395-397.

14. Nunn, M. F., Seeberg, P. H., Moscovici, C. and Deusberg, P. H. (1983) Nature 306, 391-395.

15. Nunn, M., Weiher, H., Bullock, P. and Duesberg, P. H. (1984) Virology 139, 330-339.

16. Bister, K., Nunn, M., Moscovici, C., Perbal, B., Baluda, M. A. and Duesberg, P. H. (1982) Proc. Natl. Acad. Sci. U.S.A. 79, 3677-3686.

17. Southern, E. M. (1975) J. Mol. Biol. 98, 503-517.

18. Nash, W. G. and O'Brien, S. J. (1982) Proc. Natl. Acad. Sci. U.S.A. 79, 6631-6635.

19. O'Brien, S. J. & Nash, W. G. (1982) Science 216, 257-265.

20. Watson, D. K., McWilliams-Smith, M. J., Nunn, M. F., Duesberg, P. H., O'Brien, S. J. and Papas, T. S. (1985) Proc. Natl. Acad. U.S.A. 82, 7294-7298.

21. de Taisne, C., Gegonne, A., Stehelin, D., Bernheim, A. and Berger, R. (1984) Nature 310, 581-583.

22. Watson, D. K., McWilliams-Smith, M. J., Kozak, C., Reeves, R., Gearhart, J., Nash, W., Modi, W., Duesberg, P. H., Papas, T. S and O'Brien, S. J. (1985) Proc. Natl. Acad. Sci. U.S.A. In Press.

23. O'Brien, S. J., Seuanez, H. N. and Womack, J. E. (1984) in Evolutionary Biology (Plenum Press, New York). In Press.

24. Roderick, T. H., Lalley, P. A., Davisson, M. T., O'Brien, S. J., Womack, J. E., Creau-Goldgerg, N., Echard, G. and Moore, K. L. (1984) Cytogenet. Cell Genet. 37, 312-339.

25. Nadeau, J. H. and Taylor, B. A. (1984) Proc. Natl. Acad. Sci. U.S.A. 81, 814-818.

26. O'Brien, S. J., Bonner, T. I., Cohen, M., O'Connell, C. and Nash, W. G. (1983b) Nature 303, 74-77.

27. O'Brien, S. J., Simonson, J. M. and Eichelberger, M. A. (1982) in Techniques in Somatic Cell Genetics. Shay, J. W. (Ed.), (Plenum Press, New York) pp. 342-370.

28. Kocova, M. et al. (1985) Cancer Genet. and Cytogenet. 4, 21.

29. Arthur, D. C. (1982) Blood 59, 96.

30. Esseltine, D.W., Vekemans, M., Seemayer, T., Reece, E., Gordon, J. and Whitehead, V.M. (1982) Cancer 50, 503.

31. Morse, H.G., Heideman, R., Hays, T. and Robinson, A. (1982) Cancer Genet. Cytogenet. 7, 165.

32. Van de Berghe, H., David, G., Broeckaert-Van Orshoven, A., Louwagie, A., Verwilghen, R., Casteels-Van Daele, M., Eggermont, E. and Eeckels, R. (1979) Hum. Genet. 46, 173.

33. Nagasaka, M., Maeda, S., Maeda, H., Chen, H.L., Kita, K., Mabuchi, O., Misu, H., Matsuo, T. and Sugiyama, T. (1983) Blood 51, 1174.

34. Prigogina, E.L., Fleishman, E.W., Puchkova, G.P., Kulagina, O.E., Majokova, S.A., Balakire-Frenkel, M.A., Khvatova, N.V. and Peterson, I.S. (1979) Hum. Genet. 53, 5.

35. Parkin, J.L., Arthur, D.C., Abramson, C.S., McKenna, R.W., Kersey, J.H., Heideman, R.L. and Brunning, R.D. (1982) Blood 60, 1321.

36. Geist, W., et al. (1985) Blood 66, 33.

37. Stong, R.C. and Kersey, J.H. (1985) Blood 66, 439.

38. Rowley, J.D. (1973) Ann. Genet. 16, 109; Rowely, J.D. and Testa, J.R. (1983) Adv. Cancer Res. 36, 103.

39. Summitt, R.L. (1981) in Trisomy 21 (Down's Syndrome). Research Perspectives. de la Cruz, F.F. and Gerald, P.S. (Eds.)(University Park Press, Baltimore) p. 157.

40. Alimena, G. et al. (1985) Cancer Genet. and Cytogenet. 16, 207.

41. Stong, R. et al. (1985) Blood 65, 21.

42. Sacchi, N. et al. (1986) Science 231, 379-382.

43. Salahuddin, F.A. et al. (1982) Leukemia Res. 6, 729.

44. Jones, C. et al. (1981) Somatic Cell Genet. 7, 399.

45. Davidson, J.N. et al. Advances in Gene Technology: Human Genetic Disorders. Proceedings of the Sixteenth Miami Winter Symposium, Short Reports. Ahmad, F., Black, S., Schulz, J., Scott, W.A. and Whelan, W.J. (Eds.) Vol. 1, pp. 148-149.

46. Drabkin, H.A. et al. (1985) Proc. Natl. Acad. Sci. U.S.A. 82, 466.

47. ibid (manuscript in preparation).

48. Le Beau, M. et al. (manuscript in preparation).

49. Diaz, M. O. et al. (1986) Science 231, 265-267.

50. Sandberg, A. A. (1980) "The Chromosomes in Human Cancer and Leukemia", Amsterdam, Elsevier/North Holland Biomedical Press. Mitelman, F. (1983) Cytogenet. Cell Genet. 36, 1-515. Fourth International Workshop on Chromosomes in Leukemia (1984) Cancer Genet. and Cytogenet. 11, 1. Abe, R. and Sandberg, A. A. (1984) Cancer Genet. and Cytogenet. 13, 121.

51. Rowley, J. D. (1984) Cancer Res. 44, 3159.

52. Naharro, G., Robbins, K. C. and Reddy, E. P. (1984) Science 223, 63-66.

53. Van Beveren, C., Enami, S., Curran, T. and Verma, I. M. (1984) Virology, 135, 229-243.

54. Van Beveren, C., van Straaten, F., Curran, T., Muller, R. and Verma, I. M. (1983) Cell 32, 1241-1255.

55. Mitelman, F. (1984) Nature 310, 325.

56. Rowley, J. D. (1980) Proc. Natl. Acad. Sci. U.S.A. 76, 5729.

57. Yunis, J. J. and Soreng, A. L. (1984) Science 226, 1199.

58. Croce, C. M. et al. (1979) Proc. Natl. Acad. Sci. U.S.A. 76, 3416. Erikson, J. et al. (1981) Nature 294, 173. McBride, O. W. et al. (1982) J. Exp. Med. 155, 1480. Malcolm, S. et al. (1982) Proc. Natl. Acad. Sci. U.S.A. 79, 4957.

59. Croce, C. M. et al. (1985) Science 227, 1044. Collins, S. et al. (1986) J. EMBO 3, 2347. Le Beau, M. et al. (1985) Cell 41, 335.

60. Croce, C. M. and Nowell, P. C. (1985) Blood 65, 1.

61. Shtivelman, E. et al. (1985) Nature 315, 550. Heisterkamp, N., et al. (1985) ibid, 758. Konopka, J. et al. (1984) Cell 37, 1035. Konopka, J. et al. (1985) Proc. Natl. Acad. Sci. U.S.A. 82, 1810.

13

Properties of the _met_ Oncogene

George F. Vande Woude[+], Michael Dean[+], Mary Gonzatti-Haces[+], Anand Iyer[+], Karen Kaul[+], Terrell Robins[+], Morag Park[+], and Donald G. Blair[++]

[+]LBI-Basic Research Program
NCI-Frederick Cancer Research Facility
Frederick, Maryland 21701, USA

[++]Laboratory of Molecular Oncology
National Cancer Institute
Frederick, Maryland 21701, USA

INTRODUCTION

Using the NIH/3T3 cell focus assay, transforming genes have been detected in gene transfer experiments in many different chemically-induced tumors and in cells transformed in vitro by chemical carcinogens. Most of the transforming genes identified in these studies are members of the ras family of oncogenes (see chapter Barbacid, this book). For example, the cellular homolog of Harvey sarcoma virus (rasH) has been shown to be activated in chemically-induced squamous cell carcinomas and papillomas in mice[1,2], chemically-induced mammary carcinomas in rats[3], and guinea pig cells transformed in vitro by chemical carcinogens[4]. Similarly, the rasK family member has been shown to be activated in methylcholanthrene-induced mouse sarcomas[5] and in mouse fibroblasts transformed in vitro by chemical carcinogens[6] while rasN was activated in a chemically induced thymic lymphoma[7].

In contrast to the abundance of studies on chemically-transformed rodent cells, human cells appear to be refractory to transformation by carcinogens[8-10] and there are only a few examples of human cells transformed by direct treatment in vitro with chemicals[11-13]. The transformation of human fibroblasts[11] and the nontumorigenic human osteogenic sarcoma (HOS) cells[16] by chemical carcinogens in vitro has been reported[11,13]. We have examined three chemically transformed HOS cell lines in gene transfer experiments[14,15a,b] and found that only one possesses the transferable transforming gene which we have called met[15b].

The activated met oncogene was detected in a morphologically altered derivative of HOS cells obtained after prolonged treatment with N-methyl-N'-nitronitrosoguanidine (MNNG-HOS)[13]. The MNNG-HOS cells are tumorigenic in nude mice while the parental HOS cells are not. Our results showed that DNA prepared from MNNG-HOS cells could transform NIH/3T3 cells[15a,b] and produce tumors in the nude mouse tumor assay[14] while DNA from 7,12-dimethylbenzy(a)-anthracene (DMBA) transformed HOS cells[12b], parental HOS cells[15a,b] or 4-nitro-quinoline-1-oxide transformed human fibroblasts (Hut 14) did not[14]. These results are summarized in Table 1. In these assays DNA from a Kirsten sarcoma virus transformed HOS cell derivative served as a positive control.

Molecular Cloning of the met Transforming Locus

We first determined that the MNNG-HOS transforming gene was not a member of the ras family[15a,b] and experiments with sucrose gradient sized DNA fractions partially digested with Sau3A restriction enzyme indicated that the size of the active fraction was greater than 25 kilobases (kb) (Table 2). Southern analysis[17] of DNA from MNNG-HOS NIH/3T3 transformants and nude mouse tumors revealed DNA fragments of similar size in the individually derived secondaries when probed with isotopically labeled human Alu se-

Table 1

Detection of Transforming Gene in HOS Cells[a]

		Focus Assay	Tumor Assay
HOS	MNNG	+	+
	DMBA	-	-
	KMSV	+	NT
	HOS	-	-

[a]DNA was prepared from each cell line and tested as described in either the NIH/3T3 focus assay[16] or the nude mouse tumor assay[15].

quences[14,15a,b]. A series of eight overlapping lambda recombinants were isolated from a genomic library prepared from NIH/3T3 transformant DNA partially digested with Sau 3A and cloned into the bacteriophage EMBL3[15b] (Fig. 1). While the entire biologically active met transforming gene has not been isolated, the isolated lambda recombinants served to define the size of the met locus when used as probes in Southern analyses against independent met secondary NIH/3T3 transformants[15b]. The NIH/3T3 transformant

Table 2

Estimate of the Size of the met Oncogene[a]

		Foci/10 µg	Tumors in Nude Mice
Undigested DNA	>50 kb	8	12/15
Sau3A partially digested DNA	>30 kb	14	21/30
	26-30 kb	5	5/9
	17-26 kb	1	0/3
	12-17 kb	0	0

[a]The transforming activity of DNA from an MNNG-HOS secondary NIII/3T3 transfectant was partially digested with Sau3A and sedimented on a sucrose gradient. The DNA size in kb was estimated by agarose gel electrophoresis and focus forming activity was determined in NIH/3T3 cells as described[16].

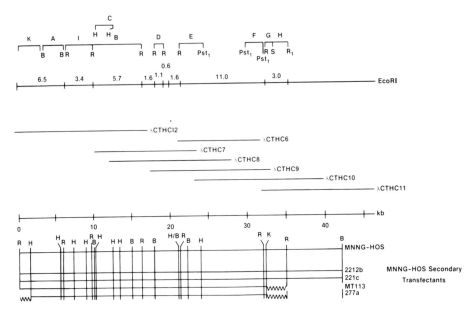

Figure 1. A partial $\underline{Sau}$ 3A digest of DNA prepared from a $\underline{met}$ secondary NIH/3T3 transformant was screened first with a human/Alu family probe to isolate the seven overlapping clones (λCTHC6-12)(16). Specific restriction fragments (A-F) were subcloned into pBR322 and used as probes in Southern transfer experiments to map the locus in MNNG-HOS DNA and in $\underline{met}$ secondary transformants 2212b, c, MT113 and 277a. R, EcoRI; B, BglII; Pst$_1$, PstI; S, SalI.

from which the $\underline{met}$ locus was cloned (2212b, Fig. 1) contains additional human sequences when compared to other transformants (MT113 and 277a, Fig. 1), presumably in excess of what is required for expression of the activated $\underline{met}$ oncogene[15b] (Fig. 1). The estimated size of the $\underline{met}$ locus by this criteria is 25-35 kb and is consistent with the size estimated from transfection of partially digested, size selected, cellular DNA containing the $\underline{met}$ oncogene (Table 2).

Analysis of met RNA Transcripts

Using 15 probes from the $\underline{met}$ locus, three different classes of RNA transcripts have been detected (Park $\underline{et\ al.}$, manuscript submitted). We have demonstrated that a novel 5 kb RNA transcript is expressed only in $\underline{met}$-transformed mouse cell lines and in MNNG-HOS cells from which the activated $\underline{met}$ oncogene was isolated. This transcript was not detected in other HOS cell lines or in any other human cell lines tested and its expression is thus associated with the $\underline{met}$ transforming activity.

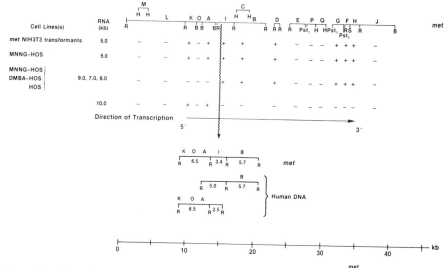

Figure 2. The direction of transcription is indicated and the position of rearrangement in the activated met gene compared to normal human DNA is indicated. The respective EcoRI restriction fragments are shown.

Probes (K,A,I,C,D,G,F,H) from the met locus in Northern analyses hybridize to the 5 kb met transcript expressed in met transformed cells and MNNG-HOS cells, but only six of these probes (I,C,D,G,F,H) detect a transcript (9.0 kb) in fibroblasts and epithelial cell lines (Park et al., manuscript submitted). Additional transcripts of 6 and 7 kb in size are detected in HOS cells with these six probes (Fig. 2). In contrast, probes K and A detect a unique 10 kb transcript in all human cell lines tested (Park et al., manuscript submitted; not shown). These data are summarized in Figure 2. The direction of transcription for all transcripts is from left to right (Park et al., manuscript submitted). Both the 9 kb class and 5 kb class of RNA transcripts appear to be 3' co-terminal while the 10 kb and the 5 kb transcripts use the same in probe K (Park et al., manuscript submitted). These data strongly suggest that the 5 kb transcript is a fused hybrid RNA with 5' sequences derived from the 10 kb class of RNA and 3' sequences from the 9 kb class of RNA (Park et al., manuscript submitted). The promoter for the 5 kb transcript probably lies within the K fragment and it is possible that it is the promoter used for the expression of the 10 kb RNA transcript (see below).

Mechanism of met Activation

The complexity of the 5 kb transcript first identified the 3.4 kb EcoRI I restriction fragment (Fig. 1) as a region containing a possible DNA rearrangement. Probes mapping to either side of this fragment detect different transcripts of 9 and 10 kb in human cells and only the 5 kb met oncogene RNA appears to share sequences in common with these two classes of transcripts. One model for met activation could be that the promoter region of the 10 kb RNA transcript class is nested within the 3' end of the 9 kb RNA transcript class. MNNG causes G to A transitions[18] and a base change within the first G of a splice donor consensus site is known to abolish or severely inhibit splicing for a variety of RNA species[19,20]. Since the 10 kb RNA is transcribed from the same DNA strand as the 9 kb class of RNA (Park et al., manuscript submitted), it is possible that the hybrid 5 kb RNA is generated by an MNNG induced alteration in splicing. However, since MNNG has also been shown to be clastogenic and a potent inducer of sister chromatid exchange[28,29], it is also possible that met is activated as a result of a deletion, insertion or a translocation. Hybrid transcripts have been found in translocations involving the bcr locus and c-abl sequences[21,23] in leukemic cells from patients with chronic myeloid leukemia (i.e., the Philadelphia chromosome translocation t(9:22)). The fused transcript encodes a hybrid protein containing 5' bcr sequences and 3' abl sequences[25,26] and the product possesses increased tyrosine kinase activity[27] compared with the normal c-abl protein.

While early attempts to detect rearrangments in the met locus were negative[15b], with the suggestion from the RNA analyses that the 3.4 kb I fragment (Fig. 1) may a site of a putative rearrangement, we probed DNA from met transformed NIH/3T3 cells and MNNG-HOS cells, HOS cells, and human placental DNA by Southern analyses[17] using fragment I as probe. These results, summarized in Figure 2, show that the 3.4 kb I fragment was present in met transformed NIH/3T3 cells and in MNNG-HOS cells (Park et al., manuscript submitted). However, in the latter DNA we observed additional 5.0 and 2.5 kb EcoRI restriction fragments and these were the only two EcoRI restriction fragments observed in all other human DNA samples tested. These data indicated that the met locus was rearranged in MNNG-HOS cells (Park et al., manuscript submitted).

Chromosomal Localization of met

Using probe E (Fig. 1) met was first assigned to chromosome 7 (7p11.4-7qter)[15b]. Recently, probe F was used for in situ mapping studies and met was more specifically localized to 7q21-q31[30]. By the criteria of the RNA analyses the region of the met locus corresponding to probes C-H should map to this region on chromosome 7. On the other hand, preliminary analyses have shown that probes K and A are located on another chromosome (Park et al., manuscript submitted). These data suggest that met may be activated via a translocation in a manner analogous to the Philadelphia translocation observed in CML patients involving the bcr and abl loci[23],[26]. The majority of the met locus appears to be derived from the 9 kb RNA transcript class (Park, et al., manuscript submitted)[30]. Nucleotide sequence analyses of this 3' portion of met shows that it is a member of the tyrosine kinase family of growth factor receptors and oncogenes[30].

The met Oncogene is a Member of the Tyrosine Kinase Family

We have begun nucleotide sequence analysis of the 3' portion of the met oncogene[30]. Several complementary DNA (cDNA) copies of met RNA transcripts, approximately 2 kb in size, were shown to contain only untranslated sequences derived from the extreme 3' end of the messenger RNA (M. Park, unpublished data). As an alternative approach, a 9 kb SalI fragment excised from λ CTHC10 (Fig. 1) was cloned into a retrovirus vector derived from Moloney sarcoma virus[31]. These vectors have been shown to process segments of genomic DNA, generating intronless genes or cDNA-like copies of messenger RNA[31]. Through use of this vector we recovered a clone processed through a retrovirus intermediate which in S1 nuclease analyses, protected a fragment 150 bases longer (M. Dean and T. Robins, unpublished data) than the corresponding segment of genomic DNA (Fig. 3). Nucleotide sequence analyses of the recovered clone and the corresponding portions of genomic DNA (Fig. 3b) revealed an open reading frame 126 amino acids long[30] (Fig. 4b). This amino acid sequence shows striking homology with several tyrosine kinase oncogenes and growth factors (Fig. 4b). Sequence analysis of a 1.1 kb D fragment from the middle of the met oncogene (Fig. 1) which is known to hybridize to met RNA transcripts (Fig. 2) contained an open reading frame (bounded by putative splice acceptor and donor signals) which also showed strong homology with other members of the tyrosine kinase family (Fig. 4a). For example, this putative exon is identical in 19/23 residues with amino acid sequence of human insulin gene[34],[41] and 18/23 residues with murine v-abl[42]. This region is highly conserved among all members of the tyrosine kinase family[43] and moderately conserved between other kinases such as mos[44], raf [45], the yeast CDC28 protein[46] and cyclic AMP-dependent kinase[47]. Although the two exons at the c-terminus of met contain a region which is less well conserved among kinases[43], certain portions are conserved among all members of the family including met (Fig. 4b).

The homology of met with members of the tyrosine kinase family strongly

246

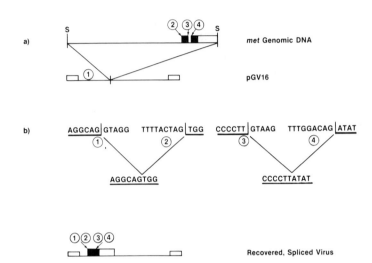

Figure 3.   Use of a retrovirus vector to remove intervening sequences.

a. The 9-kb SalI fragment was cloned into pGV16 which was modified to accept SalI fragments by inserting a SalI linker. Virus was rescued from this plasmid by co-transfection with an equal amount of pMOV-3 plasmid into NIH/3T3 cells. Infected NIH/3T3 cells were subsequently selected for resistance to G418 using 500 µg ml[-1] Geneticin (Gibco). The viral DNA from the transfected cells was recloned by fusing G418-resistant NIH/3T3 cells with COS cells using polyethylene glycol as described previously. Hirt supernatants were prepared after 72 h and used to transform Escherichia coli strain HB101 (BRL) using the procedure described by Hanahan and selected on kanamycin (35 µg ml[-1]). Only colonies which hybridized to the G fragment probe (see text) were analyzed. S, SalI.

b. Sequences of splice acceptor and donor sites (1), cryptic MuLV splice donor site; (2), first met acceptor; (3), met donor; (4), second met acceptor site. Bottom line shows the sequenced sites in the recovered virus that resulted from in vivo splicing.

suggests that its activation may be analogous to the v-erbB transforming gene of avian myeloblastosis virus which is decapitated and encodes only the c-terminal portion of the epidermal growth factor receptor, also a member of the tyrosine kinase family[32,34]. Thus if the met proto-oncogene transcript is the 9 kb RNA transcript as detected in fibroblasts and epithelial cells, the alteration of 5' sequences yielding a hybrid 5 kb met oncogene transcript would be analogous to the "decapitation" activation of v-erbB. However, the

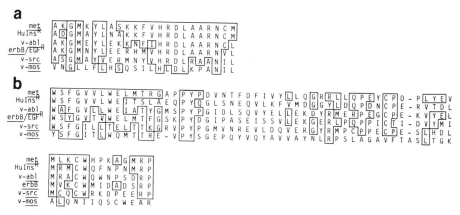

Figure 4. Open reading from a partial nucleotide sequence of the met oncogene. Comparison of the met amino-acid sequence with corresponding regions of the human insulin receptor (Hu Ins[R])[7], viral abl oncogene[8], human EGF receptor[32], and viral src and human mos proto oncogenes[10].

fusion of the 10 kb RNA transcription locus to the 5' end of met may be more analogous to c-abl activation in CML if coding sequences are provided by the former. Transcripts containing both bcr and abl sequences express a hybrid protein which can influence, for example, the cellular location of the product and influence its transforming activity[25,26].

Preliminary experiments show that a new in vitro phosphorylation activity is present in the cytosol of cells containing the activated met oncogene and this phosphorylation is resistant to alkali consistent with a putative tyrosine kinase activity (A. Iyer, unpublished data). Moreover, preliminary studies using antibodies prepared to the c-terminal peptide, predicted by the putative met amino acid sequence (Fig. 4b), show that cells containing the activated met oncogene express an immunoprecipitable in vitro kinase activity that is successfully competed with the homologous peptide (M. Gonzatti-Haces, unpublished data).

Chromosomal Abnormalities in Human 7q and Acute Nonlymphocytic Leukemia (ANLL)

Interestingly, met was activated in the HOS cell line after prolonged treatment with MNNG[12b,15b] and increasing evidence now relates the development of ANLL in patients subjected to chemotherapy treatment for a primary malignancy and in patients exposed to occupational carcinogens[35,36]. It is notable that recurring abnormalities involving chromosome 7 are common in such pa-

Table 3

met Oncogene Restriction Fragment Length Polymorphisms
in Human DNA

	Allele	kb	Frequency
D[a] (TaqI)[a]	1	7.2	.54
	2	5.2	.46
H (TaqI)	1	7.5	.56
	2	4.0	.44
H (MspI)	1	6.5	.07
	2	2.3	.50
	3	1.8	.43

[a]met fragment used as probe (restriction enzyme used
in Southern Analysis) from Dean et al., Nature 318:
385-388, 1985; White et al., and Nature 318:382-384,
1985; (Park et al., manuscript submitted).

tients[35-37]. The localization of met to 7q21-q31 by in situ hybridization[30] is just proximal of interstitial deletions of 7q observed in some patients with ANLL[38,39]. We have not yet analyzed samples from these ANLL patients but for purposes of mapping possible alterations in met restriction fragment length polymorphism (RFLP) probes were developed[40] (M.Dean, unpublished data).

The met Locus on 7q is Tightly Linked to Cystic Fibrosis

Two probes (D and H, Fig. 1) detect restriction fragment length polymorphisms in the 7q locus of met (Table 3). Probe D is a 1.1 kb EcoRI fragment while H is a 1.6 kb SalI/EcoRI fragment. RFLPs can be detected when human DNA is subjected to Southern analysis[17] after digestion with TaqI and probed with D or with TaqI or MspI and probed with H. These analyses can reveal a 7.2 kb (allele 1) fragment or a 5.2 kb TaqI fragment (allele 2) at frequencies of .54 and .46 with probe D; a 7.5 kb (allele 1) or a 4.0 kb (allele 2) TaqI fragment at a frequency of .56 and .44, respectively with probe H; and a 6.5 (allele 1), 2.3 (allele 2), or a 1.8 kb fragment (allele 3) with MspI at frequencies of .07, 0.50, and .43, respectively with probe H[40] (M. Park, manuscript submitted; S. Woodward, unpublished data). The TaqI and MspI polymorphisms detected with the latter probe have been shown to be in disequilibrium, but D and H RFLPs, approximately 10 kb apart, are in equilibrium.

We provided these probes to R. White and his collaborators at the Howard Hughes Medical Institute at the University of Utah Medical School to test whether met RFLPs show linkage with cancer prone families that are under study in that laboratory. During the course of these investigations the met probes were extended to the analysis of cystic fibrosis families[40]. The latter studies revealed that met RFLPs are tightly linked to the hereditary disease cystic fibrosis and are potentially useful in prenatal diagnostics in CF families with sibships known to be at risk. The in situ chromosomal mapping of met at 7q21-q31 is an immediate fall-out of this linkage and localizes the CF locus in man[30,40].

In initial studies by White et al.[40] using only probe H, a LOD score of 8.65 was achieved with 13 CF families tested which corresponds to odds of $4 \times 10^8:1$ favoring the hypothesis of linkage association. More recent unpublished data with over 200 meiosis from CF families and sibships tested have detected two recombinants in two separate families (S. Woodward and R. White, unpublished data). Thus, an upper limit of 1-2 centimorgans is suggested as the genetic distance between the CF locus and met which places the oncogene within 1000-2000 kb of the CF locus. The met locus linkage is so tight that it can obviously be considered for use in prenatal diagnostics with a 98% accuracy. Cystic fibrosis is one of the most common recessive genetic disorders in the northern European population. The carrier state may be as high as 1 in 20 in some populations with a resultant affected offspring of 1 in 1600. Affected individuals rarely live beyond their mid-twenties and the disease is characterized clinically by chronic obstructive lung disease, pancreatic insufficiency, and elevated sweat electrolytes. The disorder itself is speculated to involve an ion channel imbalance[48]. While met may not be the CF gene, we note that tyrosine kinase receptor activation has been linked to the regulation of the sodium ion-proton antiport[49] and it is conceivable that met, as a member of this family, could influence chloride ion exchange. It has also been proposed that a cluster of genes with receptor-like motif may reside in this region of chromosome 7[40].

ACKNOWLEDGMENTS

Research sponsored in part by the National Cancer Institute, DHHS, under contract NO. N01-CO-23909 with Litton Bionetics, Inc. A. Iyer is a recipient of the Lady Tata International Leukemia Research Fellowship.

250

REFERENCES

1. Balmain, A. and Pragnell, I.B. (1983) Nature 303, 72-74.
2. Balmain, A., Ramsden, M., Bowden, G.T. and Smith, V. (1984) Nature 307, 658-660.
3. Sukumar, S., Notario, V., Martin-Zanca, D. and Barbacid, M. (1983) Nature 306, 658-661.
4. Sukumar, S., Pulciani, S., Doniger, J., DiPaolo, J.A., Evans, C.H., Zbar, B. and Barbacid, M. (1984) Science 223, 1197-1199.
5. Eva, A. and Aaronson, S.A. (1983) Science 220, 955-956.
6. Parada, L.F. and Weinberg, R.A. (1983) Mol. Cell. Biol. 3, 2298-2301.
7. Guernero, I., Caleada, P., Mayer, A. and Pellicer, A. (1984) Proc. Natl. Acad. Sci. USA 81, 202-205.
8. Henry, S.A. (1947) Br. Med. Bull. 4, 389-401.
9. USPHS Publ. (HEW) 79-50066 (1979) U.S. Dept. of Health, Education and Welfare, Washington, D.C.
10. Renwick, A.G. and Drasan, B.S. (1976) Nature 263, 234-235.
11. Kakunaga, T. (1978) Proc. Natl. Acad. Sci. USA 75, 1334-1338.
12a. Rhim, J.S., Kim, C.M., Arnstein, P., Heubner, R.J., Weisburger, E.K., Nelson-Rees, W.A. (1975) J. Natl. Cancer Inst. 55, 1291-1294.
12b. Rhim, J.S., Park, D.K., Arnstein, P., Huebner, R.J. and Weisburger, E.K. (1975) Nature 256, 751-753.
13. DiPaolo, J.A. (1983) J. Natl. Cancer Inst. 70, 3-8.
14. Blair, D.G., Cooper, C.S., Oskarsson, M.K., Eader, L.A. and Vande Woude, G.F. (1982) Science 218, 1122-1125.
15a. Cooper, C.S., Blair, D.G., Oskarsson, M.K., Tainsky, M.A., Eader, L.A., and Vande Woude, G.F. (1984) Cancer Res. 44, 1-10.
15b. Cooper, C.S., Park, M., Blair, D.G., Tainsky, M.A., Huebner, K., Croce, C.M. and Vande Woude, G.F. (1984) Nature 311, 29-33.
16. McAllister, R.M., Gardner, M.B., Green, A.E., Bradt, C., Nichols, W.W. and Landing, B.H. (1971) Cancer 27, 397-402.
17. Southern, E.M. (1975) J. Molec. Biol. 98, 503-517.
18. Margison, C.P. and O'Connor, P.J. (1979) in Chemical Carcinogenesis and DNA, Vol.1, Grover, P.L. ed., CRC Press, Boca Raton, Florida, pp. 111-159.
19. Treisman, R., Orkin, S.H. and Maniatis, T. (1983) Nature 302, 591-596.
20. Wieringa, B., Meyer, F., Reiser, J. and Weissmann, C. (1983) Nature 301, 38-43.
21. deKlein, A., van Kessel, A.G., Groslveld, G., Bartram, C.R., Hagemeijer,

A., Bootsma, D., Spurr, N.K., Heisterkamp, N., Groffen, J. and Stephenson, J.R. (1982) Nature 300, 765-767.

22. Collins, S.J. and Groudine, M.T. (1983) Proc. Natl. ACad. Sci. USA 80, 4813-4814.

23. Groffen, J., Stephenson, J.R., Heisterkamp, N., deKlein, A., Bartram, C.R. and Grosveld, G. (1984) Cell 36, 93-99.

24. Gabe, R.P. and Canaani, E. (1984) Proc. Natl. Acad. Sci. USA 81, 5648-5652.

25. Shtivelman, E., Lifshitz, B., Gale, P.P. and Canaani, E. (1985) Nature 315, 550-554.

26. Heisterkamp, N., Story, K., Groffen, J., deKlein, A. and Grosveld, G. (1985) Nature 315, 758-761.

27. Konopka, J.B., Watanabe, S.M. and Witte, O.N. (1984) Cell 37, 1035-1042.

28. Perry, P. and Evans, H.J. (1975) Nature 258, 121-125.

29. Sasaki, M.S. and Tonomura, A. (1973) Cancer Res. 33, 1829-1836.

30. Dean, M., Park, M., Le Beau, M.M., Robins, T.S., Diaz, M.O., Rowley, J.D., Blair, D.G. and Vande Woude, G.F. (1985) Nature 318, 385-388.

31. Robins, T., Jhappan, C., Chirikjian, J. and Vande Woude, G.F. Gene Anal. Techniques, in press.

32. Downward, J., Yarden, Y., Mayes, E., Scrace G., Totty, N., Stockwell, P., Ullrich, A., Schlessinger, J. and Waterfield, M.D. (1984) Nature, 307, 521-527.

33. Liu, C.R., Chen, W., Kruiger, W., Stolarsky, L., WEber, W., Evans, R.M., Verma, I.M., Gill, G.D. and Rosenfeld, M.G. (1984) Science 224, 843-848.

34. Ullrich, A., Coussens, L., Hayflick, J.S., Dull, T.J., Gray, A., Tam, A.W., Lee, J., Yarden, Y., Libermann, T.A., Schlessinger, J., Downward, J., Mayes, E.L.V., Whitte, N., Waterfield, M.D. and Seeburg, P.H. (1984) Nature 309, 418-425.

35. Rowley, J.D., Golomb, H.M. and Vardiman, J.N. (1981) Blood 58, 759-767.

36. Mitelman, F., Nilsson, P.G., Brandt, L., Alimenia, G., Gastaldi, R. and Dalla-Piccola, B. (1981) Cancer Genet. Cytogenet. 9, 197-214.

37. Fourth International Workshop on Chromosomes in Leukemia, 1982 (1984) Cancer Genet. Cytogenet. 11, 300-303.

38. Yunis, J.J. (1984) Cancer Genet. Cytogenet. 11, 125-137.

39. Rowley, J.D. and Testa, J.R. (1982) Adv. Cancer Res. 36, 103-149.

40. White, R., Woodward, S., Leppert, M., O'Connell, P., Hoff, M., Herbst, J., Lalover, J., Dean, M. and Vande Woude, G. (1985) Nature 318-382-384.

41. Ebina, Y. et al., (1985) Cell 40, 747-758.
42. Reddy, E.P., Smith M.J., Srinivasan, A. (1983) Proc. Natl. Acad. Sci. USA 80, 3623-3627.
43. Hunter, T. and Cooper, J.A. in The Enzymes (eds Boyer, P.D. & Krebs, E.) (Academic, New York, in the press).
44. van Beveran, D. Van Straaten, F., Galleshaw, J.A. & Verma, I. M. (1981) Cell 27, 97-108.
45. Bonner, T.I. et al., (1985) Molec. Cell. Biol. 5, 1400-1407.
46. Lorinez, A.T. and Reed, S.I., (1984) Nature 307, 183-185.
47. Shoji, S. et al., (1981) Proc. Natl. Acad. Sci. USA 78, 848-851.
48. van Heyningen, V. (1984) Nature 311, 104-105.
49. l'Allemain, G., Paris S. and Pouyssegur, J. (1984) J. Biol. Chem. 259, 5809-5815.

14

ONCOGENES: MOLECULAR PROBES FOR CLINICAL APPLICATION

IN MALIGNANT DISEASES

Richard Ascione, Nicoletta Sacchi, Dennis K. Watson,
Robert J. Fisher, Shigeyoshi Fujiwara, Arun Seth[†] and Takis S. Papas

Laboratory of Molecular Oncology and LBI-Basic Research Laboratory[†]
National Cancer Institute, Frederick, Maryland 21701-1013

Research supported in part by contract no. N01-CO-23909
with Litton Bionetics, Inc.

Retroviral Oncogenes and Proto-Oncogenes

Transforming genes of all oncogenic retroviruses are known to be derivatives of cellular genes which have been termed cellular or proto-oncogenes (c-onc)[1]. Typically, these viral oncogenes (v-onc) are truncated hybrids of a specific subset of one or more proto-onc gene(s) linked to the genomic elements of the retrovirus vector that has captured or transduced it[2]. These retroviruses belong to a group of viruses that possess an enzyme reverse transcriptase, which confer upon them the capacity to convert their genomic information in the form of RNA to the more stable and typical form, DNA[3]. Thus, these viruses have the significant capability of adding a stretch of genetic information to their infected hosts[4]. Those retroviruses, containing nucleotide sequences homologous to normal cellular proto-oncogene and capable of expressing all or even a portion of the encoded protein, are generically classified as acute transforming retroviruses; they are able to cause leukemias or solid tumors very rapidly in infected animals hosts[1]. These rapid tumor-inducing retroviruses are rather unusual, primarily because most of them are replication defective; they lack one or more retroviral essential genes needed for their multiplication. It became evident that these acute transforming retroviruses transduced certain proto-oncogene sequences (c-onc) whose expression could result in malignancy in animals or cell transformation in vitro[5]. Subsequently it was found that a variety of such acute transforming retroviruses could be isolated, each containing an altered version of a c-onc gene[1]. The rapidly transforming retroviruses have been isolated from at least six different varieties of vertebrate hosts, ranging from the evolutionary lower avian species to the higher species of Mammalia[6]. The number of distinct oncogenes (v-onc) thus far identified as retroviral captives number slightly over 20 different genes[1]; so although the cell has thousands of potentially active genes, only a limited few dozen such cellular genes appear to qualify as proto-oncogenes[7].

Up to this point, the discovery of viral oncogenes has served to focus research and provide molecular evidence for specific genes as causative (genetic) determinants capable of mediating malignancy particularly in experimental animal systems. However, another parallel development within recent years, has been the revelation of nonretroviral related transforming sequences in tumors[7]. This approach may be relevant because most human tumors are not known to be caused by viruses. A significant exception, of course, is the T-cell leukemia causing retroviruses, particularly those infecting specific human cell populations. It is not, however, within the scope of this review to include this category of retroviruses which has recently been covered elsewhere[8]. Once the normal cellular residence of the v-onc homologous, c-onc sequences, had been established, it was reasonable to search out such sequences in the genome of tumor cells and ascertain if the effect of the tumor cell DNA would dominate and transform a normal cell into a malignant one. This process of transferring DNA from tumor cell to recipient cells, termed "transfection", was indeed found to cause cellular transformation in tissue culture[9]. Cells so transformed could be shown to contain the transfected human onc-gene homologous sequence and then, upon transfer into live test animals, to cause tumors at high frequency[10]. Occasionally, it was found that DNA extracted from a variety of tumors could transform "normal" appearing cells, like NIH 3T3 cells, into transformed ones. A particularly significant finding was that many, but not all, of those cellular oncogene sequences obtained from such tumors are homologous and nearly identical to those originally characterized as components of the acute transforming retroviral genomes[11].

Molecular hybridization studies using viral oncogenes as DNA probes have become the main method for identification of homologous and c-onc genes[12]. Thus in conjunction with recombinant DNA cloning methods which were utilized to augment the nucleic acid sequences under scrutiny[13], the ability to hybridize with viral oncogenes has been the sine qua non for identification of cellular onc genes[1,12]. For example, a DNA sequence containing an avian viral myc onc-gene can, under defined annealing conditions, form a hybrid with a human cellular oncogene-"myc"like sequence because the latter human gene shares partial, yet substantial homology with the former sequences[14]. By utilizing Southern transfer analysis[15] to screen for homologous genes, from any of the 50,000 or more genes present in the human or mammalian genome, it proved possible to sort through this mass of genetic information, and identify specific oncogenes in a variety of cells from a multitude of different species[1]. Similarly, a procedure referred to as a Northern analysis[16], is quite useful to determine if specific oncogenes are expressed in tumor cells. Thus, by employing labeled molecular v-myc specific probes, the messenger RNA transcribed from a cellular myc oncogene could readily be detected in a number of malignant cells for the first time[17].

Numerous studies employing molecular v-onc probes have revealed that all known v-onc genes have thus far, with only one exception (v-rel), a normal cellular oncogene counterpart[1]. It is now clearly established that the homologies observed between the v-onc and c-onc sequences are definitive ones; they have been substantiated by direct nucleotide sequencing[1].

Further, even the taxonomy of oncogenes and their evolutionary interrelationships defined by their initial hybridization to viral probes are confirmed through direct analysis of their molecular sequences[18]. What has emerged for these oncogene sequences, especially those found in the acute transforming retroviral genomes, are unique domains or regions of specific homology especially discernible at the predicted amino acid level[2].

The deduced amino acid sequences have, therefore, been useful to define some surprising relationships of oncogenes to known cellular proteins as well as to define at least three groups of oncogenes (Table I)[19]. One of the most evolutionarily conserved family of oncogenes, is that of the ras family, defined originally by molecular hybridization probes derived from the Harvey and Kirsten sarcoma viruses[1]. This grouping of oncogenes has been further subdivided into three different subcategories. Two of these (c-ras^H and c-ras^K or Harvey cellular ras and Kirsten cellular ras, respectively) were first recognized as homologs of the transduced murine sarcoma viruses bearing their names[1]. The third subgroup of ras, N-ras (or ras^N) was isolated from the DNA of neuroblastoma tumor cells as a biologically transforming gene in the transfection assay and has never been observed thus far in a retrovirus[20]. The mammalian and viral ras genes encode a 21,000 dalton membrane associated protein that can bind GTP and exhibit GTPase activity. This class of protein is also capable of autophosphorylation activity and is believed to interact in some as yet undiscovered way with the regulator proteins modulating adenyl-cyclase activity[21]. "Activated" ras genes are known to be present in numerous cell lines derived from tumors including a variety of leukemias, sarcomas as well as neuroblastomas[7] and have been subsequently sequenced. It has consequently been discovered from these studies ras family members associated with malignant transformation are usually activated by having a single point mutation which somatically alters its p21 ras gene protein[22]. Other homologous altered c-ras genes detected by molecular probe studies, have also been isolated and molecularly characterized from fresh tumors and biopsies obtained from lung, bladder and pancreas specimens[7].

The largest oncogene grouping or family, originally identified and classified by molecular hybridization studies to the viral src transforming gene[1] of the Rous Sarcoma Virus; its members are defined by comparison of their catalytic protein kinase domain and its relationship to the predicted membrane associated protein, pp60^{v-src} which has been characterized as a tyrosine phosphokinase[1]. Parenthetically included in this family are those

Table I. Oncogenes: Group; Relationships; Origin; and Disease and Activity

Group Oncogene: Origin [viral(cell)]	Disease	Activity v-onc(c-onc)	Ref.
(A) src family			
Kinases src Rous sarcoma virus (chicken)	Sarcoma	Tyrosine protein Kinase (PK)	[75]
fps Fujinami sarcoma virus (chicken)	Sarcoma	Tyrosine PK	[75]
fes Feline sarcoma virus (cat)	Sarcoma	Tyrosine PK	[76]
yes Yamaguschi sarcoma virus(chicken)	Sarcoma	Tyrosine PK	[75]
fgr Gardner-Rasheed virus (cat)	Sarcoma	Tyrosine PK	[77]
ros UR2 sarcoma virus (chicken)	Sarcoma	Tyrosine PK	[75]
fms McDonough sarcoma virus (cat)	Sarcoma	Tyrosine PK (CSF/receptor homology)	[75] [76, 27]
abl Abelson leukemia virus (mouse)	Leukemia, lymphoma	Tyrosine PK	[76]
(B) Limited sequence homology to src family			
mos Moloney sarcoma virus (mouse)	Sarcoma	Protein Kinase domain homology	[78]
raf 3611-Murine sarcoma virus (mouse)	Sarcoma	Protein Kinase domain homology	[79]
mht(mil)[a] MH2 avian virus (chicken)	Same as for myc	Domain homology with raf	[80]
erb-B[b] Erythroblastosis virus (chicken)	erythro-blastosis and Sarcoma	Domain homology to Tyrosine PK (truncated EGF receptor homology)	[25, 81]
rel[c] Reticuloendotheliosis virus	reticulo-endotheliosis	unknown	[82]
met (Carcinogen treated human osteosarcoma cell)	unknown (isolated by transfection)	Tyrosine PK	[83, 84]
(C) ras family			
Ha-ras Harvey sarcoma virus (rat)	Sarcoma and erythro-leukemia	Protein Kinase (PK) (GTPase binding)	[85]

*Table I continued on next page.

Table I (cont.)

Group	Oncogene: Origin [viral(cell)]	Disease	Activity v-onc(c-onc)	Ref.
	Ki-ras Kirsten sarcoma virus (rat)	Sarcoma and erythro- leukemia	PK (GTP biding)	[85]
	N-ras (Human tumor DNA)	(in vitro 3T3-cell transforma- tion only)	Distinct homology Ha- and Ki-ras	[86]
Growth Factor and Receptor	(D) sis family			
	sis Simian sarcoma virus (wolly monkey)	Sarcoma	Homology to PDGF (gene for PDGF-B)	[87, 88]
	neu (neuroblastoma isolate rat)	in vitro cell transform- ation only	Homology to EGF receptor	[89]
Nuclear	(E) myc family			
	myc MC29 myelocytomatosis virus (chicken)	Sarcoma Carcinoma Myelocytoma	unknown	[75]
	myc^a MH2 avian virus (chicken)	Sarcoma Carcinoma Myelocytoma	unknown (DNA binding)	[80]
	N-myc (neuroblastoma, retinoblastoma, human)	unknown	unknown (limited homology to c-myc)	[67, 90]
	L-myc (anaplastic lung car- cinoma human)	unknown	unknown (very limited homology to c-myc)	[69]
	(F) myb family			
	myb Avian myelo- blastosis (chicken)	myelo- blastosis	unknown (DNA associated)	[91]
	myb^d E26 virus (chicken)	myelo- blastosis and erythroblastosis	unknown	[92]

*Table I continued on next page.

Table I (cont.)

Group	Oncogene: Origin [viral(cel)]	Disease	Activity v-onc(c-onc)	Ref.
	(G) Unique family			
	fos FBJ osteosarcoma virus (mouse)	osteosarcoma	unknown	[93]
	ski SK770 virus (chicken)	squamous carcinoma	unknown	[94]
	ets[d] E26 virus (chicken)	myelo-blastosis and erythroblastosis	unknown	[92]
	erb-A[b] Erythroblastosis virus	erythro-blastosis and sarcoma	Homolog to the glucocorticoid receptor	[95, 96]
	bcl 1, bcl 2	B-cell neo-plasms (isolated by transfection)	unknown	[53, 54]
	tcl 1, tcl 2	T-cell neo-plasms	unknown	[97, 98]

[a]Dual oncogenes of MH2 virus.
[b]Dual oncogenes of Avian Erythroblastosis virus.
[c]Very distant homology to src.
[d]Dual oncogenes of tripartite E26 virus genome.

oncogenes such as <u>neu</u> and v-<u>erb</u> B, since they are structurally related to the cytoplasmic portion of the epidermal growth factor (EGF) receptor[23]. Although no direct kinase activity has been demonstrated for this receptor-like moiety, recent experiments utilizing antibodies against synthetic oligopeptides derived from this receptor, suggest that the v-<u>erb</u> B encodes a domain homologous to those which activate tyrosine phosphokinase[24]. In fact, a recent report indicates that the v-<u>erb</u> B protein in avian ery-throblastosis virus (AEV) transformed chicken embryo fibroblasts (CEF) not only shares homology with the <u>src</u> family of proteins and EGF receptor pro-tein but additionally this protein possesses a tyrosine-specific protein kinase activity[25]. Quite recently, a good deal has been learned about another candidate member of this family; the gene product encoded by the <u>fms</u> oncogene (c-<u>fms</u>). This cellular proto-oncogene was detected by using the viral transforming oncogene (v-<u>fms</u>), a gene related analogously to the tyrosine phosphokinase domain of <u>erb</u> B[26]. Thus, it was of considerable interest, that there is a close structural relationship (based upon the oncogene sequence identity) to that of a growth factor receptor - the one known as the colony stimulating factor (CSF-1)[27]. Also of interest is the demonstration that anti-sera against v-<u>fms</u> product binds to CSF-1 and recognizes a membrane protein of macrophages, both appropriate features of a putative CSF-1 receptor. The current hypothesis now suggests that v-<u>fms</u> confers its malignant potential upon fibroblasts by providing these cells with CSF-1 receptor sites. Since fibroblasts do not normally contain these receptors, such infected cells expressing v-<u>fms</u> product would then become "abnormally auto-responsive" to CSF-1 growth factor which they auto-logously synthesize[26,27].

Unrelated in terms of "kinase-like" activity is another oncogene encoded product similarly involved in growth regulation. Sharing a growth stimula-tion activity, this oncogene product was predicted from the known sequence of the viral oncogene, v-<u>sis</u>, a transforming gene detected in the simian sarcoma virus genome[28]. After nucleotide sequence analysis, the <u>sis</u> gene was found to be an almost perfect match to the human normal platelet derived growth factor (PDGF) gene, one whose unregulated expression could also induce cellular transformation[29]. PDGF is a known growth factor substance for many normal cells in culture as well as for natural tissues and cells of mesenchymal origin[30].

There remains uncategorized some "maverick" protein-kinase type oncogenes which appear not to be either membrane associated or capable of phosphoryl-ation. These oncogenes can be related however, by being able to phosphorylate proteins, but at the amino acids, serine and threonine. This capacity, if unregulated, could lead to malignant transformation[24]. For the time being, these oncogenes can be considered "relatives" of the tyrosine phosphokinases, and may possibly effect their oncogenity through a cascade mechanism that destabilizes the governance of cellular regulation.

The remaining group of oncogenes may be somewhat difficult to categorize structurally, but they interrelate largely on the basis of their cellular location. The familial status of these oncogenes is therefore controversial as their members show little, if any, nucleotide homology or predictable protein sequence similarities. This group of oncogenes encodes products that are localized in the nucleus (c.f., Table I)[21]. Many members of this group bind to DNA, associate functionally with the nuclear substrates and may regulate DNA expression. In certain instances, these onc-genes can even transform cells in culture[6]. It is assumed then that this family of oncogene-encoded proteins, being localized in the nucleus, must act there. These oncogenes may serve regulatory functions at the DNA inter-active level, i.e., having a direct effect on transcription[31]. Much work remains, however, to elucidate functions for this family in particular. The seemingly large diversity of oncogenes can be reduced in its complexity by this type of categorization into these descriptive groups in spite of the fact that the cellular interrelationships of oncogenes, or what may be their actual functional roles, is quite far from being understood[32].

By weaving the disciplines of molecular biology, retrovirology, carcino-genesis, cell biology and immunology, a comprehensive tapestry is formed, all sharing a common thread - an interest in proto-oncogenes; the study of which might lead to molecular explanations of how normal cells modulate their growth and why neoplastic cells are unable to regulate theirs. So far, the role of proto-oncogenes in normal cells is not precisely known; they do play some important role in cellular growth and differentiation, as evidenced by their high degree of conservation throughout the phylogenetic spectrum, but their mechanism and cellular targets remain to be defined.

Proto-Oncogenes as Markers of Specific Neoplasia
A. Proto-oncogenes, Nonrandom Cytogenetic Abnormalities, and Generation of New Tumor Markers.

In this section of the review, the relevance of oncogenes and oncogene products as possible markers to neoplasia and tumor progression will be evaluated. Proto-oncogenes are amenable to study as relevant markers of neoplasia and tumor progression, quite apart from their natural (etiological) role as important normal genes. That several proto-oncogenes map in the vicinity of breakpoints involved in chromosomal abnormalities associating with a variety of mammalian and human tumors[33] is well documented[34]. Collectively, these abnormalities, revealed by cytogenetic analysis, include nonrandom chromosomal translocations as well as inversion, deletions or fine chromosomal changes, each of which may lead to the involvement of proto-oncogenes[7,35]. The analysis of structural chromosome aberrations that occur as the only chromosome anomaly has indicated that the breakpoints involve a significantly small number of chromosome regions (61 out of 329 bands of the standard human karyotype), and that these regions contain genes of primary importance for the growth and the differentiation, like the cellular proto-oncogenes (Table II), the immunoglobulin, and the T-cell receptor genes. In some cases, the availability of molecular clones of these genes has prompted the molecular analysis of those chromosome lesions that may play a role in the development and/or maintenance of some neoplasias[35]. The interrelationship between chromosomal abnormalities and cancer is not clearly understood, because it is still being debated whether some of the chromosome changes observed in the neoplastic cells are the pristine cause, a necessary change, or a mere consequence of the neoplastic process. Although the random multiple-heterogenous, cytogenetic abnormalities may be viewed as epiphenomena to tumorigenesis, the nonrandom chromosome changes may be more directly involved in the process of malignancy and may thus be useful as specific and unique markers of certain leukemias, lymphomas, and solid tumors. The "chromosome hypothesis of oncogenesis" suggests that karyotypic changes that occur in the oncogenic process, even if they are not the primary event, may be mechanistically responsible for the occurrence of that particular neoplastic condition[36]. Subtle chromosome changes have been noted in inherited embryonic cancers of children; they represent one of the most tantalizing finding of tumor biology. In retinoblastoma[37] and Wilm's tumors[38,39] the lesion observed are deletions of varying size involving two chromosomal regions, the 13q14 and 11p13 regions, respectively. These deletions provide clues as to the chromosomal regions that might be involved in tumor formation. For these malignancies, a second genetic event (two-hit hypothesis) is necessary in order to observe the effects of the primary lesion (e.g., deletion/submicroscopic deletion). There is now strong molecular evidence that the expression of the predisposing lesion at the 11p13 or 13q14 sites is determined by abnormal chromosome

Table II. Chromosomal Location of Human Homologs of Viral Transforming Genes[1,7].

Abbrevation (proto-onc)	Species origin	Virus	Human chromosome	References
myb	Chicken	AMV	6q22-24	[99]
mos	Mouse	Mo-MSV	8q22	[100,101]
myc	Chicken	MC29	8q24	[100]
fes	Cat	ST-FeSV	15q25-26	[99]
sis	Woolly monkey	SSV	22q12.2-13.3	[102,103]
src	Chicken	RSV	20q12, 34-36]	[104]
abl	Mouse	A-MuLV	9q34	[105]
fms	Cat	SM-FeSV	5q34	[106]
Ha-ras-1	Rat	Ha-MSV	11p14.1, p15.1-15.5	[107]
Ha-ras-2	Rat	Ha-MSV	X	[108]
Ki-ras-1	Rat	Ki-MSV	6p23-q12	[109]
Ki-ras-2	Rat	Ki-MSV	12p12.1 or q24.2	[110]
ets-1	Chicken	E26	11q23-24	[48,112]
ets-2	Chicken	E26	21q22.1-22.3	[48]
N-ras	Human	None	1p(21 cen)	[111]
raf-1	Mouse	3611-MSV	3p25	[112]
raf-2	Mouse	3611-MSV	4	[112]
N-myc	Human	None	2p23ter	[113]
erbA	Chicken	AEV	17p11-q21	[114]
erbB	Chicken	AEV	7pter-q22	[114]
ski	Chicken	SK770	1q12-qter	[115]
fos	Mouse	FBJ-MSV	14q21-q31	[116]
bcl 1	Human	None[a]	11q13	[117]
met	Human	None[a]	7p11.4qter	[82]
neu	Rat	None[a]	17q21	[89]
bcl 2	Human	None[a]	18q21	[117]

[a]Not related to any known viral oncogene.

segregation events. These events induce the loss of the normal allele by mechanisms that include the elimination of the whole chromosome (by non-disjunction, duplication events of the altered chromosome, mitotic recombination, and translocations). Such mitotic events result in the production of a cell homozygous for the deleted (or mutated) allele, allowing expression of the recessive lesion(s) predisposing them to these tumors. The development of somatic homozygosity at the 11p13 region is also noted as the common pathogenetic mechanism for two other embryonic tumors, the hepatoblastoma and rabdomyosarcoma[38]. Other tumors like neuroblastomas and the familial kidney carcinomas seem to have a similar genetic basis, having deletions that involve the 1p31-35 and 3p14 regions, respectively. Genes like the ones discussed have been classified as "tumor suppressors" or "anti-oncogenes"[33]. The eventual isolation and identification of these genes, and the ability to determine which parental chromosome carries the mutant allele should have enormous potential in the genetic counseling of families having an occurrence of these tumors.

Reciprocal chromosomal translocations have been known to characterize hematopoietic tumors. One of the best described examples is the (8;14) chromosomal translocation in Burkitt's lymphoma, observed in 90% of the tumors presenting such chromosomal aberrations[40]. This event juxtaposes the human proto-oncogene c-myc from the long arm of chromosome 8 into the vicinity of the heavy chain locus of the immunoglobin (Ig) gene on chromosome 14 [41]. Concomitant with this chromosomal transposition is a notable dysregulation of transcription of the c-myc oncogene, thought to be due to the effect of the nearby Ig enhancers[42]. Some 10% of the remaining Burkitt lymphomas alterations are translocations involving the critical chromosomal number 8, containing the c-myc oncogene, exchanging locations to chromosome numbers 2 or 22 in the proximity of the light chain Ig loci, presumably to be activated by a similar mechanism[33].

Recently, another abnormality associated with chronic myeloid leukemia (CML) has been identified as having a distinctive Philadalphia (Ph) translocated chromosome (22q-) as a cytogenetic marker. This disease correlated with a novel rearrangement involving the proto-oncogene locus, c-abl[43]. These studies have revealed a reciprocal exchange between the oncogene c-abl, normally located on chromosome 9, but notably translocated to chromosome 22. The resultant (Ph) chromosomal recombinant is observed in over 95% of all patients presenting with CML. Because only a small region of chromosome 9 that contains the c-abl locus translocates to chromosome 22 [44,45], the abnormally shortened chromosome 22q- (or Ph) can be readily observed by cytogenetic methods. Interestingly, the rearrangement has been described molecularly and has been shown to involve the linkage of a region of chromosome 22 denoted as a breakpoint cluster region, bcr, at the 5' end fused to a truncated c-abl gene located at the 3' end. This head-to-tail fusion of bcr (locating at q11 on chromosome 22) with the c-abl (derived from q34 on chromosome 9) results in a chimeric mRNA consisting of: 5'-bcr-c-abl-3' sequences. Consistent with this observation is the finding of a c-abl protein of abnormal size, 210,000 daltons, in CML-Ph leukemic cells that unmasks a cryptic tyrosine kinase activity not found associated with the normal 145,000 dalton c-abl protein[46]. Although the oncogenic potential of the fusion bcr-abl product remains to be determined, the c-abl portion of the genome retained is homologous to the v-abl transforming region a gene that induces a rapid B-cell lymphoma in mice[34]. Because this peculiar chromosomal abnormality is only noted in CML, which is associated with the malignant proliferation of hematopoeitic cell, it may be reasonable to suggest that the bcr gene is regulated only during stem cell differentiative processes, which trigger the expression of the hybrid bcr-abl protein[47]. This "abnormal" protein then effects an aberrant activity within cells so afflicted with this translocated-induced gene. There seems to be a reasonable body of evidence to incriminate the (9;22) translocation as a critical event in the development of CML. Thus, this association of an altered oncogene with a known human neoplasia, should afford researchers an opportunity to discover unique markers, ones capable of detecting activation of such an oncogene by immunologically identifying the abnormal fusion bcr/c-abl protein. For diagnostic purposes, such reagents could be used to monitor various treatment protocols as well as to quantitate the level of remaining cells expressing such proteins.

Investigations in our lab on the human homologs of the ets region derived from the transforming gene of the avian erythroblastosis virus, E26, have shown this proto-oncogene to be composed of two distinct domains located on separate chromosomes[48]. We have subsequently cloned and analyzed the nucleotide sequences of the human ets-related genes, and we have further found that the human ets-1 gene is transcriptionally active and encodes a single mRNA species of 6.8 Kb, whereas the human ets-2 gene encodes three distinct mRNA species of 4.7, 3.2, and 2.7 Kb, respectively[49].

Because a number of leukemias of the monomyelocytic lineage show chromosome abnormalities in the very regions where the human-ets genes reside, we have used our human ets probes to examine specific translocations occurring in these acute leukemias[50]. In particular, we focused on the (4;11) chromosome translocation. This cytogenetic marker characterizes a leukemia observed more frequently in infants and young adults, having a rapid course and poor prognosis; in infants, this leukemia may be congenital. The (4;11) blasts may be considered as the malignant counterpart of a very undifferentiated precursor cell of the myelomonocytic lineage or of a common lymphoid/myeloid precursor cell. The 11q23 region, where the human ets-1 gene is located, is known to participate also in a number of translocations involving a second variable chromosome in acute myeloid leukemias, and for this reason, it is believed to contain critical myeloid transformation gene(s). The usual and recombinant chromosomes of the t(4;11) leukemic cells were examined in a chinese hamster cell background by means of somatic cell hybridization. Such studies permitted the identification of the human ets-1 gene as 3.0 kb PstI and 6.2 kb EcoRI fragments, using ets-1-specific probe[49]. In fact, this gene was present in hybrids containing either the intact 11 or the recombinant 4q⁻ chromosomes only. Although such experiment suggested that ets-1 may be involved in the formation of a chimeric gene sequence on the 4q⁻ chromosome, it still left unresolved whether the chromosomal breakpoint is within or outside of the human ets-1 gene.

Similarly, by somatic cell hybrid fusions we studied the translocation (8;21)(q22;q22) observed in acute myelogenous leukemia with morphology M2. This region (21q22) is also implicated in Down's Syndrome (DS); patients with three (or more) chromosome 21 show a marked predisposition toward acute leukemia, particularly an increased incidence of acute non-lymphoblastic leukemia (ANLL). Southern blot data of DNA from somatic cell hybrids containing either the normal 8 and 21 chromosomes or the recombinant derivatives of the t(8;21), 8q⁻ and 21q⁺ were tested using ets-2 specific probes. We were able to conclude from these sets of experiments that at least 20.3 Kb of the human ets-2 gene had been translocated to chromosome 8. Independent t(8;21) AML-M2 patient samples showed no human ets-2 gene rearrangements using Southern-blot analysis with a variety of restriction enzymes. Nevertheless, studies with a ³H-labeled human ets-2-specific probe (H33), found it to hybridize specifically to the 8q⁻ chromosome of fresh leukemic cells from t(8;21) AML-M2 patients. This finding confirms the translocation of ets-2 gene from 21 to 8 is a general phenomena[51]. In situ hybridization analysis using a v-ets probe on fresh leukemic cells having a different translocation (9;11)(p21;q23), involving the 11q23 region, supplied additional evidence for the translocation of the ets sequences from chromosome 11 to chromosome 9 in t(9;11) acute myelomonocytic leukemia (AMMoL-M4) and acute monocytic leukemia (AMoL-M5)[52].

When total RNA was isolated from leukemic samples obtained from patients with both translocations and compared to normal human lymphocyte RNA using the Northern-blot technique, the t(4;11) patient and the RS4;11 cell line showed low levels of ets-1-specific mRNA. Similarly, experiments using two t(8;21) AML-M2 leukemic specimens, yielded RNA that did not have all of the human ets-2 mRNA species seen in the normal control lymphocyte samples and which are known to be present in other tissues and cell lines of human origin. In particular, the 4.7 Kb and 3.2 Kb ets-2 mRNA species were notably absent in one sample and the 4.7 Kb species, only, was absent in the other patient sample. The expression of the human ets-2 gene in the t(8;21) cells was also much lower than levels observed in the control lymphocytes. So far, it is not possible to conclude whether the different expression patterns of ets-1 and ets-2 specific mRNA in leukemic samples compared to the normal peripheral lymphocytes is the result of the specific translocations; further studies are warranted to elucidate the exact role of the ets genes in these translocations.

Cloning and molecular analysis of other nonrandom chromosomal breakpoints have identified novel sequences like bcl-1 [53] and bcl-2 [54] and the 18q21 [55] element. These genes are derived from chromosomes present in the t(11;14) and t(14;18) associated to the chronic lymphocytic leukemia (CLL) and human follicular lymphomas, respectively. Recently, the p53 tumor antigen located in the 17q21-22 was found transposed to the 15q$^+$ critical recombinant chromosome in t(15;17), a feature of 40% of all acute promyelocytic leukemia (APL)[56], which further supports the association between proto-oncogenes and specific breakpoints in hematopoietic tumors. The research impetus, to clone and molecularly define the new chimeric regions resulting from disease associated translocations, is of paramount importance. For example, if we consider the Ph chromosome of CML cells, we find that the bcr-abl chimeric gene is indeed a unique genetic marker. As previously described in CML patients, there are two potential markers resulting from the fusion of the bcr (exon 2 or 3) and c-abl (exon 1) genes. These gene rearrangements, therefore, can be viewed as nucleotide sequences coding for unique antigens in CML cells containing these fused genes. Because the sequences of the bcr/abl junctions are known, two distinct putative oligopeptides can be deduced and synthesized and used to generate specific antibodies against bcr/abl-associated tumor antigens. It is satisfying to think that this approach, using the complete molecular characterization of a cytogenetic anomaly associated with a known leukemia, may yield a significant reward. Such reagents may have direct application in the routine screening and detection of Ph-containing CML cells in patients receiving various treatment protocols, as well as an application for the detection of relapse[57].

In particular, a number of patients with CML in the chronic stage, having had allogenic bone marrow transplantation (BMT), seem to be having most encouraging responses[58]; some 50-65% of such patients, respectively, undergo remission and are surviving, still free of Ph positive cells. Most patients with leukemias usually present between 10^{12}-10^{13} leukemic cells when first diagnosed; to qualify as a remission for conventionally treated leukemias, it is generally acceptable for marrow to contain from 10^4-10^5 leukemic cells[59]. For patients that qualify for BMT, it would be necessary to purge the marrow of leukemic cells even more drastically to prevent relapse. An idealized goal, therefore, would be to eliminate these residual leukemic cells as much as possible. Having more specific molecular markers to identify residual leukemic cells, would make it possible to monitor and apply specific treatment protocols before BMT.

Along similar lines recent studies by Huebner et al.[60] using cDNA-encoding granulocyte macrophage colony stimulating factor (GM-CSF) as a molecular probe localized this gene to the human chromosome region 5q21-5q23. A truncated GM-CSF allele was found in the HL60 human promyelocytic leukemic cell line and in association with a candidate 5q⁻ marker chromosome. This truncated GM-CSF allele may, therefore, prove valuable for 5q⁻ deletions, a chromosomal abnormality associated with various blood disorders, some often detected in patients with acute myelogenous leukemia (AML)[61]. Additionally, the proto-oncogene c-fms, which has a known homology to the gene coding for the CSF-1 receptor[62], has also been shown to be deleted in the 5q⁻ syndrome. It remains to be demonstrated that the absence of these markers bears a direct and causal relationship to the hematologic disorders. However, as markers, this growth factor gene and the c-fms proto-oncogene may allow the correlation of specific chromosomal abnormalities to specific known disease associations when used as molecular probes. Such information, if substantiated by sufficient cytogenetic and molecular analysis, may yet prove to have prognostic value. In particular, probes utilizing these genetic markers could be used to detect individuals at risk for certain hematologic malignancies and perhaps even those predisposed toward AML.

B. Proto-oncogenes as Indicators of Tumor Progression.

Alteration in the expression of certain specific proto-oncogenes associated to other nonspecific chromosomal abnormalities seems to correlate with
clinical behavior in human tumors[7]. Amplified myc, myb, and Ha-ras have
been present in critical chromosomal regions like double minutes (DMs),
homogenously staining regions (HSRs) and abnormally banded regions (ABRs)[63].
It has been proposed that these amplifications represent one of the mechanisms of activation of proto-oncogenes[33], but there is as yet no clear
evidence for this. Seemingly, it would appear that amplification of certain
proto-oncogenes confers a selective advantage upon the tumor cell and may
represent a genetic event accompanying the accelerated evolution of the
tumorigenic cell[64] toward malignancy. Because this phenomena is not limited
to specific neoplastic conditions, it may be reasonable to suspect that the
amplified genes are more involved in cellular growth than cellular differentiation. Amplification of proto-oncogenes has been observed in human tumors
of varying histological composition including colon and lung carcinomas
as well as leukemias and lymphomas[7]. In support of the concept of amplification as a parameter of tumor progression, it may be signficant to note
that the chromosome regions containing amplified proto-oncogenes are inter-
convertable during tumor evolution. These regions show a degree of plastic-
ity both when undergoing transposition from extrachromosomal (DMs) to intra-
chromosomal (HSRs) locations and when going from one chromosome to another
with preferential integration in the sites predisposed to breakage (i.e.,
fragile sites)[65,66].

N-myc, a gene which is related to the myc family has been found amplified[67] in cell lines derived from neuroblastomas. The amplification of
N-myc gene expression occurs only in late-stage neuroblastomas, whereas
early stages of these tumors are devoid of any amplification[68]. This is
an example of how the level of expression of a protooncogene (or its product)
may serve as a useful marker for monitoring the progression of a particular
malignant disease. The same marker may be useful to monitor the efficacy
of various chemotherapeutic regimens. Of particular interest is the finding
that human small-cell lung carcinoma (SCLC), with a high degree of c-myc
DNA amplification (20-70 fold) and greatly increased levels of c-myc RNA,
resides in the varient class of SCLC (SCLC-V). This varient class is
characterized by altered morphology lack of expression of some SCLC differentiated functions, and more malignant behavior than the "classic" SCLC.
This observation suggests that a correlation exists between a high level of
c-myc gene expression and malignant behavior of human lung cancer[69].

Classic and variant type of SCLC also show a differential expression of intermediate filament proteins using immunocytochemical techniques. Classic SCLC types contain cytokeratin proteins but no neurofilaments, whereas variant SCLC types do not contain any detectable cytokeratin protein but only partly express neurofilament and vimentin[70]. Taken together these observations show that the concomitant application, on fresh biopsy specimens, of antibodies to intermediate filament proteins as well as the determination of proto-oncogene expression - may be of clinical relevance.

It is interesting in view of the functional correlation between oncogene proteins and growth-factor receptors that some tumors show amplification of genes coding for growth factor receptors, i.e., the epidermal growth factor (EGF) receptor[71]. Data demonstrating amplified EGF receptor in human tumors suggest also that the anomalous expression of the receptor may play a role in the tumor progression[71-74]. Notably, the viral erb B oncogene is known to transform cells through the expression of a truncated EGF receptor.

It becomes more and more apparent that an accurate diagnosis of malignancy, particularly in the case solid tumors, will require the development of a battery of immunological and molecular reagents for an appropriate characterization and classification. Since neoplastic cells retain their tissue-specific intermediate filament proteins, the combined use of antibodies to these proteins, i.e., keratin, vimentin, and desmin, will become indispensable for a correct histopathological classification. Additionally, antibodies to proto-oncogene products, growth factors and hormone-receptors will more precisely allow the staging and monitoring of tumor progression. A better diagnostic procedure would then determine more effective therapeutic protocols and help in the prognostic evaluation of cancer patients.

Even if the ultimate challenge for the molecular oncologist is the comprehension of the role of cellular or proto-oncogenes in the etiology of cancer, the systematic study cataloging and correlating oncogene-associated alterations may represent an important collateral development of diagnostics with clinical potential. For now, the goal to use oncogenes as diagnostic and prognostic markers of neoplasia, as well as to monitor various treatment protocols, seems both realistic and feasible.

271

REFERENCES

1. Gilden, R. V., Rice, N. R. and McAllister, R. M. (1984) Gene Anal. Tech. 1, 23-33.
2. Papas, T. S., Kan, N. K., Watson, D. K., Flordellis, C. S., Psallidopoulis, M. C., Lautenberger, J., Samuel, K. P. and Duesberg, P. (1984) "myc-related genes in viruses and cells." In Vande Woude, G. F., Levine, A. J., Topp, W. C. and Watson, J. D. (Eds.) Cancer Cells: Oncogenes and Viral Genes, Cold Spring Harbor Laboratory, Cold Spring Harbor, NY. 2, 153-164.
3. Baltimore, D. (1985) Cell 40, 481-482.
4. Linial, M. and Blair, D. (1982) "Genetics of retroviruses." In Weiss, R., Teich, N., Varmus, H. and Coffin, J. (Eds.) Op. cit. 1, 649-784.
5. Teich, N., Wyke, J., Mak, T., Bernstein and Hardy, W. (1982) "Pathogenesis of retrovirus-induced disease." Ibid 1, 785-998.
6. Bishop, J. M. (1985) Cell 42, 23-38.
7. Marshall, C. (1985) "Human Oncogenes." In Weiss, R., Teich, N., Varmus, H. and Coffin, J. (Eds.) Op. cit. Supplement 2, 487-558.
8. Wong-Staal, F. and Gallo, R. C. (1985) Nature 317, 395-403.
9. Cooper, G. M. (1982) Science 217, 801-806.
10. Blair, D. G., Cooper, C. S., Oskarsson, M. K., Eader, L. A. and Vande Woude, G. F. (1982) Science 218, 1122-1125.
11. Eva, A., Tronick, S. R., Gol, R. A., Pierce, J. H. and Aaronson, S. A. (1983) Proc. Natl. Acad. Sci. U.S.A. 80, 4926-4930.
12. Papas, T. S., Kan, N. C., Watson, D. K., Lautenberger, J. A., Flordellis, C., Samuel, K. P., Rovigatti, U. G., Psallidopoulos, M., Ascione, R. and Duesberg, P. H. (1985) "Oncogenes of avian acute leukemia viruses are subsets of normal cellular genes." In Neth, R., Gallo, R. C., Greaves, M. F. and Janka, G. Haematology and Blood Transfusion, Modern Trends in Human Leukemia III: Springer-Verlag, Berlin.
13. Maniatis, T., Fritsch, E. F. and Sambrook, J. (1982) "Molecular cloning: A laboratory manual." Cold Spring Harbor Laboratory, Cold Spring Harbor, NY.
14. Watson, D. K., Psallidopoulis, M. C., Samuel, K. P., Dalla-Favera, R. and Papas, T. S. (1983) Proc. Natl. Acad. Sci. U.S.A. 80, 3642-3645.
15. Southern, E. M. (1975) J. Mol. Biol. 98, 503-517.
16. Alwine, J. C., Kemp, D. J. and Stark, G. R. (1977) Proc. Natl. Acad. Sci. U.S.A. 74, 5350-5354.

17. Eva, R., Robbins, K. C., Andersen, P. R., Srinivasan, A., Tronick, S. R., Reddy, E. P., Ellmore, E. W., Galen, A. T., Lautenberger, J. A., Papas, T. S., Westin, E. H., Wong-Staal, F., Gallo, R. C. and Aarsonson, S. A. (1982) Nature 295, 116-119.

18. Van Beneden, R., Watson, D. K., Chen, T. and Papas, T. S. (1986) Proc. Natl. Acad. Sci. U.S.A. In Press.

19. Gilden, R. V. (1984) "Oncogenes." In Oncos, Oncor, Inc., Gaithersburg, MD 1, 1-4.

20. Hall, A., Marshall, C., Spurr, N. and Weiss, R. (1983) Nature 303, 396-404.

21. Weinberg, R. A. (1985) Science 230, 770-776.

22. Reddy, E. P., Reynolds, R. K., Santos, E. and Barbacid, M. (1982) Nature 300, 149-152.

23. Kris, R. M., Libermann, T. A., Avivi, A. and Schlessinger, J. (1985) Biotechnology 3, 135-140.

24. Hunter, T. (1984) Nature 311, 414-416.

25. Gilmore, T., DeClue, J. E. and Martin, G. S. (1985) Cell 40, 609-618.

26. Newmark, P. (1985) Nature 316, 681.

27. Sherr, C. J., Rettenmier, C. W., Sacca, R., Roussel, M., Look, A. T. and Stanley, E. R. (1985) Cell 41, 665-676.

28. Devare, S. G., Reddy, E. P., Law, J. D., Robbins, K. C. and Aaronson, S. A. (1983) Proc. Natl. Acad. Sci. U.S.A. 80, 731-735.

29. Igarashi, H., Gazit, A., Chiu, I. M., Srinivasan, A., Yaniv, A., Tronick, S. R., Robbins, K. C. and Aaronson, S. A. (1985) In Feramisco, J., Ozanne, B. and Stiles, C. (Eds.) Growth Factors and Transformation: Cancer Cells, Cold Spring Harbor Laboratory, Cold Spring Harbor, NY. 3, 159-166.

30. Antoniades, H. N., Pantazis, P., Graves, D. T., Owen, A. J. and Tempst, P. (1985) Ibid, 145-151.

31. Ralston, R. and Bishop, J. M. (1983) Nature 306, 803-806.

32. Duesberg, P. H. (1985) Science 228, 669-677.

33. Klein, G. and Klein, E. (1985) Nature 315, 190-195.

34. Croce, C. M. (1985) Hospital Practice 20, 41-48.

35. Mitelman, F. (1984) Nature 310, 325-327.

36. Sandberg, A. A. (1983) Cancer Genet. Cytogenet. 8, 277-285.

37. Cavenee, W. K., Dryja, T. P., Phillips, R. A., Benedict, W. F., Godbout, R., Gallie, B. L., Murphee, A. L., Strong, L. C. and White, R. L. (1983) Nature 305, 779-784.

38. Koufos, A., Hansen, M. F., Copeland, N. G., Jenkins, N. A., Lampkin, B. C. and Cavenee, W. K. (1985) Nature 316, 330-334.

39. Orkin, S. H., Goldman, D. S. and Sallan, S. B. (1984) Nature 309, 172-174.

40. Croce, C. M. and Nowell, P. C. (1985) Blood 65, 1-7.

41. Dalla-Favera, R., Bregni, M., Erikson, J., Patterson, D., Gallo, R. C. and Croce, C. M. (1982) Proc. Natl. Acad. Sci. U.S.A. 79, 7824-7827.

42. Hayday, A. C., Gillies, S. D., Saito, H., Wood, C., Winman, K., Hayward, W. S. and Tonegawa, S. (1984) Nature 307, 334-340.

43. Gale, R. P. and Canaani, E. (1985) British J. of Haemat. 60, 395-408.

44. de Klein, A., Geurts van Kessel, A. and Grosveld, G. (1982) Nature 300, 765-767.

45. Adams, J. M. (1985) Nature 315, 542-543.

46. Stam, K., Heisterkamp, N., Grosveld, G., de Klein, A., Verma, R. S., Coleman, M., Dosik, H. and Groffen, J. (1985) N. Engl. J. Med. 313, 1429-1433.

47. Konopka, J. B., Watanabe, S. M. and Witte, O. N. (1984) Cell 37, 1035-42.

48. Watson, D. K., McWilliams-Smith, M. J., Kozak, C., Reeves, R., Gearhart, J., Nash, W., Modi, W., Duesberg, P. H., Papas, T. S. and O'Brien, S. J. (1985) Proc. Natl. Acad. Sci. U.S.A. In Press.

49. Watson, D. K., McWilliams-Smith, M. J., Nunn, M. F., Duesberg, P. H., O'Brien, S. J. and Papas, T. S. (1985) Proc. Natl. Acad. Sci. U.S.A. 82, 7294-7298.

50. Sacchi, N., Watson, D. K., Geurts van Kessel, A. H. M., Hagemeijer, A., Kersey, J., Drabkin, H. D., Patterson, D. and Papas, T. S. (1986) Science 231, 379-382.

51. Le Beau, M. M. (Personal Communication).

52. Diaz, M. O., LeBeau, M. M., Pitha, P. and Rowley, J. D. (1986) Science 231, 265-267.

53. Tsujimoto, Y., Yunis, J., Onorato-Soave, L., Erikson, J., Nowell, P. C. and Croce, C. M. (1984) Science 224, 1403-1406.

54. Tsujimoto, Y., Finger, L., Yunis, J., Nowell, P. C. and Croce, C. H. (1984) Science 226, 1097-1099.

55. Bakshi, A., Jensen, J. P., Goldman, P., Wright, J. J., McBride, W., Epstein, A. and Korsmeijer, S. J. (1985) Cell 41, 899-906.

56. LeBeau, M. M. and Rowley, J. D. (1985) Nature 316, 826-828.

274

57. Grosveld, G. C., Bootsme, D., de Klein, A., Heisterkamp, N., Stam, N. and Groffen, J. (1986) In "Detection and Treatment of Minimal Residual Disease in Acute Leukemia." In Press.
58. McCredie, K. B., Kantarjian, H., Keating, M. J., Hester, J. P. and Freireich, E. J. (1985) In Neth, R., Gallo, R. C., Greaves, M. F. and Janka, G. (Eds.) Haematology and Blood Transfusion, Modern Trends in Human Leukemia VI, Springer-Verlag Publishers, Berlin 29, 51-52.
59. Clarkson, B. (1985) In Neth, R., Gallo, R. C., Greaves, M. F. and Janka, G. (Eds.) Haematology and Blood Transusions, Modern Trends in Human Leukemia VI, Springer-Verlag Publishers, Berlin 29, 96-101.
60. Huebner, Isobe, M., Croce, C. M., Golde, D. W., Kaufman, S. E. and Gasson, J. C. (1985) Science 230, 1282-1285.
61. Rowley, J. D. (1980) Ann. Rev. Genet. 14, 17-39.
62. Nienhuis, A. W., Bunn, H. F., Turner, P. H., Gopal, T. V., Nash, W. G., O'Brien, S. J. and Sherr, C. J. (1985) Cell 42, 421-428.
63. Schwab, M. (1984) In "Cancer Cells", Cold Spring Harbor Laboratory, Cold Spring Harbor, NY. pp. 215-220.
64. Sager, R., Gadi, J. K., Stephens, L. and Grabowy, C. T. (1984) Proc. Natl. Acad. Sci. U.S.A. 82, 7015-7020.
65. Yunis, J. J. (1983) Science 221, 227-236.
66. Wolman, S. (1985) Cancer Genet. Cytogent. 17, 133-141.
67. Schwab, M., Alitalo, K., Klempnauer, K., Varmus, H., Bishop, J. M., Gilbert, F., Brodeur, G., Goldstein, M. and Trent, J. (1983) Nature 305, 245-248.
68. Brodeur, G. M., Seeger, R. C., Schwab, M., Varmus, H. E. and Bishop, J. M. (1984) Science 224, 1121-1124.
69. Nau, M. M., Brooks, B. J., Battey, J., Sausville, E., Gazdar, A. F., Kirsch, I. R., McBride, O. W., Bertness, V., Hollis, G. F. and Minna, J. D. (1985) Nature 318, 69-73.
70. Broers, J. L. V., Carney, D. N., DeLey, L., Vooijs, G. P. and Ramaekers, F. C. S. (1985) Proc. Natl. Acad. Sci. U.S.A. 82, 4409-4413.
71. Hunts, J., Vede, M., Ozawa, S., Abe, O., Pastan, I. and Shimizu, N. (1985) Gann 76, 663-667.
72. Gusterson, B., Cowley, G., McIlhinney, J., Ozanne, B., Fisher, C. and Reeves, B. (1985) Int. J. of Cancer 36, 689-695.
73. Gullick, W. J., Marsden, J. J., Whittle, N., Ward, B., Bobrow, L. and Waterfield, M. D. (1985) Cancer Res. 46, 285-293.

74. Lax, I., Kris, R., Sasson, I., Ullrich, A., Hayman, M. J., Buy, H. and Schlessinger, J. (1985) EMBO J. 4, 3179-3183.

75. Bister, K. and Duesberg, P. H. (1982) In Klein, G. (Ed.) Advances in Viral Oncology, Raven Press, NY, 1, 3-42.

76. Stephenson, J. R. and Todaro, G. J. (1982) In Klein, G. (Ed.) Advances in Viral Oncology, Raven Press, NY, 1, 59-82.

77. Naharro, G., Robbins, K. C. and Reddy, E. P. (1984) Science 223, 63-66.

78. Papkoff, J., Verma, I. M. and Hunter, T. (1982) Cell 29, 417-426.

79. Rapp, U. R., Goldsborough, M. D., Mark, G. E., Bonner, T. I., Groffen, J., Reynolds, F. H., Jr. and Stephenson, J. R. (1983) Proc. Natl. Acad. Sci. U.S.A. 8, 4218-4222.

80. Kan, N. C., Flordellis, C. S., Garon, C. F., Duesberg, P. H. and Papas, T. S. (1983) Proc. Natl. Acad. Sci. U.S.A. 80, 6566-6570.

81. Downward, J., Yarden, Y., Mayes, E., Scrace, G., Totty, N., Stockwell, P., Ullrich, A., Schlessinger, J. and Waterfield, M. D. (1984) Nature 307, 521-527.

82. Stephens, R. M., Rice, N. R., Hiebsch, R. R., Bose, Jr., H. R. and Gilden, R. V. (1983) Proc. Natl. Acad. Sci. U.S.A. 80, 6229-6233.

83. Cooper, C. S., Park, M., Blair, D. G., Tainsky, M. A., Huebner, K., Croce, C. M. and Vande Woude, G. F. (1984) Nature 311, 29-33.

84. Dean, M., Park, M., LeBeau, M. M., Robins, T. S., Diaz, M. O., Rowley, J. D., Blair, D. G. and Vande Woude, G. F. (1985) Nature 318, 385-388.

85. Ellis, R. W., Lowy, D. R. and Scolnick, E. M. (1982) In Klein, G. (Ed.) Advances in Viral Oncology, Raven Press, NY, 1, 107-126.

86. Shimizu, K., Goldfarb, M., Suard, Y., Perucho, M., Li, Y. Kamata, T., Feramisco, J., Stavnezer, E., Fogh, J. and Wigler, M. (1983) Proc. Natl. Acad. Sci. U.S.A 80, 2112-2116.

87. Robbins, K. C., Devare, S. G., Reddy, E. P. and Aaronson, S. A. (1982) Science 218, 1131-1133.

88. Chiu, I. M., Reddy, E. P., Givol, D., Robbins, K. C., Tronick, S. R. and Aaronson, S. A. (1984) Cell 37, 123-129.

89. Coussens, L., Yang-Feng, T. L., Liao, Y. C., Chen, E., Gray, A., McGrath, J., Seeburg, P. H., Libermann, T. A., Schlessinger, J., Francke, H., Levinson, A. and Ullrich, A. (1985) Science 230, 1132-1139.

90. Kohl, N. E., Kanda, N., Schreck, R. R., Bruns, G., Latt, S. A., Gilbert, F. and Alt, F. W. (1983) Cell 35, 359-367.

91. Klempnauer, K.-H., Ramsay, G., Bishop, J. M., Moscovici, G. M., Moscovici, C., McGrath, J. P. and Levinson, A. D. (1983) Cell 33, 345-355.

92. Nunn, M. F., Seeburg, P. H., Moscovici, C. and Duesberg, P. H. (1983) Nature 306, 391-395.

93. Curran, T. and Teich, N. M. (1982) J. Virol. 42, 114-122.

94. Stavnezer, E., Gerhard, D. S., Binari, R. C. and Balazs, I. (1981) J. Virol. 39, 920-934.

95. Weinberger, C., Hollenberg, S. M., Rosenfeld, M. G. and Evans, R. M. (1985) Nature 318, 670-672.

96. Hayman, M. J., Ramsay, G. M., Savin, K., Kitchener, G., Graf, T. and Beug, H. (1983) Cell 32, 579-588.

97. Erikson, J., Williams, D. L., Finan, J., Nowell, P. C. and Croce, C. M. (1985) Science 299, 784.

98. Croce, C. M., Tsujimoto, Y. and Nowell, P. C. (1986) Gene Amp. Anal. In Press.

99. Harper, M. E., Franchini, G., Love, J., Simon, M. I., Gallo, R. C. and Wong-Staal, F. (1983) Nature 304, 169-171.

100. Neel, B. G., Jhanwar, S. C., Changanti, R. S. K. and Hayward, W. S. (1982) Proc. Natl. Acad. Sci. U.S.A. 79, 7842-7846.

101. Prakash, K., McBride, O. W., Swan, D. C., Devare, S. G., Tronick, S. R. and Aaronson, S. A. (1982) Proc. Natl. Acad. Sci. U.S.A. 79, 5210-5214.

102. Swan, D. C., McBride, O. W., Robbins, K. C., Keithley, D. A., Reddy, E. P. and Aaronson, S. A. (1982) Proc. Natl. Acad. Sci. U.S.A. 79, 4691-4695.

103. Dalla-Favera, R., Gallo, R. C., Giallongo, A. and Croce, C. M. (1982) Science 218, 686-688.

104. Sakaguchi, A. Y., Naylor, S. L. and Shows, T. B. (1983) Prog. Nucl. Acid Res. Mol. Biol. 29, 279-283.

105. Bartram, C. R., de Klein, A., Hagemeijer, A., van Agthoven, T., van Kessel, A. G., Bootsma, D., Grosveld, G., Ferguson-Smith, M. A., Davies, T., Stone, M., Heisterkamp, N., Stephenson, J. R. and Groffen, J. (1983) Nature 306, 277-280.

106. Groffen, J., Heisterkamp, N., Spurr, N., Dana, S., Wasmuth, J. J. and Stephenson, J. R. (1983) Nucl. Acid Res. 11, 6331-6339.

107. Jhanwar, S. C., Neel, B. G., Hayward, W. S. and Chaganti, R. S. K. (1983) Proc. Natl. Acad. Sci. U.S.A. 80, 4794-4797.

108. Huerre, C., Despoisse, S., Gilgenkrantz, S., Lenoir, G. M. and Junien, C. (1983) Nature 305, 638-641.

109. O'Brien, S. J., Nash, W. G., Goodwin, J. L., Lowy, D. R. and Chang, E. H. (1983) Nature 302, 839-842.

110. de Taisne, C., Gegonne, A., Stehelin, D., Bernheim, A. and Berger, R. (1984) Nature 310, 581-583.

111. Hall, A., Marshall, C. S., Spurr, N. K. and Weiss, R. A. (1983) Nature 303, 396-400.

112. Papas, T. S., Watson, D. K., Sacchi, N., O'Brien, S. J. and Ascione, R. (1986) In Hagenbeek A. and Lowenberg, B. (Eds.). Minimal Residual Disease in Acute Leukemia: 1986. Dodrecht/Boston, Martinus Nijhoff Publishers, pp. 23-42.

113. Kohl, N. E., Kanda, N., Schreck, R. R., Bruns, G., Latt, S. A., Gilbert, F. and Alt, F. W. (1983) Cell 35, 359-367.

114. Spurr, N. K., Solomon, E., Jansson, M., Sherr, D., Goodfellow, P. N., Bodmer, W. F. and Vennstrom, B. (1984) EMBO J. 3, 159-163.

115. Balazs, I., Grzeschik, K. H. and Stavnezer, E. (1984) Cytogenet. Cell Genet. 37, 410-411.

116. Barker, P. E., Rabin, M., Watson, M., Breg, W. R., Ruddle, F. H. and Verma, I. M. (1984) Proc. Natl. Acad. Sci. U.S.A. 81, 5826-5830.

117. Tsujimoto, Y., Gorham, J., Cossman, J., Jaffe, E. and Croce, C. M. (1985) Nature 229, 1390.

Index

Activation of oncogene, 22, 208-209

Acute leukemia virus, 129t, 138

   myc containing, 125-127

Abelson murine leukemia virus (abl),
   13, 83

Ab-MuLV-transformed cells, 168

Abnormally banded regions (ABRs), 269

ABLS tumors, 105

ABPC tumors, 105

ABPL tumors, 104-106, 107

Acquired immunodeficiency syndrome
   (AIDS), 144

Acute lymphocytic leukemia (ALL),
   224, 225t

Acute nonlymphocytic leukemia (ANLL),
   224, 225t

   chromosome abnormalities, 223,
      247-248

Acylation, p21, 58

Adenylate cyclase, G-protein, 57, 68

Amino acid, 40

   changes, 220

   residues, 17, 139

   sequence, 2, 256

      c-sis gene, 165

      gag specific, 82

      homology between p28sis and
         human platelet-derived
            growth factors, 162,
               163-164

      Hu-ets-1, 218

      Hu-ets-2, 218

      insulin gene, 245

      met oncogene, 245, 247, 247f

      myc oncogene, 126

   of ras protein, 56, 57f, 58

   of src protein, 3, 10, 15-16

   v-sis gene, 165

   substitution, 127

   v-sis coded, 166

Amino terminal

   in myc gene product, 105

      mutation, 6-10

   pp60src, 14

   v-sis coded, 166

AML-M2, 227, 266

AMV, See Avian myeloblastosis virus

Antibodies

   anti-BP-2, 86

   anti-myb, 87

   anti-peptide, 121

Antigens

   BP-2, 87

   myelomonocytic, 221, 224

   polyoma middle T, 16

"Anti-oncogenes," 264

Antisera

   anti-p1, 77

   anti-p2, 77

   anti-p4, 77

   anti-peptide, 64

4AP, 200, 201t

Arginine-12, 66

Asparagine-116, 64

ATP binding, 34

ATPase activity, 54

Autokinase activity, 62f, 63f, 63, 64

Avian acute leukemia virus, 129t, 138

Avian carcinoma virus, MH2, 257t, 258t,
   See also MHs virus

c-$\underline{ras}^K$, 57

c-$\underline{sis}$, 172

H-$\underline{ras}$-1, 25

proto-$\underline{myc}$, 118

Extracellular growth factor (EGF), 13

    receptor-related oncogenes, 34

FBJ osteosarcoma virus, 259t

Feline $\underline{ets}$-1, 213-214

$\underline{fgr}$ protein, 13

Fibrinopeptides, 165

Fibroblast, transformation, 80, 167

Fibroblast growth factor (FGF), 179,

    185, 186, 188, 190, 191

Fibrosarcoma, 34, 174

Flanking sequences, v-$\underline{sis}$ gene, 165

$\underline{fms}$ proteins, 13

$\underline{fms}$ proto-oncogenes

  c-$\underline{fms}$, 260, 268

  v-$\underline{fms}$, 260

$\underline{fos}$ gene, 180, 259t

  c-$\underline{fos}$, 199-200, 203-204

$\underline{fps}/\underline{fes}$ protein, 13

Fractionation, subcellular, 79

Fusion protein, 60f

G-protein, 55, 64, 68

    chemical properties, 66

    GTP binding domain, 65

    N-terminal sequence, 61f

$\underline{gag}$ oncogene, 13-14, 77, 81

  $\underline{gag}$-$\underline{myb}$-$\underline{ets}$, 209

  $\underline{gag}$-$\underline{myc}$ gene, 133

$\underline{gag}$ region, MH2, 128

GDP, binding, 64

Gene

    amplification, 22, 91-93

    induction, 197-206

transcription, 199

transfection, 110

transfer assay, 22, 186-191

Genetic cloning, recombinant, 110

Glioblastoma, 174

Glycine-12, mutation at, 64

Granulocyte macrophage colony stimula-

    ting factor (GM-CSF), 268

Growth, control, 49, 67

Growth factors, 22

    calcitonin, 226

    epidermal, See Epidermal growth

      factor

    extracellular, See Extracellular

      growth factor

    fibroblast, See Fibroblast growth

      factor

    independence, 191

    insulin-like, 179

    peptide, 178, 179

    platelet-derived, See Platelet-

      derived growth factor

    receptors, 22, 270

    requirements

      loss of, 185-186

      $\underline{onc}$-genes relieving, 186-191

    role in E26 transformation, 82-83

    $\underline{sis}$/PDGF-2, 166, 168

    T-cell, 198

GTP

    binding, 62, 63f, 63, 66-67

    binding domain, 59, 64-67, 68

GTPase, 62, 63f, 63

Guanine, 68

    binding properties, with p21, 57

Ha-$\underline{ras}$ gene, 257t

    /CAT vector, 47-49

Subclones
    pRD6K, 219
    pRd700, 219
SV40, 49, 50

T-cell
    activation, 197-206
    receptor, 154-157, 158
T-cell leukemia (T-ALL), 154, 156f,
    254
T-cell neoplasia, 157-158
    oncogene activation in, 156-157
3T3 cells, See NIH/3T3 cells
TAG, 118
TaqI fragment, 248, 249
Taxonomy of oncogenes, 256
Temperature shift, 80-81
Terminal deoxynucleotidyl transferase
    (TdT), 221
Terminal differentiation, 79
Tetrapeptide, 59
TGA, 118
Threonine-59, 66
Thymidine, 27, 182
TPA, 34
Transcription termination signals, 136
Transduced sequences, 81
Transfection, 255, See also under
    specific heading
Transfer analysis, Southern, 255
Transferrin, 188
Transforming genes, See Proto-onco-
    genes
Translocation, reciprocal, See
    Reciprocal translocation
Transmembrane
    receptor, 67
    signalling, 198, 204

Trout (Ft-c-myc) gene, 117f
Truncation, 90
Ts mutant, of RSV, 7
Tumor, progression, 262, 269-270
Tumor markers
    new, generation of, 261-268
    proto-oncogenes as, 261-270
Tumor promoter
    SV40, 49, 50
    TPA, 34
Tumor suppressors, See Anti-oncogenes
Two-hit hypothesis, 262
Tyrosine, phosphorylation, 2, 16
Tyrosine kinase, 10, 11f
    activity, 2
        src gene, 13, 17
    family, 245-248
    src related, 83

V α genes, 155t
Valine, 42
VDJ joining enzyme, 153, 154
Vectors
    CAT-based, 47-49
    containing Ha-ras gene, 42f, 43
    pBR322, 132
    pBR325, 131
    retrovirus, 245, 246f, 248
    RSV, 4-5
Verapamil, 200, 201t
v-erb gene, 14, 74
    v-erb A, 232
    v-erb-B, 232, 260
V-ets gene, 232
    dispersion, 218-220
v-fma gene, 260
v-mht gene, 130, 130f, 135, 136, 232
v-myb gene